Ayurveda

A Comprehensive Guide to Traditional Indian Medicine for the West

FRANK JOHN NINIVAGGI, M.D.

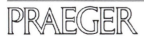

Westport, Connecticut
London

Library of Congress Cataloging-in-Publication Data

Ninivaggi, Frank John.
   Ayurveda : a comprehensive guide to traditional Indian medicine for the West /
Frank John Ninivaggi.
      p. ; cm.
   Rev. ed. of: An elementary textbook of Ayurveda / Frank John Ninivaggi. c2001.
   Includes bibliographical references and index.
   ISBN 978–0–313–34837–2 (alk. paper)
      1. Medicine, Ayurvedic. I. Ninivaggi, Frank John. Elementary textbook of Ayurveda. II. Title.
III. Title: Comprehensive guide to traditional Indian medicine for the West.
      [DNLM: 1. Medicine, Ayurvedic. 2. Attitude to Health. 3. Life Style. 4. Medicine,
Ayurvedic—history. WB 50.1 N715a 2008]
   R605.N49 2008
   615.5'38—dc22   2007029917

British Library Cataloguing in Publication Data is available.

Library of Congress Catalog Card Number: 2007029917
ISBN-13: 978–0–313–34837–2

First published in 2008

Praeger Publishers, 88 Post Road West, Westport, CT 06881
An imprint of Greenwood Publishing Group, Inc.
www.praeger.com

Printed in the United States of America

∞™

The paper used in this book complies with the
Permanent Paper Standard issued by the National
Information Standards Organization (Z39.48–1984).

10 9 8 7 6 5 4 3 2 1

MEDICAL DISCLAIMER
This text is primarily a reference guide introducing the theoretical principles of Ayurveda. It is not
intended to create a physician-patient relationship or to supplant any actual clinical assessment, consultation, examination, evaluation, or treatment planning. Information in this book is not intended to
diagnose, treat, or cure. This text does not intend to replace, and cannot replace, proper patient-
provider medical care.

CONTENTS

PREFACE

My previous work on Ayurveda had as its principal purpose introducing the fundamental elements of this age-old medical tradition. Since then, several other aims have emerged and taken shape in this book.

Ayurveda: A Comprehensive Guide to Traditional Indian Medicine for the West not only incorporates the fundamental elements of Ayurveda, but also expands to present itself as a course book, a reference guide, and a personal self-help tool. New material is introduced throughout this text. In addition, a chapter that discusses the cultivation of consciousness and another that presents the novel *BioPsychoSpiritual* perspective, the alignment of Ayurveda and modern Psychiatry, are presented. It is a consciousness-based, phenomenological model. Practical guidelines for the practice of psychotherapy have been addressed. Attention to the integration of relevant aspects of Buddhism and Taoism is included. The expansive Glossary can be used as a virtual dictionary.

Besides incorporating a history of medicine and orienting Ayurveda within the world's healing traditions, this work has attempted to achieve understandability in its presentation. For example, the entire conception of digestion, which is central to Ayurveda, has been reworked and compared to the Western view. Not only does this illustrate differences in physiological emphases, but it aptly illuminates differences that illustrate philosophical and existential tenets that imply a qualitatively different Weltanschauung, that is, Ayurveda as a 6,000-year-old perspective on everyday living. The latter has become more integrated within and an integral part of Western thought and health-oriented practices in recent years.

The composition and arrangement of work in this book has been the sole effort of the author. This work on Ayurveda has remained a singular pursuit over the last 30 years. It is one man's grasp of Ayurveda as a worldview and as a way of life. It is hoped that these expansions will usefully enlarge the scope of this book making it a useful contribution not only to Western medicine but also to Western culture.

Frank John Ninivaggi, M.D.
Yale University School of Medicine

INTRODUCTION

Ayurveda, life wisdom, is an ancient yet living discipline. Its theories and methods combine the ordinary with the extraordinary. Some regard it as more than a medical tradition; it is a comprehensive life-style, a way of life with choice and deliberation that reflects values and actions toward achieving optimal health in body, mind, and spirit. Adherents of Ayurveda believe that its origins extend back at least 6,000 years. There is some inferential evidence to support this contention. Others say that a 3,000-year-old legacy is clearly verifiable. It would not be an understatement to regard Ayurveda as a world-class system of health and well-being. Health promotion and wellness are prime values. If this is true, one then wonders why its recognition as such in the West has been so delayed. Ayurveda, an ancient Sanskrit word (*Ayus*/living and *Veda*/revealed wisdom), derives from the traditions of the ancient Indian *rishis* (sages) and denotes the enlightened knowledge of all aspects of optimal, healthy, everyday living, and longevity. Its adherents consider it a "fortress of wisdom."

A factor responsible for the slow recognition of Ayurvedic wisdom in the West may be the intentional ambiguity in form and content that has characterized its prehistory, history, and development. Its practical relevance for the Westerner may also be unclear. Eastern ideas have always been clothed in fluid boundaries, and their content may have appeared amorphous, intangible, impractical, and speculative, if not fanciful, to Western thinkers. A solid emphasis on self-inquiry and self-development, perhaps with a strong introspective, private, and very personal quality, has always been central.

Among Ayurveda's primary values are the concepts of *Sattva* and of *Dharma*. The Sanskrit word *Sattva* refers to the ongoing attainment of ever-greater degrees of purity, harmony, balance, and goodness in one's life. For Hindus, the Sanskrit word *dharma,* an equally broad notion, refers to an individual's recognition of inherent lawfulness in the universe, assuming personal responsibility, and taking charge of one's own life in the world. In the

Buddhist tradition, which emerged out of Hinduism in the sixth century B.C., the term *dharma* has come to refer to the entire body of teachings, the corpus of enlightened life wisdom, ascribed to the Buddha. This denotes the cosmic law, itself, and also the words that the Buddha used to express it.

In fact, one of the great luminaries of Ayurveda, Nāgārjuna (c. second century A.D.), was both an Ayurvedic physician and a Buddhist priest. The breadth of his wisdom not only enriched the Ayurvedic Materia Medica in a pragmatic way with the introduction of iatrochemistry (mineral-based medicine), but advanced the scope of Buddhism with contributions having profound philosophical and psychological significance. The inestimable significance and living historicity of Nāgārjuna's contributions attest to his continuing to be a creative Ayurvedic presence, a golden thread stretching back two millennia.

The range of Ayurvedic thinking covers thousands of years of ideas, practical experience, and theory building. It is hoped that this book will not inadvertently oversimplify the profound depth of this ancient medical system but, instead, present its basic elements in an intelligent, yet reverent and compassionate, fashion to the serious reader.

An attempt has been made not to overly intellectualize or to present the material in a stringently academic, experience-distant manner, as is found in many serious books on Indological subjects. The beating pulse or consciousness—the living spirit at the heart of Ayurveda—is intentionally kept in the forefront. Ayurveda is truly in a class of its own. It is not similar to a Western medical subspecialty like Internal Medicine or Psychiatry; it is an overarching worldview encompassing the health and disorders of body, mind, and spirit—at times, in one breath.

After my first book on Ayurveda, *An Elementary Textbook of Ayurveda: Medicine with a Six Thousand Year Old Tradition* (2001), many have said that that text was much more than merely elementary. It encompassed a significant measure of the breadth of Indian thinking and culture both past and present in one small volume. While it may be said that the present text represents Ayurveda in its more classical tradition, one derived from its historical roots, it also attempts to incarnate Ayurveda in its more modern form as generally understood and practiced today. Such a contemporary American translation offers Westerners a comprehensive guide not only to theory, but also to practical guidelines made understandable and usable.

In many ways, the current book has now emerged as an advanced, encyclopedic distillation of the theoretical and clinical range of Ayurvedic medicine. Hence, its title more aptly reflects this: *Ayurveda: A Comprehensive Guide to Traditional Indian Medicine for the West.* Since this modern practice continues to retain its uniquely Eastern orientation, translation into Western terms continues to be a challenge, one that is often harshly criticized by Western standards. In order to orient the reader and to facilitate a greater sense of familiarity in, at least, a few important areas, material in Chapter 4 and in Chapter 8, for example, offers an attempt at some correlations between the manner in which foods and herbs are processed physiologically both from the Ayurvedic point of view and from that of Western science. Issues such as pharmacodynamic and pharmacokinetic mechanisms key to Western research scientists are outlined, at least in a partial manner. In addition, a short course in Western pharmacology is offered in terms understandable to those without specific biochemical or medical training. This material, especially that dealing with the complex processes of digestion, is a formidable area of study. Undoubtedly, it will be seen as difficult to understand, but its central place within theoretical and clinical Ayurveda makes its detailed presentation a fundamental necessity.

Clear-cut nutritional suggestions are given. The explosion of concern with health and weight management and the alarming rise in the incidence of prediabetes, the Metabolic Syndrome, coronary artery disease, and blood lipid irregularities make Ayurvedic nutritional interventions a welcome and refreshing addition to current health-promoting strategies. In addition, an attempt has been made to place Ayurvedic nutrition alongside Western nutritional concepts in a practical manner. This cross-correlation may provide readers with a much clearer understanding of the way in which Ayurveda and Western medicine share many noncontradictory and, for that matter, even compatible approaches.

Ayurveda is currently referred to as Traditional Indian Medicine (TIM). Yet, Ayurveda truly is more than merely Indian medical science. It is, in fact, a universally applicable way of life that addresses all aspects of living both in health and in disease. Practitioners of this art frequently refer to it as being proven over time. Ongoing experience, however, has and will continue to suggest, short of hard scientific proof, degrees of validity in the Ayurvedic worldview. Ayurveda may be aptly viewed as real science in the context of discovery.

Ayurveda as narrated in this book has emerged out of the history and development of Indian culture. This context is famous for introducing and entertaining a multiplicity of widely divergent worldviews. Disputes abound concerning the nature and meaning of the individual's place in the world, of personal identity, of pluralism versus monism, and of a personal Deity or a more transcendent Absolute. For Ayurveda, reality consists of a universe of animate and inanimate beings, all of which are grounded in a primordial matrix of immaterial consciousness, the substratum of all that exists. The Sanskrit term that covers the entire range of all that exists is *Brahman,* the one absolute reality. The ancient Vedic scriptures repeatedly stressed the point that ontologically, "everything is *Brahman*" (*sarvam khalvidam Brahma*) and "all is *Brahman*" (*kham Brahm*). This view especially pertained to man; his essence was seen to be identical with *Brahman* (*Tat Tvam Asi*). This unifying monism is central to Ayurveda and transcends the scientific particularization required in any attempt at a written exposition. Moreover, in like fashion to most other philosophical, religious, spiritual, humanistic, and healing ideologies, Ayurveda centers its attention almost entirely on man and the meaningfulness of his existence in the world. Man's place in the universe is an essential theme. The role of man on earth, in society, within the family, interpersonally, and with himself, per se, is viewed as a proper and necessary concern, and not as an archaic, anthropomorphic, and fanciful self-indulgence.

The Ayurvedic system delineates a wide-ranging way of life for human beings, which enables them to address all aspects of self-development. Self-inquiry, self-realization, and self-actualization are central themes. A strong emphasis is put on the individual's mandated responsibility (*dharma*) for himself; one must take active charge of one's own well-being. The interpersonal and social aspects of this reside in the belief that when one fulfills one's own *dharma* (personal and social duties), one also benefits the immediate and extended social group in very direct ways. In addition, Ayurveda sees the surrounding natural world (animals, minerals, seasons, and so forth) as being sacred and uses aspects of it in an ecologically respectful manner to further the welfare both of man and of nature. Not only appreciating the indigenous perfection already extant in creation, Ayurveda seeks to continue the ongoing work of further perfecting the world, starting with the individual self.

Ayurveda is world-embracing; in many ways, the only thing that is renounced is renunciation itself. Any form of escapism is eschewed. This conception of the intrinsic connectedness between man and nature is mirrored in the Ayurvedic theory of the five Elements, a delineated matrix of five material principles within nature that make up all animate and inanimate bodies. I have referred to this by coining the term *eco-corporeality*. In addition, the more subtle Ayurvedic ontic entities in nature termed *Prana* (life force), *Tejas* (flame of intelligence), and *Ojas* (enduring immunity) are intrinsic constituents of human psychological functioning. I have referred to this commonality as an individual's *eco-psychological* mental disposition.

Self-care and personal change are among Ayurveda's central concerns. This covers change both in the psychological and in the physical domains. Both aspects are pressing since they repeatedly present the individual with an apparently rebellious and persistent tendency to go awry, produce malaise, and then spark an impulse toward correction. Personal change both materially and emotionally, however, is usually exceedingly difficult; most persons not only resist but also appear to be resistant to change. This again attests to the provocatively rebellious nature that we all experience as a central aspect of ourselves. One of the main reasons for this may be related to a commonly encountered clinical presentation in the field of rehabilitative medicine, that is, the universal tendency "to accommodate to the deformity."

In order to overcome this resistance to change, man's will, his conative or volitional faculty, is preeminent in implementing the energy for self-activation in order to produce change in everyday, conventional existence. All change, in fact, is considered self-change. This idea has two levels of meaning: (1) the abstract cognitive recognition of personal distress and disharmony along with the experience of the impulse to change and (2) an individual's integrated efforts aimed at producing the material occurrence of actual, concrete change. Some comparisons between Ayurveda and Western medicine may be useful to demonstrate some similarities and differences since issues of disorder and strategies for change are major features of both.

Whereas Western medicine strives for accuracy by using the scientific method and accumulating statistically significant data about health and disease, Ayurveda tends more toward naturalism, that is, an empirical approach closer to nature. This entails a strong, almost exclusive reliance on clinical examination and diagnosis and the virtual absence of any formal laboratory investigations. The linear thinking and logic of Western medicine is highly analytic, categorical, and uses a classification system of discrete disease entities as a basic template to guide the direction of treatment. Most pathological conditions in this view are primarily conceived of as coarse manifestations of actual gross disease processes. By comparison, the central paradigm in Ayurveda is the maintenance of optimal health by daily proactive care. The individual is seen in a comprehensive way as an integral *BioPsychoSpiritual* being who strives for an optimal quality of life by adhering to daily health routines (Ninivaggi, 2001, 2005a, 2005b). These include diet, exercise, lifestyle choices, and psychological work, all of which must be continually modified according to age and seasonal changes. The individual participates in a systems continuum, microcosm within macrocosm. Ayurveda presents a comprehensive way of life that encourages balance in all aspects of living. It proactively treats the subtle, almost imperceptible, trends toward imbalance and their inevitable diatheses toward formal illness using routine prophylactic maintenance. The individual, in part, is believed to have an innate capacity for potential self-correction and for primary self-healing.

Chapter 11, "The Cultivation of Consciousness," addresses many contemporary issues, which have been formally raised and are currently debated, for example, within various branches of cognitive science. These very concerns have been recognized and coherently addressed within Ayurveda and Buddhism for, at least, the last 2,500 years. Correlations, for example, between epistemological debates thus take on a clearer, perhaps a fresher, perspective. Chapter 12 introduces the novel conception of the *BioPsychoSpiritual* perspective in clinical Psychiatry. Such an Ayurvedically oriented psychological delineation offering concrete therapeutic strategies may be particularly useful as adjunctive considerations in psychotherapy settings. This also has great relevance to all forms of counseling and guidance. A developmental perspective is at the core of Ayurveda. An important extension of this is the significance of Ayurvedic principles in the well care of children and adolescents. A mental health example of this would be offering parental guidance in *envy management skills* that would be a regular part of family health values and modeling. Families may benefit immeasurably by incorporating dietary, lifestyle, and even meditative strategies. Since Ayurveda is not a "one size fits all" intervention, parents must diligently examine the nuances of the material, psychological, and spiritual dimensions of their children and create unique environments that dynamically change over time.

While Western medicine treats discrete disease entities, Ayurveda treats, most often proactively, the subtly experienced states of dysphoria and malaise whose insidiously disruptive trends may only later develop into discrete disease entities. The technological approach of Western medicine, therefore, strives for scientific objectivity and verifiability. Disease and disease states are seen as discrete entities that are superimposed, for the most part, on man. Medical interventions have a relatively more ahistorical and "experience-distant" basis. Ayurveda, on the other hand, is preeminently "experience near" and holds *pratyaksha,* a direct grasp of the multisensory perceptive understanding of each individual patient, as its foremost diagnostic tool. This essential feature reflects the astute attention, listening, and concern that the Ayurvedic practitioner gives each patient. The patient is central, and the chart or medical record is ancillary. Disease and illness are understood to be dynamic imbalances (*dosha* imbalances) that organically emerge out of man's innate constitution as it interacts with the environment over time. An individual's perception and use of the environment is emphasized. The role that the interpersonal environment plays, especially in infancy and childhood, on an individual's development cannot be emphasized enough. All of this reflects Ayurveda in its role as a science whose leading context is dynamic discovery.

The question regarding an attempt to correlate Western technomedicine and Ayurveda or Traditional Indian Medicine is an important one to consider. A deliberate and conscious choice has been made not to attempt such a large undertaking in the limited space of this book. Such a serious study would deserve consideration in the form of an entire book. The principal goal of this work is to introduce Ayurveda in as authentic a manner as the use of Western concepts and terminology may permit. Whether or not this can be done without corruption remains an open question. Eastern and Western conceptions and practices are often qualitatively different. For example, in Ayurveda, the subtle energies and the spiritual qualities behind an idea and its clinical application probably defy ordinary observation and measurement using parameters for validity and reliability so crucial in Western science. Whether the philosophical and psychological underpinnings of each are light-years away or can be recognized to exhibit intermittent convergences is a weighty topic. In the author's best judgment, such questions are best reserved for a different forum that may give such considerations the ample and extensive diligence that they deserve. The present work does not lend itself to that additional and challenging endeavor.

A fair question then becomes, Why consider using Ayurveda when Western medicine has so much to offer? A satisfactory answer is fraught with the complexities that both healing systems intrinsically contain along with the fact of their differing cultural origins. While it may be reasonable to consider that the two health-care systems, if viewed as strictly alternative, probably may not be capable of immediate theoretical integration at this time, some compatibility, in fact, does exist. Their complementary and adjunctive clinical application seems both reasonable and justifiable, if used intelligently and realistically. Positive, negative, or uncertain outcomes need to be reviewed periodically. In the future, these two approaches may become increasingly integrative.

The applicability of Ayurveda as a design for healthy living with a high modicum of quality can easily be understood from a Western perspective if the entire range of stress and stress response is considered. The recently expanding fields of psychoneuroimmunology, stress and the immune system, for example, and psychoneuroendocrinology, the hypothalamic-pituitary-thyroid axis, for example, within medicine explores the links between the mind, the nervous system, hormones, and immune responses in health and disease. Stressors or stressful life events are typical. The manner in which an individual adapts to these determines in large measure the benign or deleterious effects that may result. Studies have shown that chronic stress has negative consequences (Harris, Wolkowitz, & Reus, 2005). For example, one's overall immune response may fall far below its normal baseline; proinflammatory cytokines may increase and lead to pervasive endothelial dysfunction of the lining of all blood vessels. In turn, this may contribute to atherosclerosis, cardiac disease, and diabetes. Chronically increased cortisol levels may impact the hippocampus with resultant memory impairments and depression. In addition, the long-term increase of corticotrophin releasing factor on amygdala structures has been shown to increase fear and anxiety; and dopamine depletion in the ventral tegmentum and nucleus accumbens results in anhedonia, low motivation, and the incapacity to experience pleasure and satisfaction.

Recent studies (Russo-Neustadt, 2003) have demonstrated that "brain-derived neurotrophic factor" (BDNF), a protein found in brain structures, helps support the survival of existing neurons and also encourages the growth and differentiation of new neurons. This factor is active in the hippocampus, cerebral cortex, and basal forebrain in areas that are vital to learning, memory, and higher cognitive processes. Chronic exposure to stress and the stress hormone, corticosterone, in rats, for example, has been shown to decrease the expression of BDNF and leads to hippocampal atrophy, which is associated with clinical depression in humans. Stress when managed appropriately also contributes to diminishing the likelihood of the development of blood glucose irregularities and insulin resistance, risk factors for diabetes. In addition, the hippocampus is dense in insulin receptors. The proper functioning of insulin, therefore, may also be significantly involved with learning and memory. Ayurvedic diet and life-style offer a major means of dealing with everyday, acute stress reactions. Its proactive strategies and practices may prevent the much more deleterious effects of chronic stress responses. Even small, intentional efforts toward change in one's manner and style of living can yield meaningful benefits.

If Ayurveda and Western medicine are used together, pragmatically, their reciprocal interaction could be synergistic and create a greater degree of clinical efficacy. This remains an interesting and open question and will rest heavily on the skill, ingenuity, and good will of health providers of differing disciplines. Of course, therapeutic results from either one or both health systems will naturally result in differential beneficial response rates due to the heterogeneity of patients, diseases, and other intervention variables. Ayurveda, in general, is geared more toward health maintenance rather than disease treatment. Its primary emphasis is health promotion, namely, reducing and attempting to eliminate health-related risks, especially by advancing lifestyle wellness values. It is a system of diet and lifestyle choices whose aim is to enhance the quality of life by dealing with the subtle trends that might lead to actual disease. It is, therefore, a method for living life in a more fulfilled manner. Quality of life is a high priority.

Another important consideration would take into account the fact that Ayurveda might not be a useful choice or rather may appear incompatible with the beliefs, values, and motivations of those whose outlooks preclude such naturalistic, spiritual, and consciousness-oriented approaches. Natural and alternative approaches often require intentional and sustained self-discipline, perseverance, and taking an active, personal role in matters of health and overall lifestyle choices. This self-help approach has not been a part of the traditional Western medical model. In recent times, however, this is changing. In addition, substantive change requires guidance and monitoring from a highly qualified Ayurvedic specialist. This, in itself, may be viewed as arduous since it necessitates commitment over time. Insofar as consciousness and spirituality are inclusive domains within Ayurveda, some may prefer to focus only on the psychological aspects that are an inseparable part of these; others may choose to use only the health practices. These partial approaches are certainly useful and worthwhile. Ayurveda, it will be seen, is compatible with virtually all points of view, that is, health, philosophical, religious, and spiritual, for example. It can even provide one with a more enhanced mind-set and state of physical well-being, thus affording more success in any particular way of life that is already in place. Ayurveda encourages people to remain in their native habitat—geographically and psychologically—at least in the initial stages of the journey toward change.

Ayurveda, like Western medical science, developed subspecialties to address particular medical and health needs. The *Asthanga Ayurveda* (eight branches or limbs of Ayurveda) are the following:

1. *Kayachikitsa,* Internal Medicine
2. *Shalyatantra,* Surgery
3. *Shalakyatantra,* Otolaryngology, Ophthalmology
4. *Kaumarabhritya,* Obstetrics, Gynecology, and Pediatrics
5. *Agadatantra,* Toxicology

6. *Bhutavidya,* Psychiatry

7. *Rasayana,* Antiaging and rejuvenation

8. *Vajikarana,* Reproductive and aphrodisiac medicine

Ayurveda: A Comprehensive Guide to Tradition Indian Medicine for the West concentrates on the presentation of the theoretical propositions and clinical principles that make up the fundamental Ayurvedic corpus. It is primarily intended for students of Ayurveda, and its optimal use is as a companion in a classroom, seminar, or clinical setting with a qualified teacher. The formal discussions in this reference work cover an extensive range of topics uniquely salient to Ayurveda in its larger Hindu, Buddhist, and cultural contexts, especially its complex history. Hence, the breadth of these discourses as has been alluded to may appear advanced rather than merely elementary. Yet, this comprehensive guide is presented in such a way that anyone—professional, lay person, or health-minded citizen—can use it or parts of it in a practical way since each section is written in a self-explanatory fashion.

It is worthwhile reiterating that the principal goal of this text is to present a representative range of authentic Ayurveda in the spirit of its Eastern roots. The author has intentionally refrained from attempting to add more commentary than necessary to this end. It is also important to underscore that no attempt has been made to synthesize what are already highly complex ideas —Eastern and Western—whose ramifications are clearly beyond the scope of this introductory compendium. This has been a conscious and deliberate choice.

Sanskrit terms are rendered in a simplified and anglicized manner as is commonly found in nontechnical English transliterations. Phonetic pronunciations reflected in spelling preferences rather than strict Sanskrit ones are used in order to be more cordial and user-friendly to the Western tongue. Particular spellings, formats of phrases, capitalization, and so forth, have been chosen, to some degree arbitrarily, for the sake of uniformity and to emphasize special significance. A broad glossary of selected terms, inclusive but not exhaustive, has been provided that contains the basic vocabulary necessary to achieve an adequate grasp of the subject. Not every Sanskrit term used in the text is included in the glossary, either because its significance as a term per se is considered nonessential to an understanding of basic Ayurveda or because it is more properly related to a different specialized field, for example, Yoga. Following current conventions when presenting Ayurvedic concepts in English-speaking circles, this text attempts to use either the appropriate Sanskrit term or its English meaning in a relatively uniform, though not rigid, fashion. As mentioned earlier, since the breadth of detail in Ayurveda is formidable, only selected essential areas will be covered here. These areas and the level of detail presented are, in fact, representative of the substantive matrix of basic Ayurveda. It should also be mentioned that time frames and dating, especially of the B.C. era, are approximate; they should be regarded as provisional since archeological discoveries continue to unearth new findings.

Much important material, of necessity, has been intentionally left out. Two large areas of omission are (1) a detailed account of the herbomineral armamentarium of Ayurvedic Materia Medica and (2) an exhaustive outline of particular disease states, their remediation, and more than merely a small sampling of brief clinical examples. Since it is not in the tradition of Ayurvedic texts to include case examples and their treatments, I have respected this custom. A latter work, perhaps, can be specifically devoted to this area, which is certainly important and of special interest to Western practitioners. Proper and rational treatment is a highly complex field that requires not only theoretical expertise but also "hands-on" and closely supervised clinical training over time. The discourses in this book provide an orientation; they do not purport to substitute for actual clinical work under supervision. Some popular as well as scholarly publications covering these areas are currently available in English; some of these will be cited in the references. However, key herbs and medicinal substances, as, for example, those used for the critical processes of *Ama pachana* (detoxification) and *Agni dipana* (optimal digestive enhancement) have been included and highlighted.

The author has made extensive use of one of Ayurveda's indisputably foundational medical compilations, the *Charaka Samhita*. Thanks to the Yale medical and university libraries, an original and highly annotated English translation in four volumes has provided the backbone for the present work (Kaviratna, 1902–1925).

Finally, as a Western trained medical doctor and psychiatrist, I have tried to write a book that both intelligently and accurately embodies the essence and spirit of Ayurveda in a form that is logical, plausible, and *understandable to Western thinkers*. My training and my ongoing appointment in Child and Adolescent Psychiatry at the Yale University School of Medicine since 1975 have afforded me a broad range of experience both intellectually and in treating patients from early childhood into later life. The psychoanalytic contributions of Sigmund Freud and Melanie Klein have served as both theoretical frameworks and therapeutic instruments. Diligent and sensitive observation of mental processes and their expressions in speech, in emotional displays, and in behavior have continued to be high priorities.

Buddhism, moreover, has deeply influenced my understanding of human psychology and the problem of meaning and of meaningfulness. For me, this path has opened blockages to a freer experience of the integration of consciousness or spirituality within both body and mind. Spiritual hunger and existential loneliness underlie the malaise of a life without meaning. In this sense, spirituality connotes a sense of renewal and a sense of the sacred. Within this consciousness are feelings, ideas, and intuitions that, in special ways, are set apart from ordinary experience. These apperceptions constitute what is inferred to be intangible, subtle, pure, restorative, integrating, and good. One's individual share of consciousness in the broadest sense may be viewed as the quintessential activity of all information processing. The experience of such consciousness partakes both of corporeal (genetic, chromosomal, cellular, and the body as a whole) and of mental/psychological data and processes. Consciousness-enhancing ideas and practices as presented in this text, it is hoped, may act to integrate all material and immaterial dimensions that touch consciousness. This connectivity is presumed to enhance more optimal self-awareness and healthy adaptation. Ultimately, this apparent integration of previously split experiential phenomena becomes an awakening to and a recovery of the fundamental unity that has always been present at least implicitly although not consciously recognized.

The current text, it is my hope, will bring Ayurveda and its practices into contemporary focus not merely with scholarship, but also with an appealing understandability. An important aim is to help advance a proper and more formal recognition of this "life wisdom" that will auspiciously facilitate its achieving status as a significant part of world medicine for the third millennium.

Frank John Ninivaggi, M.D.
Yale University School of Medicine
New Haven, Connecticut

Vesak Festival
May 2007

1

BACKGROUND, HISTORY, AND DEVELOPMENT

AYURVEDA WITHIN THE CONTEXT OF WORLD CULTURE

Lord Dhanvantari was regarded, in ancient India, as a deity and patron of classical medicine. He continues to hold that honor among Ayurvedic physicians today. Most depictions and statuary show him holding in his left hand a bowl of *amrit,* the nectar of life; his right hand holds a medical text, an herb, a leech, and a knife. These items, symbolizing the whole range of medicine and surgery, serve as a model of inspiration spanning past and present. The opening passages of the *Sushruta Samhita* (Acharya & Pandurang, 1945; Bhishagratna, 1968; Trikamji & Ram, 1980), an ancient Indian medical text, describe Ayurveda's mythological origins in the following way:

> "O, Sire, it grieves us much to find men, though otherwise well befriended by their kin and relations, falling prey to diseases, mental, physical, coming to them from outside or from their inner being, and piteously wailing in agony like utterly friendless creatures on earth; and we supplicate thee, O Lord, to illumine our minds with the truths of the Eternal Ayurveda so that we may faithfully discharge the duties allotted to us in life, and alleviate the sufferings of humanity at large. Bliss in this life and hereafter is in the gift of this Eternal Ayurveda, and for this, O Lord, we have made bold to approach thee as thy humble disciples." To them thus replied the holy Dhanvantari, "Welcome to all of you to this blissful hermitage. All of you are worthy of the honor of true pupilship or tutelage."

Ayurveda is a Sanskrit word meaning the knowledge, wisdom, or science of life in the sense of the optimal measure of all aspects of high-quality and healthy living. It has its origins in the distant past before the historical period of written documentation and is believed to have been received and formulated by the ancient sages (*rishis*) of India who were considered individuals with the stature of mental giants. The accurate dating of the historical origins of Ayurveda, like that of Traditional Chinese Medicine, is uncertain. The portraits in this chapter—historical surveys—are painted with broad strokes intentionally omitting finer details. My aim is to convey understandability by means of fractal levels of orientation. Dating, therefore, may be considered only an approximation, in part derived from surviving documents, and in larger measure from tradition. Historical accuracy becomes more objectively verifiable during and after the advent of Buddhism in the sixth century B.C., and with the historical writings of the Greek historian Herodotus (c. 490/ 80–425 B.C.), considered by some as the father of Western history. His commentaries, especially on the Greek and Persian wars, reflect a very active international exchange of conflict, conquest, and ideas.

The significance of this documented, early (c. 550 B.C.) contact between Persia and Greece lies in the fact that the Persian Empire constituted the geographical, if not cultural, link between India and territories to the west—the Near East and the Roman Empire. The ancestors of the Persians (modern-day Iranians) were derived, in part, from the same Proto-Indo-Iranian peoples who, it is believed, significantly contributed to the *Vedas,* ancient wisdom texts of India, in the second millennium B.C. (Biardeau, 1989). In addition, Cyrus the Great captured Babylon in 539 B.C. This conquest gave Persia control over Mesopotamia and the entire Babylonian Empire that then reached to the borders of Egypt. Historical sources testify to the fact that the Persian Empire, at this early date, borrowed heavily from the cultures of Assyria, Babylonia, Egypt, and Greece. To what extent Persia absorbed parts of India's culture and Ayurveda is not clearly documented. Some Indian influence may have occurred and contributed to the development of Persian medicine. An Ayurvedic influence becomes clearer much later and is reflected in the prolific work of the Persian physician Avicenna in the tenth century A.D.

After Cyrus, the subsequent Persian ruler, Darius (c. 522 B.C.), entered India (Figure 1.1) and annexed the Sind (the ancient Mohenjo-daro area; present-day Sind, southeast Pakistan) and, perhaps, the Punjab region (ancient Harappa; present-day Sahiwal in western Pakistan). Later, Alexander the Great (c. 334 B.C.) not only conquered the Persians, but in 327 B.C. entered India and there defeated the Indian king Poros. Aspects of Hellenic culture, therefore, were introduced into India and some aspects of Indian culture including Ayurveda were surely absorbed by the Greeks and the Persians. Bloodshed and an active need for medical and surgical skill no doubt accompanied these invasions and military conflicts. The exchange of medicosurgical knowledge among the cultures—India, the Middle East, and the Greek and Roman West—especially via this route, is an implied certainty (Wohlberg, 1990).

WRITTEN HISTORY AND ORAL TRADITION

Written history is relatively recent. Oral tradition is certainly much older and the primary source of much of what can only be properly termed "historical speculation" regarding the ancient roots and developments within cultures

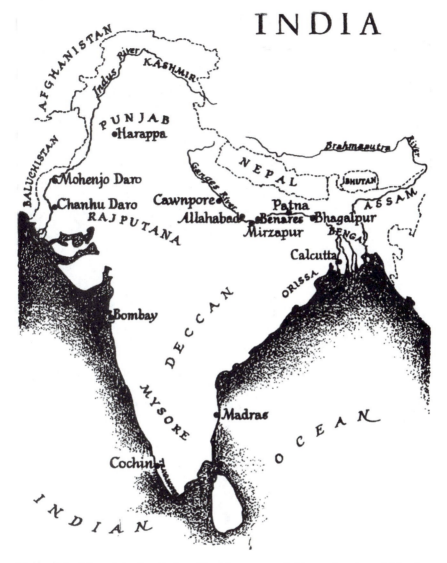

Figure 1.1 Map of Ancient India with older names of cities and regions. Mohenjo-daro was in the Sind region. Harappa was in the Punjab region. Ancient Taxila was on the Indus River, north of Harappa in the Kashmir region, now modern Pakistan. The Hindu Kush Pass was northwest of Harappa. Benares was also called Varanasi.

[Map of India (p. 118–119) from *History of Medicine Vol 2: Early Greek, Hindu and Persian Medicine* (1961) be Sigerist HE. By permission of Oxford University Press.]

and peoples. Recognizing this, only a board overview, much of which is objectively tentative, will be outlined for the primary purpose of providing an orientation to Ayurveda and Indian culture within the larger scope of human cultural development.

The primitive roots of culture are believed to have formally developed just after the last Ice Age (c. 10,000 B.C.). This first occurred in the region of the Near East. The transition from a more nomadic hunter-gatherer and pastoral life-style to an agricultural one with a food-producing economy contributed to significantly greater stability over time in a central geographical location, the stable settlement. Jericho, near present-day Jerusalem, was the site of the Natufian culture (c. 9500 B.C.). The area called Catal-Huyuk in present-day Turkey was the home of another complex Neolithic culture (c. 8500 B.C.). These two areas were focal points of agriculture and the domestication of animals by 7000 B.C. These two achievements along with the development of human technology, primarily the invention of tools, mark the Neolithic era (7000 B.C.–3300 B.C.). Hallmarks of civilization include literacy, organized religion, art forms, stable settlements and planned cities, agriculture, and the domestication of animals. The Mesopotamian city of Sumer is considered the first recognizable city, its origins dating back to the fourth millennium B.C. The earliest known writing is early Mesopotamian cuneiform and dates to about 3300 B.C.

Formal history begins with the written word. Written documents in various formats began to appear about the middle of the fourth millennium B.C. with hieroglyphic, cuneiform, and Minoan script. Significant medical content can be found in early writings such as the *Rig-Veda* of India (conventionally presumed origin c. 1500 B.C.), the *Codex Hammurabi* of Mesopotamia (c. 1755 B.C.), and the *Medical Papyrus Ebers* of Egypt (1570 B.C.) (Sigerist, 1951).

A legacy of written documents describing the medical systems of these eras is sorely lacking in current times. They are either undiscovered or non-existent. Scholarship, in the form of libraries and archives dedicated to collections of writings that reflect the history, literature, art, and science of the times, appears to have been launched in ancient Assyria when Ashurbanipal amassed the most complete collection available at the time in his grand library of Ninivah/Nineveh (c. 720–612 B.C.) on the northeastern shore of the Tigris River. It is inferred that this included not only local contributions but also the scientific, literary, and artistic writings that were taken from his conquest of Egypt.

In Nalanda, Northeast India, in the ancient kingdom of Magadha (present-day Bihar near Patna bordering Nepal to the north), existed what is referred to as "The Buddhist University." The famous Nalanda University is reputed by some to have been established at this site as a monastery by as early as the fifth century B.C. This center of learning was a repository of extant literature not only of Buddhism but also of medicine, astronomy, mathematics, and other sciences. The Buddha (c. 563–483 B.C.) is believed to have visited it and given sermons there. The Jain luminary, Mahavira (sixth/fifth century B.C.), is said to have attained *Moksha* (enlightenment) at Pavapuri in Nalanda.

The three major schools of Buddhism—Theravada, Mahayana, and Vajrayana—are considered to have been expounded at Nalanda. Theravada Buddhism flourished and then spread into Sri Lanka (formerly called Ceylon) c.

250 B.C., Myanmar (formerly called Burma) c. fifth–third century B.C., Thailand (formerly called Siam) c. sixth century A.D., and Cambodia (third century A.D.). Mahayana Buddhism, elucidated by the famous Ayurvedic physician and Buddhist priest Nāgārjuna, flourished at Nalanda and then spread to Vietnam, China (c. A.D. 2), Korea (fourth century A.D.), and Japan (c. A.D. 522). The development of Vajrayana Buddhism or Tibetan Buddhism stems from the ninth–twelfth century A.D. Nalanda teachers. Vajrayana is also referred to as Tantrayana, Tantric Buddhism, the Diamond Vehicle, and Lamaism. Buddhism was originally brought to Tibet by Padmasambhava ("the Lotusborn," c. A.D. 755–797) who was born in northwestern Kashmir. He established the Samye Monastery in A.D. 775 and was venerated by his followers as "the second Buddha." He is still venerated today in the Himalayan countries under the name of Guru Rinpoche (the Precious Guru).

In A.D. 1193, Turkish Muslim invaders destroyed the Nalanda University consortium. Many Buddhist monks fled to Tibet at this time, and this event is considered to have heralded the near extinction of Buddhism in India.

King Ashoka, emperor of India (c. 260–218 B.C.) was an ardent Buddhist who proselytized Buddhism to lands outside of India. These included Bactria (modern northern Afghanistan), Athens, Antioch (the ancient capitol of Syria), and Alexandria in Egypt.

The Tang Dynasty Chinese pilgrim, Xuanzang (also spelled Hsuan-tsang or San-tsang, A.D. 600–664), left detailed written accounts of the University with its one time 10,000 students in the seventh century A.D. to document Nalanda's history. He reported his experiences in his famous travel account *Ta-t'ang hsi-yu chi*, which provides important dates for research on the history, archaeology, and state of Buddhism in India at that early time. Many Buddhist priests were also Ayurveda physicians, and as Buddhism traveled outside of India, so did Ayurveda. In its new locations, Ayurveda, like Buddhism, took on the cultural face of its followers.

Ptolemy I (c. 305 B.C.) later brought together arguably the greatest and most complete library of its time in Alexandria, Egypt. Perganum (c. 200 B.C.) in Asia Minor was the site of another library said to rival that of Alexandria with an especially impressive Hellenistic influence gathered from the Roman conquests of Syracuse (c. 212 B.C.) and later of Corinth (c. 146 B.C.). Of importance is the fact that these early library collections, especially in Alexandria, with all their probable historical masterpieces were progressively destroyed beginning in 47 B.C. when Caesar was compelled to set fire to his fleet to prevent its falling into the hands of the Egyptians. What remained of the library was destroyed in piecemeal fashion at various later periods, according to historical tradition, probably culminating around 642 A.D. with the capture of Alexandria by the Muslims.

Ayurveda, sometimes referred to as Indian medical science or Traditional Indian Medicine (TIM), appears to have its discernible origins in the *Rig-Veda* and later *Vedas,* particularly the *Atharva-Veda* (presumed origin c. 1200 B.C.). These roots suggest that Ayurveda may be among the oldest systematized forms of medicine and subsequently may have contributed to or influenced later medical systems both in Asia and in the West. Ayurveda's origins lie in an oral tradition. Verifiable, written documentation is sparse and relies heavily on the *Vedas,* a group of religious and philosophical writings, and particularly the oldest one, the *Rig-Veda. Veda* is the Sanskrit word meaning science, knowledge, or wisdom. *Rig* is a Sanskrit word that connotes "stanzas of praise." Historians have found it almost impossible to date the Vedic hymns and poetry with any degree of accuracy. Their content is known to have been transmitted by word of mouth for centuries, if not millennia, before they were written down. In a similar fashion, historians acknowledge that the *Iliad* and the *Odyssey* of ancient Greece were sung by itinerant bards long before they were edited and collected in the form known to us today. The oldest known manuscript of the Vedic scriptures dates to the fifteenth century A.D. Its actual origins, however, are believed to be much older, and archaeological evidence demonstrates that these writings, in fact, do reflect aspects of the earliest Indus civilization (c. 2500–1750 B.C.).

INDIAN CULTURE

Ayurveda and Indian culture are inseparably linked (Kak, 1987). Ayurveda and Hinduism, the socioreligious underpinnings of the peoples of Bharata (India), are inextricably intertwined. Hinduism is the world's oldest extant religion. Most Hindus today live in India or Hindustan (the land of Hindus). Although subject to differences of opinion, many accept that the word "Hindu" was originally of Persian origin and denoted peoples who lived around and beyond the Indus River, which is called *Sindhu* in Sanskrit. Until about A.D. 1800s, the term "Hindu" comprised a culture, an ethnicity, and a religion of the Indian peoples. When the British began to organize legal systems and the taking of a census, then the term "Hindu" took on more of its narrower religious parameters.

It is said that the self-designation of Hinduism in Indian languages is *Vedic dharma* (the religion of the *Vedas*). Hindus often refer to their religion as *Sanatana Dharma,* the eternal religion. This appellation strongly connotes more than merely a religion; it denotes a way of life, the timeless foundations of which predate their human recognition. Although such a fierce and passionate conviction in being unique and virtually ahistorical pervades Indian thought, Ayurveda's beginnings and current emergence, especially in the West, have more universalistic rather than narrowly sectarian expression and application.

It has only been since 1921–1922 with the discovery of the ancient cultures of Harappa and Mohenjo-daro that India's ancient past has come to light in the writings of contemporary archeology. An accurate clarification of India's roots in civilization and of the specific contributions that it has made to world culture is still in their infant stages of discovery.

The origins of the *Vedas* and the contributions of various different groups of ancient cultures to them has been a source of uncertainty and ongoing debate (Shaffer, 1984; Bryant, 2001; Bryant & Patton, 2005). One group within mainstream anthropology currently holds that by about 2500 B.C. and before 1500 B.C., the Dravidians, supposedly an indigenous, dark-skinned people about whose origins little is known, inhabited India. The forebears of these varied groups are believed to be of Mehrgarh (modern-day Baluchistan) origin, that is, to have come from the earlier Neolithic cultures (7000–6000 B.C.) of Afghanistan and Baluchistan to the northwest (modern-day Pakistan). Many Indian historians consider the latter sites to have been part of ancient India.

These peoples, also referred to as the pre-Harappan or Early Indus culture, established complex urban sites in northwest India along the Indus River. It is inferred that they had an already developed culture with significant material, psychological, and spiritual dimensions. This civilization reached its peak around 2300 B.C. and trade links with Mesopotamia have been dated to this period.

The subsequently developed culture of the mature Indus Valley Civilization, or Harappan Civilization (3300–1500 B.C.), is seen in the regions called Mohenjo-daro in Sind and Harappa in Punjab (Dales & Kenoyer, 1993). It was the largest of the four ancient civilizations of Egypt, Mesopotamia, India, and China. These ancient Harappan areas are part of modern-day Pakistan in the region of the Indus River. Ongoing excavations at these sites have yielded impressive archaeological finds and are recognized as the most important and extensive Bronze Age sites. Their hieroglyphic style of writing has yet to be deciphered (Parpola, 1994). Material evidence from these sites suggests a strong cultural unity, evidence of trading links with Mesopotamia, and a high degree of uniformity of urban planning. The high level of sophistication of these cultures is solidly demonstrated by their meticulously organized city planning with complex drainage systems, the earliest known evidence of cotton cultivation, and a standardized system of weights and measures in use for commerce.

Mohenjo-daro is recognized as one of the oldest, if not the oldest, known planned city. Significant material evidence from this very early period is highly suggestive of a cultural recognition of a spiritual dimension with religious overtones. Figurines and steatite seals having god and goddesslike images have been uncovered. The famous Pasupati/Pashupati seal (Figure 1.2) has been inferred to possibly represent a prototype of the Hindu god, Shiva, the yogi and Lord of the animals, having three faces and sitting in a classic Yoga posture. This Indus culture, therefore, is thought to contain early and important elements of what later significantly contributed to, developed into, or was rooted in the Vedic tradition.

It is plausible that the most ancient roots of Indian culture are essentially indigenous to the entire Indian continent—the "continuous civilization" point of view. There continues, however, to be a hotly debated controversy

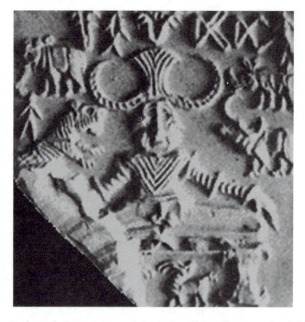

Figure 1.2   Pashupati: Terracotta seal depicting Shiva discovered at Mohenjo-daro

involving the aforementioned. It is known as the "Aryan Invasion Theory" (AIT) or the Indo-Aryan migration hypothesis. The latter proposes that sometime in the second millennium B.C. (around 2000–1500 B.C.), a new group of non-Indian people, who are thought to have come from the plains of central Asia, came into northwest India through the passes of the Hindu Kush (Pamir Mountains and most western part of the Himalayan Mountains in present-day northeast Afghanistan and Pakistan) bringing with them the domesticated horse (Fairservis, 1975). This group has been referred to as "Aryans." The precise meaning of this designation is arguable. Speculations about its connotations and its meaning include the following: stranger, potential guest, refined, noble, righteous, or a self-designation for one whose lineage and language are of ancient Persian (modern-day Iranian) descent. The hypothetical arrival of the Aryan peoples is associated with the decline of the previous indigenous Indus Valley Civilization.

It is believed that their language was Vedic Sanskrit, one of the oldest Indo-European root languages. The AIT advocates propose that these outsiders brought the sacred scriptures, the *Vedas,* into India. The *Vedas* reflect a total worldview that includes aspects of creation, metaphysics, philosophy, ethics, religion, magic, medicine, dietary rules, and guidelines for the activities of daily living. The Aryan culture (1500–500 B.C.) is believed to have eventually merged with and then dominated the pre-Aryan peoples of the Indus civilization. Although the Aryans exerted an overriding influence on the developing culture, including religion and philosophy, of India during this period, the earlier indigenous Dravidians, especially in central and southern India, Tamil, the Deccan and Mysore regions, are considered to have made important and substantial contributions to the form and content of this newly emerging Aryan evolution.

It should be mentioned that many highly regarded figures in modern Hinduism such as Sri Aurobindo (1872–1950) and Swami Vivekananda (1863–1902) hold that the so-called Aryans were, in fact, highly advanced proto-Hindu Vedics indigenous to and not coming from outside ancient India (Varma, 1968). This view represents an alternative "cultural transformation thesis." It is plausible especially since the Hindu Kush (now Afghanistan and part of Pakistan) was considered part of India at that early time. In this perspective, the descriptions of war in the *Rig-Veda* between Aryans and Dravidians are interpreted on metaphorical levels, reflecting spiritual warfare and nature poetry.

Recent speculation has continued to propose a more intimate link between Dravidian and Aryan cultures, if not an actual identity. For example, the great Sarasvati River, now dried up, that flowed from the Himalayas through the western Rajasthan Desert to the Arabian Sea was described in detail and venerated in the early *Vedas* (O'Flaherty, 1981). It was located roughly in the northwest areas near and running parallel to the modern-day Indus River. Some believe that the ancient Sarasvati River can be identified with the seasonally wet Ghaggar River in present-day India and the dried up Hakra riverbed in present-day Pakistan. Since currently accepted research postulates that the Sarasvati River dried up around 3000 B.C., the *Vedas,* which accurately described this ancient geography, must have been in existence at this early time. It is speculated that since the Sumerian Empire declined sharply around 2200 B.C. due to a climate shift that caused major droughts for several centuries, the Harappans, close to Sumer, also could have been affected by this and so abandoned the Indus cities and pushed westward. The authors of the *Vedas,* therefore, may very well have been indigenous to this region, which was part of ancient India. They may have been the Harappan, Indus Valley Civilization (3300–1500 B.C.) peoples. In other words, the seers of ancient Harappa may have been of the same lineage as, perhaps the ancestors of, the Aryans of the Vedic period (1900/1500–500 B.C.).

Last, and of note in this regard, are the relatively recent though uninterpreted findings of the rock shelters and caves at Bhimbetka. This archaeological find in the state of Madhya Pradesh in the central region, the geographic heart, of modern India attests to the earliest known traces of human life dating back to the Mesolithic period, roughly c. 30,000 B.C.–7,000 B.C. These prehistoric paintings show scenes of animals and men, hunters, horsemen, and archers. This was discovered and explored in modern times (1958–1974) by D. V. S. Wakankar, one of India's leading archaeologists. Modern-day tribal peoples called *adivasis,* who now mostly live in these central geographical areas, constitute about 8 percent of the nation's total population and may be the descendants of the Bhimbetkans.

THE ANCIENT *VEDAS*

The ancient *Vedas* or cannons of wisdom constituted the foundation of ancient Indian culture and a way of life. Modern Indology is replete with references to these virtually inscrutable texts. To this day, the *Vedas* are still considered by orthodox Hindus to be the most authoritative source and template of all knowledge (Zaehner, 1966; Zimmer, 1951). They were believed to have been revealed by the godhead, Brahma, creator of the universe, and received, in fact, heard (*sruti*) by inspired sages (*rishis*) who passed them on by word of mouth. Brahma, it is held, propounded or asserted rather than invented the content of the *Vedas,* which includes Ayurveda. *Sruti* was and is considered to be *apauruseya* (not man-made, but of divine origin). Sages were leaders of extraordinary wisdom having the unique quality of *apta* (inspiration and authority). The *Samhita Vedas,* four in number, therefore, have a twofold denotation that encompasses both revelation (*sruti*), whose content is not of human origin (*apauruseya*), and, as well, the literature reflecting this sacred knowledge that was written down many centuries later.

The *Vedas* are considered to have been composed roughly around 1500 to 1200 B.C.; this dating regarding their oral compilation is a conservative and generally accepted idea. Others speculate that the *Vedas* were received by the *rishis* much earlier, possibly 3000 B.C. or even earlier although finally redacted around 1500 B.C. Final codification (c. 600 B.C.) may have occurred just before the time of Buddha. Modern anthropology dates the Vedic Civilization from 1900–500 B.C. Early Vedic society was largely pastoral. After the *Rig-Veda,* this society became increasingly agricultural and was organized around the four *varnas* (color code) or social classes differentiated upon occupational function: *Brahmin* (priests, scholars, and philosophers whose color code was white; symbol: head), *Kshatriya* (warriors, soldiers, and royalty whose color code was red; symbol: arms), *Vaishya* (merchants whose color code was yellow; symbol: thighs), and *Shudra* (artisans and laborers whose color code was dark colors; symbol: feet). The standard Vedic form for the teaching, learning, and dissemination of the *Vedas* and the subsequent commentaries (*bhasyas*) on them, in fact, consisted of their being sung as hymns or *sutras* (aphorisms in the form of oral lyrical prose/poetry). Pupils sat across from the teacher (*up-pa-sad*) and, in an intimately solemn and interpersonal fashion, recited the *sutras* of knowledge and wisdom.

The guardians and disseminators of the *Vedas* were the priestly class called *Brahmins*. The Brahmanic tradition is virtually synonymous with the Vedic tradition. Written versions of some Vedic commentaries appeared relatively late, around the middle of the first millennium B.C. The *Vedas,* therefore, constituted an oral body of knowledge that was transmitted from generation to generation but not organized into written form until well into the second millennium A.D. The profound significance of the *Vedas* lies in their being the bedrock upon which Ayurveda rests. The continuity of this ancient relationship is clearly suggested by a recognized tradition that regards

Ayurveda as an *upaveda* or supplementary *Veda,* with some going so far as to reverently ascribe to it the standing of the "fifth *Veda.*"

The primary *Vedas* are the four mantric or hymnal texts: the *Rig-Veda,* the *Yajur-Veda,* the *Sama-Veda,* and the *Atharva-Veda.* The *Rig-Veda* (Griffith, 1973; O'Flaherty, 1981) is considered the oldest and is reputedly the source of the other three. It is made up of stanzas of adulation (*rik*) that are compiled in ten books (*mandala*), which contain 1,028 sacred mantras, chants, hymns, and verses. Ayurvedic tradition, as well as some scholarly speculation, suggests that its content reflects events occurring earlier than 6000 B.C. The *Sama-Veda* (Ganapati, 1992) contains 1,810 mantras developed into musical forms, songs (*saman*), priestly chants, and instructions on their recitation. The *Yajur-Veda* contains action or ritual formulas (*yajus*) especially composed for sacrificial rites. It consists of five *samhitas,* collections of prayers and ritual texts in verse and prose. The *Atharva-Veda* (Bloomfield, 1967; Dwight, 1984; Whitney & Lanman, 1996) contains 731 magical incantations and ritual texts with a preponderance of medically related information spanning 20 books and is the *Veda* most closely associated with later Ayurvedic texts. The *Atharva-Veda* may have been composed around 1200 B.C. Many diseases are mentioned, including fever, diarrhea, heart disease, jaundice, cough, leprosy, and mania. In addition, there are ample references to obstetric and gynecological issues and procedures, as well as to what we now recognize as mental disorders. This ancient Vedic medicine, like Greek archaic medicine, had religious and magic elements. Certainly, no early Greek texts comparable to the *Atharva-Veda* have come down to us, perhaps because there were none or because of the destruction of the libraries in ancient Alexandria that may have housed them. The *Vedas* remain repositories of principles of understanding that are heavily suffused with moral precepts and rules of conduct. The *Vedas,* therefore, stand as an extant grand monument at the very beginning of Indian literature presenting a record of what is believed to be the source of all knowledge, including medicine and science.

Later authoritative supplements and appendixes based on the primary Vedic collections (*samhitas*) were called *Brahmanas* (ritual rules and explanatory texts; c. 1000 B.C.), *Aranyakas* (ritual and interpretation texts written in the forest; c. 1000 B.C.), and *Upanishads* (self-development; spiritual texts emphasizing interiority and internalization rather than external ritual; c. 600 B.C.) (Bedekar & Palsule, 1995; Radhakrishnan, 1953). These additional three groups of writings developed the ideas contained in the *samhitas,* and they all are considered to be part of the primary Vedic corpus. They, like the four *Samhita Vedas,* are considered *sruti* (revealed scriptures with the highest authority). Each of the four main *Vedas* can be viewed as composed of four layers or categories of text corresponding to the time frame within which they were composed: *Samhita, Brahmana, Aranyaka,* and *Upanishad.*

Since the Vedic period (c. 1900 to 500 B.C.) may be considered the foundation not only of Indian culture but also of Ayurveda, some significant aspects of the Vedic worldview as expressed in daily life are addressed. Two of the most central themes around which Vedic culture was organized were that of the significance of *fire* and that of *ritual sacrifice* (Heesterman, 1993; Staal, 1983). It may be difficult for modern man to fully appreciate the centrality that the phenomenon of fire had thousands of years ago. Not only was basic survival predicated on it, but the maturation and development of civilization was also enhanced. Fire provided warmth, the ability to cook and use a variety of foods (predominantly milk, ghee, grains, and meats), sterilization of water and foods, purification and cleaning, and light by which to extend human activities into the night. Man, at that time, was dependent on fire for survival. The singular importance of fire was expressed in the Vedic reification of it. Fire was identified with the god *Agni*. The conceptual understanding of *Agni* was multilayered. It included associations with heat, the sun, part of the earth as the sacred cow, *Prisni,* with the digestive fire within the human stomach, and as being the actual fire used in sacrificial ritual. The profound significance, meaning, and value of fire to humans and their well-being in the ancient world can be equated in meaning and significance to that of electricity in the modern world.

The concept of ritual and sacrifice is an ancient one (Jamison, 1991; Vesci, 1992). Its meaning includes a ritualized process whereby man gives offerings to a higher or transcendent reality. The concept of prayer is implicit in this activity. The idea that this may result in some beneficial effect is implied but complex. By the fifth century B.C., Vedic society had an established set of guidelines that charted out a developmental sequence of life stages (*asramas*) especially for the priestly classes. The second stage entailed obligations set by the mandates of prescribed dharmic responsibilities to establish a strong central and extended traditional family unit within which a variety of intricate home-based and public-based rituals were regularly performed. For the Brahmanic priests in Vedic times, sacrifice or *homa* consisted of a ritual sequence in which a material substance such as milk, ghee, yogurt, rice, barley, an animal, or the sacred plant, *Soma,* was put into a sacred fire and immolated wholly or in part. In addition, parts of the sacrificial offering were consumed by the participants and parts were believed to be consumed by the gods (*devas*) or transcendent forces invoked. The oldest Vedic literature makes clear that ritual sacrifice is a mandate of *dharma,* the natural law of the Vedic universe that sets categorical imperatives for man but does not include an explicit promise of reward. Ritual sacrifice was a human obligation done for ritual's sake alone. Acknowledgment, awe, and praise appear to have been an integral part of the mind-set of those performing these obligatory, daily duties. The Western conception of the meaning of prayer has similar features.

The Vedic concept of sacrifice, however, remains complex in its subtleties (Staal, 1989). Having no expectation of reward was considered a virtue in fulfilling one's life choices or *dharma* in the formal Vedic literature (pre-500 B.C.). Post-Vedic literature, moreover, and commentaries on the Vedic *samhitas* expanded and extended this initial conception. One may speculate that some of the significant motivations and intentions behind the act of sacrifice reflected a psychological posture that included aspects of deference, remembrance, renewal, and gratitude. The one that engaged in the ritual sacrifice was called the *yajamana*. His actions indicated an awareness of a transcendent reality that required recognition. This strongly connotes a sense of another and is characterized by a mood of awe and reverence; in fact, this may be termed a sense of the *sacred* or the *spiritual*. This implies a level of cognitive expansion, that is, the ability to abstract from concrete, literal, and material experience to immaterial themes, that is, to meaning. Post-Vedic literature, especially the works of *Vedanta,* which drew heavily from the *Upanishads,* interiorized what had previously been acted out in the external world. There was much greater emphasis on interior contemplation and meditation.

One outstanding feature of Vedic ritual, however, was that of fostering remembrance (*smriti*), considered an antidote to the natural inclination to forget. Remembrance and a conscious awareness of the Vedic worldview are enhanced by the continued recognition of *dharma*'s rules, laws, personal and social obligations, values, and virtues. The Vedic sacrificial ritual consisted of a material offering into the sacred fire accompanied by the recitations of several Brahmanic priests who spoke and chanted Vedic axioms from the four major *Vedas*. Mandates concerning ritual, sacrifice, and lawful behavior were made explicit. The experience of the sacrificial ritual, a solemn liturgy of action and the recounting of Vedic law, done in a communal setting, reinforced remembrance on a daily and repeated basis.

The central intention behind sacrificial acts was to express the fundamental Vedic belief in the nexus between microcosm as man and macrocosm as universe. This cosmic homology was a fundamental Vedic theme. The *Vedas* rigorously adhered to the idea of man's need to preserve his harmony and alignment with the rest of nature. This coordination or correspondence was termed *bandhu* and was mediated by the transformative power of *Agni*. The sacrificial fires, by their innate powers, resulted in the acquisition of purity, health, auspiciousness, grace, and a regulation of any imbalances created by man both within himself and in the world. Ritual sacrifice, therefore, was considered vital; as such, it was organized in daily life around the natural cycles of the 24-hour period, the junctures of seasons, the cycle of the moon, and the chronological life cycle from birth to death. The observance of ritual and sacrifice, therefore, had several axiomatic themes: remembrance, ongoing need for purification, and the dharmic mandate to uphold the integrity of the human and extended universe.

The intimate identity between the external ritual sacrificial fire, *Agni,* and the internal digestive fire became explicit in later *Upanishad* commentaries (*bhasyas*) and was acknowledged early on in the work of the Ayurvedic physicians Charaka and Sushruta (c. 700 B.C.). The medical reality and practical significance of this was an essential part of Ayurveda in ancient times and, in essence, continues today. In modern times, the transmutational dynamic of ancient ritual sacrificial action is reflected in a recognition of one's duty to observe dietary and lifestyle practices that foster and optimize the transformative action of *Agni,* the digestive metabolism in the body. Paralleling what had been ritual and sacrificial duties in the past are activities practiced now in more sublimated forms: study of the ancient writings, meditation, and acts that reflect a sense of gratitude, reconciliation, and harmony between man and the greater world of which he is part. These all contribute to the theory and practice of Ayurveda in contemporary times.

The *Rig-Veda,* therefore, considered one of the oldest extant compilations reflecting the daily life of an ancient civilization, attests to a life-affirming, awe-filled celebration of all that is earthy and material. These ancient canons show that this ancient culture experienced all aspects of the world in tangible ways using visual acuity, a developed sense of sound, tactile awareness, olfactory sensation, and taste. Every sense organ of these ancient peoples savored in reverence the experience of the senses as they interacted with the material world around. At this early Vedic period, nowhere is found any indication of a sense of renunciation of the physical world or of its being qualitatively subordinate to anything else. There is a simultaneous poignant awareness of a spiritual dimension, demonstrated by pervasive ritual and sacrifice. This, however, is not displayed in a delimited or circumscribed fashion. The spiritual aspect of Vedic life, an awareness of a consciousness intrinsic in nature and of powers having limited but possible access to humans, imbues all activities of daily living. It is this wide and all-encompassing perspective that echoes throughout the origins and development of the ancient Vedic worldview and finds current expression in Ayurveda today.

THE CLASSICAL EPIC AND PURANIC PERIODS

The Vedic period ended about 500 B.C. The Classical and Puranic periods followed. Subsequent texts deriving from the primary Vedic *samhitas* laid more emphasis on the *dharma* of self-development but with considerably more explicit spiritual, mystical, and philosophical content (Hiltebeitel, 1999). These later writings, commentaries, and interpretations of the *Vedas, Brahmanas,* and *Aranyakas* are known as *Upanishads.* They are considered *sruti* (revealed scripture). *Sruti,* it must be emphasized, denoted that the information received was heard and experienced in a direct manner. This method of transmission is elevated to the highest level of accuracy and meaning that knowledge can attain in Hinduism.

The *Upanishads* (c. 600 B.C.–A.D. 200–1600) have the distinction of containing original metaphysical contributions that antedate even the beginnings of Greek philosophy. Precise dating is ambiguous but believed to have its beginnings with most works dating around 800–600 B.C.; its ending is very speculative. It is considered the primary source for the subsequent schools called *Vedanta* (c. 400 B.C.–A.D. 200) upon which later Vedantists further elaborated. *Vedanta,* meaning "end of the *Vedas,*" is also called *Uttara-Mimamsa* (c. 400 B.C.–A.D. 200), the later or last discussions of attaining truth. *Vedanta* is a *darshana* (worldview) used in and very important within the fabric of Ayurveda. In addition, the six orthodox *darshanas* and Buddhism emerged during this classical period of *sutras* and complementary worldviews.

The *Upanishads* are considered to contain deeply philosophical and spiritual insights derived from the *Vedas.* Some have likened them metaphorically to creeping plants (*valli*) that lean on the preceding sections of the *Vedas* to which they belong yet retain a sort of independence from priestly dogma. This almost paradoxical anaclitic clinging has given the *Upanishads* a unique place within Indian spiritual traditions. The central theme of the *Upanishads* (literally meaning "to sit down near"), initially imparted in the intimate relationship of teacher/guide and student, was an ongoing consideration of the significance of *atman* (individual spirit) and *Brahman* (the Absolute). The *Upanishads* put great emphasis on relocating external ritual observance to the more internal field of meditation. True sacrifice then became the fire oblation on the breath (*prana-agni-hotra*), a sacrifice of the self within the self in the presence of *Brahman* and OM, *Pranava.*

Other significant texts, considered, however, of secondary importance to the large group of the *Vedas,* were in the form of epic poems. The *Ramayana,* the *Mahabharata,* and the *Bhagavad Gita,* a section of the *Mahabharata,* were first written down (final redaction c. 500 B.C.–200 B.C.) during the *Vedanta* period but, like the *Vedas,* appear to be set much earlier, between 1000 and 700 B.C. (Buitenen, 1973–1978, 1981; Johnson, 1994; Narasimhan, 1997; Prabhupada, 1997). This important literature is considered *smriti* (secondary revelation). The *Ramayana* and the *Mahabharata* are collectively referred to as *Itihasa* (history) and the "Great Epics."

Later commentaries on the *Upanishads* were forthcoming in the A.D. era. *Vedanta* is the term used to encompass the two *darshanas, Purva-Mimamsa* (typically termed only *"Mimamsa"*) and *Uttara-Mimamsa* (typically termed only *"Vedanta"*). *Vedanta* commentaries draw from many earlier texts, the most notable of which are the *Brahma Sutra,* the *Upanishads,* and the *Bhaghavad Gita.*

Significant contributions to *Vedanta,* regarded by many as the philosophical paradigm of Hinduism par excellence, were made by three important figures: Shankara (A.D. 788–820) in his conception of *Advaita-Vedanta* (nondualism), Ramanuja (A.D. 1017–1137) in his conception of *Vishishtadvaiata-Vedanta* (qualified nondualism), and Madhva (c. A.D. 1238) in his conception of *Dvaita-Vedanta* (dualistic *Vedanta*). All of these great religious and philosophical giants are considered major spiritual figures in Indian culture. They addressed the problem of "the one and the many" or the nature of the individual spirit (*atman*) within the fabric of the universal Absolute (*Brahman*). The foundations of Indian philosophy, religion, and culture are rooted in these ancient works.

Mention should be made of an important group of literature called *Puranas*. They were written from about A.D. 320–520 and have been continuously amended up to medieval times (c. A.D. 1500). These "stories of the ancient past" are narratives that contain genealogies of deities and kings, cosmologies, law codes, descriptions of rituals, and pilgrimages to holy places. These expositions related specific details of religious systems that centered on deities such as Vishnu, Shiva, and Devi. Devi is also known as *Shakti* and is considered the feminine consort of Shiva. This last classical period produced much of what constitutes the religious literature of India's current and diverse contemporary spiritual sects (Kripal, 1998; Lipner, 1994; Narang, 1984; Oberoi, 1995; Sivaraman, 1973). Beginning at this time around the fourth century A.D. and up to the present day, those (usually Brahmins) who followed the Puranic literature (*smriti*) and who held deities such as Vishnu, Shiva, Devi, Ganesha, and Surya as central and more primary than the *Vedas* (*sruti*) were known as the *Smartas*. Modern-day *Smartas* are said to believe in the essential unity of all reality although accepting that it may have simultaneous manifestations in the multiple faces of the apparently differing aspects of the aforementioned deities.

THE DEVELOPMENT OF EARLY MEDICINE AND AYURVEDA

Evidence shows that scientific or rational medicine, the allopathic medicine of the West as it exists today, had its beginnings in Greece with the school of Hippocrates in the fifth century B.C. (Sigerist, 1961). Before that, the main streams of the healing arts came from Minoan culture (2200–1450 B.C.), Egyptian culture (2700 B.C.), the Indus Valley/Harappan culture (3300–1500 B.C.), and the Mesopotamian/Babylonian priestly tradition (2300 B.C.).

Ayurvedic medicine is rooted in very ancient traditions, most of which were oral. As it began to appear in written form, Ayurveda owes a great debt to the advent of Buddhism in the sixth century B.C. Many great Ayurvedic physicians became Buddhists, and many Buddhist monks began to chronicle the development of Ayurveda within India and later in foreign lands such as Ceylon (Sri Lanka), Tibet, and China, paralleling their missionary excursions.

AYURVEDA AND BUDDHISM

The historical Buddha (c. 563–483 B.C.) was born in the foothills of the Himalayas near present-day Nepal. His first name was Siddhartha, his family name Gautama. In order to distinguish the historical Buddha from the transcendent Buddhas of all epochs, Siddhartha Gautama is generally called

Buddha Shakyamuni. It is said that he is the seventh Buddha of the present, six others preceding him in earlier epochs; some sources describe a total of 24 Buddhas, the first being called Dipamkara.

During the lifetime of the Buddha and for a time thereafter, Indian culture experienced a Golden Age of development during which learning and trade expanded until the twelfth century A.D. when Muslim forces entered India and ruled until about 1700. The development of Buddhism and that of Ayurveda became closely entwined (Clifford, 1984).

Ayurveda emerged out of the ancient *Vedas* and retained allegiance to its authority as did most developing Indian systems, much later referred to as *Hindu*. Buddhism, however, perhaps in an attempt to purify, reform, and reorient (making available for all) the older Vedic traditions, in effect, appeared to abandon them, at least concerning their detailed ritualistic mandates.

Buddhism, moreover, was comfortable adopting Ayurveda as a medical and therapeutic program. Ayurveda, to be sure, also had and continues now to embrace Buddhism. During the fifth to fourth centuries B.C., the University at Taxila, north of ancient Harappa, whose present site is modern Pakistan, was a major node of higher learning. Jivaka, one of Taxila's outstanding Ayurvedic physicians, was the royal doctor and son of King Bimbisara (544 B.C.–491 B.C.) of the kingdom of Magadha south of the Ganges River in northeast India. He was also Buddha's personal physician. Jivaka is reputed to have been expert in many subspecialties of medicine and a variety of surgical techniques. He was considered the most skilled physician of his time, trained at the University of Taxila (ancient Gandhara). Stories about his achievements abounded in all the Buddhist territories, namely Magadha in northeast India, Benares, and Peshawar near the Khyber Pass (between modern western Pakistan and Afghanistan) in northern Asia near China.

The association between Buddhist doctrine, with its emphasis on moral and ethical behavior, and its espousal of Ayurveda became renowned during this time. It led King Ashoka, emperor of most of the Maurya kingdom of northern India from 272 to 236 B.C., to become a convert to Buddhism in the third century B.C. Ayurvedic medicine became widely disseminated through this ruler's establishment of a number of charitable hospitals with extensive medical, surgical, and psychiatric components to treat both humans and animals. This reflected the pragmatic implementation of the Buddhist virtue of compassion for all sentient beings. This was an attempt to reach all, not merely the Brahmin Hindus within India. There are extant documents cut in rock that display Ashoka's edicts directing embassies to be erected in foreign lands and ordering Buddhist missionaries to travel within and outside of India to disseminate the teachings. It is believed that Ayurveda and Theravada Buddhism, an early Buddhist perspective that laid great emphasis on renunciation, self-discipline, and individual self-development outside of mainstream society, reached Sri Lanka at this time. The Bower Manuscript, written in the fourth century A.D., that was found in Central Asia attests to the fact that

Buddhist medical missionary work continued and expanded at this time. The introduction of Ayurveda into Tibet took place around A.D. 650 with the translation of Buddhist Ayurvedic texts into Tibetan. The history of the spread of Buddhism throughout the East, therefore, may be seen as paralleling the expansion and impact that Ayurveda had outside of its home in India. Nāgārjuna and Vagbhata were Buddhists and Ayurvedic scholars.

The last Indian-born, 28th patriarch of Buddhism in India was Bodhidharma (c. 470–543 A.D.). Toward the end of his very long lifetime, he traveled to China and arrived at the Shao-lin Monastery on the north side of the western peak of the Sung-shan Mountain in Lo-yang, north China where he founded Chinese Buddhism, called Ch'an/Chan Buddhism. He is considered the first (Indian born) patriarch of Ch'an or Chinese Buddhism. The Shao-lin Monastery was originally founded in 495 A.D. by the Indian-born Buddhist monk Batuo after he traveled from India to China in 464 A.D. This monastery and temple were the repository of written treatises not only on health issues and mental/physical disciplines such as Kung Fu (Shahar, 2001), but also on the health practices, for example, Ayurveda and Yoga, that were brought in by missionary traveler monks from India who settled in China.

The sixth patriarch of Ch'an, and the last major figure in Chinese Buddhism, was the Chinese-born Hui-neng (c. 638–713 A.D.). He represented the "southern school" of Ch'an. Hui-neng advocated the doctrine of "sudden awakening," which held that the Buddha mind arises in a flash of insight, not gradually as is held in some schools. Enlightenment is achieved, in part, through meditation (see Chapter 11), especially the elimination, or at least suspension, of discursive and conceptual thought. This is referred to as the "no mind" state (*wu nien*).

AYURVEDA AND VETERINARY MEDICINE

In reviewing the history of Buddhism, especially the laudatory work of the Buddhist King Ashoka, third century B.C., the role of Ayurveda in relation to animals has an interesting history. It is believed that domestication of dogs, buffalo, elephants, and fowl occurred in India between 6000 and 4500 B.C. (Somvanshi, 2006). Cattle husbandry was well developed during the Rig-Veda period, and the cow (*kamdhenu*) was held in high esteem. It is believed that the first veterinarian in history was an Indian named Sahlihotra who specialized in the care of horses and wrote a text devoted to that subject, *Haya Ayurveda*. Another veterinary text, *Gaja Ayurveda,* is attributed to Palakapya, a veterinarian who specialized in the care of elephants. Even as far back as the Mahabharata period (c. 1000 B.C.), the two Pandeva brothers, Nakula and Sahadeva, are reputed to have been experts in horse and cattle husbandry. The closeness of Ayurveda to nature, especially to the care of animals, has strong historical roots and persists to the present.

ANCIENT AYURVEDIC MEDICAL TEXTS: *CHARAKA SAMHITA* AND *SUSHRUTA SAMHITA*

The ***Charaka Samhita*** (Kaviratna, 1902–1925; Mehta, 1949; Ray & Gupta, 1965; Sharma, 1995), a major Ayurvedic compendium of medical theory and practice, may have been formulated around 1000 B.C. or earlier, but is believed to have been redacted by the famous Ayurvedic physician Charaka of Kashmir (modern-day India) at the University of Taxila (the capital of eastern Punjab in antiquity) and compiled in written form around 760 B.C. Some date it between 400 and 200 B.C. It is uncertain whether this organized medical collection was the work of one man or the school of Charaka's followers. This *samhita* was composed in the form of prose and poetry with over 8,400 metrical verses in eight major sections and 120 lessons or chapters. These were memorized and lyrically recited by Ayurvedic physicians of ancient times and continue to be recited to this day by modern Ayurvedic physicians. Charaka discusses the field of internal medicine, describes the five subdoshas of *Vata* (the five bioenergetic, physiological principles that regulate the central nervous system and all movements in the body), and gives particular emphasis to the value, care, and priority of the consciousness within man. Of particular note, given the lack of the microscope at that early time, are Charaka's detailed descriptions of anatomical dissection and analysis of skin with enumeration of its six layers.

Sushruta of Varanasi (modern-day Benares in India), a great Ayurvedic surgeon, produced the other classic medicosurgical text, the ***Sushruta Samhita,*** around 660 B.C. (Acharya & Pandurang, 1945; Bhishagratna, 1968; Trikamji & Ram, 1980). This *samhita,* composed both in prose and in poetry, emphasized a surgical viewpoint. The importance of blood is extensively addressed. Sushruta includes the first description of the five subdoshas of *Pitta* (the five bioenergetic, physiological principles that regulate the body's metabolic functioning) and gives a classic definition of the concept of health. Like Charaka, using only the naked eye, he goes on to describe the layers of the skin. Together, the *Charaka Samhita* and the *Sushruta Samhita* are considered the oldest extant classic texts of Ayurvedic medicine and surgery. These two medical compendia constitute the historically documented foundations of most of Ayurvedic medicine. Modern medicine today recognizes some of the ancient Indian roots of current medical and surgical practice (Das, 1984; Kansupada & Sassani, 1997; Prakash, 1978; Savithri, 1987). Inhalation therapy can be traced back to India some 4,000 years ago (Grossman, 1994). Sushruta has been called the father of surgery since he was the first to develop acknowledgedly novel techniques in plastic and reconstructive surgery such as the use of skin grafts and procedures for total nasal reconstruction (Hauben, Baruchin, & Mahler, 1982; Nichter, Morgan, & Nichter, 1983). A timeline of the Ayurvedic oral and written tradition appears in Appendix 1.

A SHORT HISTORY OF WESTERN MEDICINE AND AYURVEDA

Hippocrates (460 B.C.) is considered the father of Western medicine (Porter, 1997; Singer & Underwood, 1962). His methods, unlike those of his predecessors, were less influenced by animist and other religious doctrines. He is reputed to have relied more on detailed clinical observation and to have had closer clinical contact when evaluating and treating individual patients. The school of Hippocrates held the humoral theory in which the body was believed to be composed of four *humors:* blood (*sanguis*), phlegm (*pituita*), yellow bile (*chole*), and black bile (*melanchole*). Humors were considered to be vaporous material substances contributing to health as well as being capable of going awry and causing illness. This notion was applied clinically to delineate constitutional and temperamental body types. Dietary therapy and the influence of the seasons on health and disease were also very prominent features of the Hippocratic tradition. To what extent these theories and practices were influenced by the much older yet very similar Ayurvedic concepts remains unknown.

Aristotle (384 B.C.), the great codifier of ancient science, using a perspective similar to that of Hippocrates, relied heavily on empirical observation and naturalistic classification. An important part of his ontology and taxonomy was a classification system using what he referred to as the four *prime qualities:* hot, cold, wet, and dry, together with four fundamental *essences* or *elements:* Air, Fire, Water, and Earth. Emphasis was placed more on anatomical description rather than on physiological functioning. As with Hippocrates's use of the humors and constitutional types, Aristotle's descriptive and explanatory use of the *qualities* and *elements* is strikingly similar to those found in the historically older Ayurvedic concepts.

When Alexander the Great invaded India in 327 B.C. and temporarily occupied the Sind and Punjab areas, historical reports describe his contact with Ayurvedic physicians whose talents he is said to have used almost exclusively to treat poisoning cases in his armies. It is plausible to believe that he and his cohort of physicians took some of this Ayurvedic knowledge back to the West, perhaps influencing the then early development of the Greek medical corpus.

Galen of Pergamon (A.D. 129–215) was an influential physician in the Western Latin world, especially in Rome. He is reputed to have been trained in Asia Minor and at the medical school in Alexandria, Egypt. The substance of his work was derived from the *Corpus Hippocraticum,* a collection of medical writings that have been transmitted through the ages and attributed to Hippocrates and his school. The form of Galen's practice was taken from the Aristotelian method. He held a rationalist view placing reason, observation, and experimentation over knowledge derived from empirical or sense-based experience. Via the Arabic tradition that developed later, Galen became the most influential physician of the ancient world. His distinctively Western style then became the theoretical basis for all of Western medical practice for the next 1,500 years until the sixteenth century A.D. Indeed, his influence persisted until the end of the nineteenth century in spite of the discoveries of seventeenth-century medicine, such as William Harvey's description of the circulation of the blood in 1615 and Anton van Leeuwenhoek's microscopic observations of cells and microbes (c. 1700).

Although Ayurveda has been introduced in a substantial way into North America only very recently, Indian culture and its spiritual traditions have their first roots in the United States in the early part of the 1890s. Special mention here is made about Swami Vivekananda's (1863–1902) visit at that time. *Swami* denotes an appellation of respect to a distinguished religious figure and is roughly equivalent to the English term "reverend." He is arguably the leading figure responsible for the globalization of Hinduism in modern times with an implicit role in bringing Ayurveda or, perhaps, its underlying framework to the West.

His conventional name was Narendranath Datta; he was born in Calcutta, India. Naren, as he was called, was a highly intelligent and handsome individual. He was drawn to spiritual pursuits from early childhood. He pondered the meaning of life, the existence of a spiritual realm, and a God behind the apparent universe of material realities. He was a disciple of Ramakrishna (1836–1886), a Bengali Indian mystic. In 1893, with the financial support of the Maharaja of Khetri, Vivekananda traveled uninvited to the World Parliament of Religions at the Columbia Exposition in Chicago. This is reputed to have been the first time that an ecumenical gathering of international spiritual leaders convened in modern times in one place. In a sense, he acted as a missionary of the East to the West. His charisma, deep spirituality, and intelligence left a lasting impression on Americans and on the West. He established the Vedanta Society in New York City. He then traveled to England, France, and Switzerland where he introduced India's spiritual worldview and culture on a large scale. On July 4, 1902, he passed away at the Ramakrishna Mission, which he helped to inaugurate in Belur Math, India. Much of the initial exposure to and lasting interest in the Hindu worldview and subsequently to Ayurveda in America is attributed to this great spiritual leader.

CHINESE TRADITIONAL MEDICINE AND AYURVEDA

In terms of further historical perspective, the oldest extant Chinese medical text, the *Huang-di Nei-jing* or *Inner Classic of the Yellow Emperor,* was compiled by unknown authors somewhere between 300 and 100 B.C.; some put the dating between 475 and 221 B.C. (Unschuld, 1979, 1985). Three subsequent works arising out of the Han Dynasty (206 B.C.–A.D. 220), the *Classic of Difficult Issues* (*Nan-Ching*), *Discussion of Cold Induced Disorders* (*Shan Han Lung*), and *Shen Nong's Materia Medica* (*Shen Nong Ben Cao*) further codified and defined Chinese Traditional Medicine in the form that has come down to us today. Although principles of shamanic healing and Confucianism are woven into its inscrutable web, the inestimable influence of Taoism founded by Lao Tzu (c. 550 B.C.) on Chinese medicine is unquestionable. Leading fundamental propositions include Yin-Yang theory, the generative and control cycles of the Five Elements, phases, and movements theory, the centrality of the five bodily substances: Vital energy (*Qi*), Blood (*xue*), Essence (*jing*), Spirit (*shen*), and Fluids (*jin ye*), and the energy flows through the meridians (*Qi jing*).

There are many striking similarities both in theory and in clinical practice between Ayurveda and Traditional Chinese Medicine, as well as some significant differences (Mahdihassan, 1985b, 1989; Wiseman & Ellis, 1985). The influence of Ayurveda, perhaps brought to China by itinerant, missionary Indian Buddhist monks, has been suggested. This influence is in addition to the independent origins of each. Some evidence for early cross-fertilization, however, can be seen in the recorded origins of pulse diagnosis. Whereas it makes its first appearance in the Ayurvedic literature around the fourteenth century A.D., it appears earlier in Chinese texts such as the *Nan-Ching* in the early part of the Han Dynasty, perhaps around A.D. 100. This may have occurred indirectly through the gradual influence of *Unani Tibb* and Tibetan medicine on Ayurveda around the twelfth century A.D.

Historically, there is evidence that migrations (176–30 B.C.) of the Chinese Yueh-chih (also called Yuezhi) tribes, the Kushans, coming from western China, occupied Benares (Varanasi) in northeast India. The Kushans had diplomatic ties with Rome, Persia, and China. They are considered to have formed a bridge, in effect, between East and West, traversing the Silk Road, which joined Babylon, ancient India, and China. The Yueh-chih were noted for their ongoing supply to China of jade. The first contacts between China and Central Asia occurred with the opening of the Silk Road in the second century B.C. The Silk Road transmission of Buddhism to China in the first century A.D. is documented historically. The University of Taxila, where the Ayurvedic textbook *Charaka Samhita* was composed, was located on the Silk Road. The Burma Road (115 B.C.) to the south also opened the exchange of material goods and ideas to and from China. Trade with the Roman Empire, at the height of its wealth, included spices, ivory, and other luxuries.

The third and greatest Kushan king, Kanishka (c. A.D. 100), whose capitals were Purushapura (now Peshawar in northern Pakistan) and Mathura in northern India, near the Khyber Pass close to ancient Taxila, was considered to be a great patron of *Mahayana Buddhism,* the Buddhist system that distinguishes itself by fostering self-development through compassion within a social context. It is in this school of Buddhist practice that the role of the *Bodhisattva,* the seeker who renounces complete entry into enlightenment until all beings are first saved, is most cherished. He ushered its entry into northern Asia and China. Records show that Buddhist monasteries were established in China by A.D. 65 and that there existed translations of Sanskrit texts into Chinese in the Luoyang region by the second century A.D. (Chen, 1984). From China, Buddhism then spread to Korea in the fourth century and to Japan in the sixth century. The Ayurvedic influence, since it existed in tandem with Buddhism for so many centuries, may have contributed to Traditional Chinese Medicine by this association.

NĀGĀRJUNA: BUDDHIST PRIEST, PHILOSOPHER, AND AYURVEDIC PHYSICIAN

The development of Ayurveda, particularly in regard to its medicinal armamentarium, was further advanced by the great Buddhist priest, philosopher, and Ayurvedic physician Nāgārjuna, born around A.D. 100 in Amravati (modern-day Guntur district of the eastern coast of Andhra Pradesh), India (Garfield, 1995; Hajicek-Dobberstein, 1995; Kalupahana, 1986; Lindtner, 1997; Mahdihassan, 1981, 1985a; Sharma, 1977; White, 1996; Williams, 1989). In the history of Indian Buddhism, Nāgārjuna is considered the 14th Patriarch (recognized spiritual leader) after Buddha Shakyamuni, the historical Buddha. He is the father of *iatrochemistry,* the science of the preparation of medicinal mineral substances. Up to this time, most medical interventions of the Charaka tradition were derived from an herbal or plant-based pharmacopoeia, while Ayurvedic physicians of the Sushruta School were more skilled in surgical approaches. Nāgārjuna's effort was to expand the therapeutic armamentarium by constructing a mineral-based repertoire of active, healing substances. Many heretofore toxic substances, like mercury, were now processed in complex ways, using the innovative techniques of the Nāgārjuna School, to render them nontoxic and suitable for human consumption. This opened a new and much broader field for development and expanded the range of therapeutic interventions that today continue to be an integral and characteristic aspect of Ayurvedic medicine. It is said that he wrote an important commentary on Sushruta's *Samhita.* The brilliance of Nāgārjuna's contributions, however, extended far beyond this and encompassed a qualitative advance in Buddhist theory and practice with an especially productive literature both in medicine as well as in philosophy and religion.

The renowned Nalanda University in the region of Bihar, northeast India near Patna, where Nāgārjuna was a prominent teacher, retained its prominence until the twelveth century. Some of the subjects taught included history, geography, literature, law, mathematics, trade, commerce, and medicine. There are descriptions in the historical archives by Chinese travelers (Xuanzang, A.D. 600–664) telling of the university's diverse culture and commenting on the estimated 10,000 students and 1,500 teachers who were involved in academic pursuits.

ASTHANGA: AYURVEDIC MEDICAL TEXTS OF VAGBHATA

The seventh century A.D. produced another great Ayurvedic scholar and Buddhist, *Vagbhata* of Sind (present-day southeastern Pakistan), northwest of modern-day India. His effort and that of his followers produced the next greatest collection of Ayurvedic medical writings, the ***Asthanga Sagraha*** (Murthy, 2005), and about 100 years later, the shorter collection known as the ***Asthanga Hridhaya*** (Harishastri, 1939; Moos, 1984; Murthy, 2004).

The *Sagraha* (collected teachings), a larger work that is 40 percent greater by verse size than the *Hridhaya* (heart of the teachings), is primarily composed in the form of poetry with only some prose narrative. The *Hridhaya,* composed of 7,800 verses, is in prose. Within these works, the first description of the five subdoshas of *Kapha* (the five bioenergetic, physiological principles that regulate and contribute to the body's structure and physical form) is presented. This significant text gave emphasis to the more material value of life than that found in *Charaka* and *Sushruta.* Even today, the *Asthanga Hridhaya* is highly regarded as a primary medical text by the Ayurvedic physicians in Kerala, southern India. The triune of texts, *Charaka Samhita, Sushruta Samhita,* and the *Asthangas* of Vagbhata, is referred to as the *Brihat Trayi,* the senior or greater triad. These three works are universally recognized as the textual foundations of Ayurvedic medicine.

THE ARAB MEDICAL TRADITION OF AVICENNA

The parallel progress of medicine can also be seen in the work of the Persian physician *Avicenna* (A.D. 980–1037). He produced the comprehensive *Canon of Medicine,* a compendium of the previous works of Hippocrates and Galen. It was to become the preeminent medical text both for the Muslim world and for the entire Latin West until the seventeenth century. Arab or Muslim medicine had been and continues to be known as *Unani Tibb* (Greek-based medicine), which connotes the very strong influence of the ancient Greek physicians on Arab medical thought.

There are historical reports that describe the interchange between Ayurveda and the Middle East. Ayurvedic physicians were invited to Jundishapur and to Baghdad in the Middle East to teach and to organize hospitals. From the seventh century A.D., Arab traders along the Malabar Coast were a vehicle for the exchange of goods and ideas, including Ayurveda, between Indian and Arab cities. The great Arab physicians of the tenth and eleventh centuries, Razes (died c. A.D. 923) and Avicenna (A.D. 980–1037), are thought to have had extensive knowledge of Indian medicine. Their voluminous and influential writings, incorporating Ayurvedic concepts along with those of the Greeks, were translated into Latin in the thirteenth century and were used as standard medical texts in medieval Europe. *Unani Tibb,* for instance, holds a theory of four bodily humors and four elements. It has a constitutional typing system and uses herbal medicines in a way similar to that in Ayurveda. The influence of each system on the other seems strong.

FURTHER AYURVEDIC MEDICAL TREATISES

Between A.D. 700 and 1100, another important Ayurvedic medical text was produced, the *Madhava Nidana* (Murthy, 1987), which was devoted to a survey of diagnostic procedures with an emphasis on the classification of disease. In the fourteenth century, another fundamental Ayurvedic text, *Sarangadhara (Sharangdhara) Samhita,* appeared. It contained the first textual reference to the unique method of Ayurvedic pulse diagnosis. The eightfold clinical examination was outlined. A systematized materia medica with pharmacological formulations was also enumerated. In the sixteenth century, a final, classic, and significant text was written, the *Bhavaprakasha*. It included a description of new herbs, minerals, dietetic advances, and rejuvenation theory. Comments were also made on newly discovered sexually transmitted diseases, particularly the clinical presentation of syphilis brought into India by foreigners. This last triune of medical texts, the *Madhava Nidana,* the *Sharangadhara Samhita,* and the *Bhavaprakasha,* is called the *Laghu Trayi,* the junior or lesser triad of fundamental texts.

The period from the twelveth to the early eighteenth century A.D. was dominated by Muslim control of India. This medieval period is considered an era of consolidation of Ayurvedic medicine. Innovative developments in Ayurveda, in general, were less prominent in deference to the strong Muslim rule. *Unani Tibb* or Greek-based medicine prevailed, especially after the Moghul Empire was established in India in 1526.

AYURVEDA IN THE NINETEENTH AND TWENTIETH CENTURIES

The influence of Great Britain played a major role in every aspect of India's economic, social, political, and medical development (Edney, 1997). The British soldier and statesman Robert Clive, in the service of the East India Company, in the 1750s eradicated the then dominant French influence and introduced British control. Later, around 1818, the British East India Company exerted a gradually more powerful influence that spread throughout all of India. In 1833, it closed virtually all the existing Ayurvedic training centers and schools. A British medical school was opened in Calcutta, and Western influence dominated the country, especially the medical field, for almost 100 years. In 1920 there arose a national revival and a resurgence of interest in traditional Indian culture, practices, and Ayurveda. In 1946 there was formal governmental recognition and reacceptance of Ayurveda and a resurgence of research, development, and modernization programs.

Today, there are many Ayurvedic or Traditional Indian Medicine training schools and clinics in India. Interestingly, in India, the current belief, however, is that this traditional healing art may be unscientific according to Western standards, if not too atavistic in general. It is, therefore, relegated to a secondary place with Western or allopathic medicine in the forefront. The Indian government officially recognizes the following as legitimate:

allopathy, homeopathy, naturopathy, *Unani Tibb,* Ayurveda, and its cousins, *Siddha* and *Yoga*. The Siddha system of Indian medicine is prevalent in southern India, especially in the Tamil region. Another form of traditional medicine called *Emchi* is distinctively Tibetan and Buddhist in its trappings, but strongly resembles Ayurveda in theory and practice.

THE LEGENDARY ORIGINS OF AYURVEDA

While the above history has placed Ayurveda in a historical context, Ayurveda also has a rich mythological history with a narrative that imparts a sense of wonder and profundity. It begins with Brahma, the creator of the universe, who is considered to be the original propounder of Ayurveda. The system, it is said, was then handed down to Daksha Prajapati, a primordial creative sage, sometimes described as a son of Brahma. From him, it was passed to the Ashwin twins, considered to be divine physicians in *Svarga* or Paradise. From the Ashwins, Ayurveda was handed to Indra, the supreme leader of the gods.

Indra then transmitted the knowledge to his disciples: Bharadvaja, Bharadvaja's disciple Atreya also known as Punarvasu, Kasyapa, and Dhanvantari. Internal medicine was revealed primarily to Atreya Punarvasu. He conveyed it to Agnivesa, his disciple, and this culminated finally in the classical Charaka tradition.

The beginning paragraphs of the *Charaka Samhita* describe the origins of Ayurveda, the science of life, in the following way. In the most ancient of prehistoric times, a group of holy *rishis* (sages), living in the Himalayan Mountains and watching over the welfare of mankind, met to discuss "the ills that flesh is heir to." The story unfolds thusly.

When diseases arose like so many impediments to the austerity, fasting, study, continence, and the vows of the embodied souls, then the great sages, the doers of good, keeping compassion for creatures foremost, met together on the sacred slopes of the Himalayas. Our bodies, which are the means of attaining the four aims of life, i.e., *dharma* (virtue), *artha* (worldly possessions), *kama* (pleasure), and *Moksha* (liberation), are subject to diseases that emaciate and weaken them, deprive the senses of their functions, and cause extreme pain. These diseases are great impediments to our worldly affairs and bring on premature death. In the face of such enemies, how can men be happy? It is necessary, therefore, to find remedies for such diseases.

Having thus posed this seemingly insoluble and enormous dilemma, they began to meditate. In that intuitive state, they all realized that the supreme leader of all the Vedic gods, Indra, was the only authority wise enough to render an adequate solution. The first *rishi* in the assemblage to speak was

Bharadvaja; he, thus, was given the mandate to approach Indra. The *Samhita* continues to say,

> Bharadvaja, the mighty ascetic, in search of (the science of) longevity approached Indra, having deemed him, the lord of the immortals, worthy of suit. Daksha Prajapati (the progenitor) first obtained the Science of Life in its entirety as promulgated by Brahma (the Great One, the Creator) and from him in turn the Ashwin twins obtained it. From the Ashwin twins the god Indra acquired it. Therefore, Bharadvaja, bidden by the sages, approached Indra.

Bharadvaja then disseminated this life wisdom to all the *rishis*. Atreya Punarvasu consolidated it and then transmitted it to his six disciples, one of whom was Agnivesa. It is Agnivesa's understanding that finally was synthesized into the standard medical compilation known as the *Charaka Samhita*.

The Sushruta tradition, more surgically oriented, has a complementary legendary base. The god Indra, it is said, revealed surgery to Divodasa, the King of Kasi and the city of Benares, while he was living in a hermitage. Divodasa is considered an incarnation of the god Dhanvantari, divine patron of Ayurveda. This lineage culminated finally in the classical Sushruta tradition of Ayurvedic surgery and medicine. While the school of Atreya and Bharadvaja, as mentioned previously by Charaka, specialized in general and internal medicine, the Dhanvantari School, according to Sushruta, specialized in surgery.

2

THEORETICAL FOUNDATIONS AND AN OVERVIEW

There was neither non-existence nor existence then; there was neither the realm of space nor the sky which is beyond. What stirred? Where? In whose protection? Was there water, bottomlessly deep?

There was neither death nor immortality then. There was no distinguishing sign of night nor of day. That one breathed, windless, by its own impulse. Other than that there was nothing beyond.

Darkness was hidden by darkness in the beginning; with no distinguishing sign, all this was water. The life force that was covered with emptiness, that one arose through the power of heat.

Desire came upon that one in the beginning; that was the first seed of mind. Poets seeking in their heart with wisdom found the bond of existence in non-existence.

Their cord was extended across. Was there below? Was there above? There were seed-placers; there were powers. There was impulse beneath; there was giving-forth above.

Who really knows? Who will here proclaim it? Whence was it produced? Whence is this creation? The gods came afterwards, with the creation of this universe. Who then knows whence it has arisen?

Whence this creation has arisen—perhaps it formed itself, or perhaps it did not—the one who looks down on it, in the highest heaven, only he knows—or perhaps he does not know.

Creation Hymn' (27 Lines) from *The Rig Veda* translated by Wendy Doniger O'Flaherty (Penguin Classics, 1981). Copyright © Wendy Doniger O'Flaherty, 1981.

This Vedic poetry, composed more than 4,000 years ago by the ancient sages of India, reflects the world-class profundity of their thought, imagination, and existential musings. Sages or *rishis* were considered to be of exceptional brilliance and holiness. They were individuals who were believed to be in almost intimate contact with the divine and extraordinary dimensions of reality, and whose wisdom reflected this divine understanding, *dharma,* universal law, and divine will. Rather than advancing categorical certainties, the wisdom of the *Vedas* shows itself to contain a series of scholarly inquiries that are logical, empirical, erudite, and awe-inspiring. Out of the towering achievements called the *Vedas,* Ayurveda emerged.

There is no universally standardized Ayurvedic body of theory and clinical technique. This may be a consequence, in part, of several factors. Ayurveda is strongly clinical and empirical in application, marked by a heavy oral tradition, and has kept itself separate from the political and economic support of the times. This clinical, oral-empirical, nonlegalistic, and independent status apparently did not lend itself to a widespread Ayurvedic literature. These factors, however, have been changing since the 1920s. Ayurveda now has been recognized and has become more integrated into mainstream Indian culture, and research and development is being supported by government funding. There is also more literature in a variety of languages and translations of works previously available only in Sanskrit. In addition, there is a small but growing body of more recent literature that outlines some theoretical and practical aspects of Ayurveda (Corcos, 1984; Dube, 1979; Frawley & Lad, 1986; Jee, 1895/1993; Lad, 1984, 2002; Lele, 1986; Manyam, 1990; Ranade, 1993; Ranade, Ranade, Qutab, & Deshpande, 1997; Svoboda, 1992).

The classical traditions of Charaka and Sushruta have long been esteemed as constituting the very core of all Ayurvedic knowledge and practice. They have been adapted to the varying times, prevailing trends, and exigencies of their day. Ayurveda, as presented here, will take a centrist position. The classical sources are considered the bedrock foundation of timeless, enduring truths. In the spirit of Ayurveda, however, these fundamentals have been and are now applied, in a flexible way, with adaptations to include accommodation to the current culture in which they now emerge. These adjustments, in fact, have been a skillful means of helping to usher Ayurveda into modern times while striving to preserve the qualitative heart of the authentic Ayurvedic system.

Ayurvedic knowledge is thus to be understood both in intuitive and in logical terms. It may be considered an empirical science since its naturalistic methodology combines a trust in the wisdom and experience of the past with an applicability that is both artful and scientific in the widest sense. As such it becomes a living, flexible reality kept fresh by reason and by the creative use of an intuitive sensitivity. It would be imprecise to view Ayurveda as a closed or dogmatic system; rather, it is one in which judicious uncertainty mixes with contemplation, reason, and time-honored guidelines.

The term *Ayurveda* is composed of two Sanskrit words, *ayus* meaning the period of life and longevity, and *veda* meaning revealed knowledge or wisdom. Ayurveda, in many contemporary contexts, has been called "the science of life." Ayurveda, however, may also be expressed by the phrase "life wisdom," which connotes its pragmatic, judicious, diligent, and mature vision. Ayurveda always had and continues to have a strong empirical and pragmatic foundation. It is scientific in that it is an organized body of theories at times used in an explanatory fashion and at other times used proposition-ally to be tested through experience.

Western science and rational medicine evolved based on a highly logical series of systematic observations made scientific by repeated tests of validity and reliability. This experimental method requires evidence, which, over time, proves consistently true and verifiable. Modern statistical analysis accompanies most of current Western science and medicine. This method of using evidence-based approaches goes even beyond the Western world and has become part of most contemporary and modern pursuits in those areas. Approaches, such as Ayurveda, have long histories, and while their propo-nents regard these approaches as having been "proven" over time, they may be regarded by others as less or even unscientific. The scientific view, so to speak, if considered from the larger historical perspective of the development of medicine, must become less exclusionary. Eastern medical perspectives that have been outside of the mainstream medicine of the West because of geographical, cultural, and language barriers need examination. Current trends not only permit but also demand such open-mindedness. The increas-ing global awareness that characterizes the beginning of the third millennium mandates lifting the constraining perspectives of the past. Ayurveda, as pre-sented here, may not fall under the aegis of being "scientific" in the accepted Western sense. Ayurveda, whether or not it may ever lend itself to more sci-entific methodologies, may accurately be seen as a parallel, alternative, or complementary system standing on its own merits and deserving serious con-sideration for historical, if not pragmatic, reasons.

DARSHANAS

In the complex history of ideological systems, India has been prolific and fruitful (Coward & Raja, 1990; Dasgupta, 1975; Jha, 1984; Kadar, 1996; Muller, 1899; Potter, 1994; Yukteswar, 1894/1990). Traditionally, most Indian or Hindu philosophical and religious schools of thought are visions (*darshanas*) that orient themselves around the authority of the *Vedas* although some remain apparently more independent. Those systems that regard the *Vedas* as primary revelation, as axiomatic, and as their authorita-tive foundation are characterized as being orthodox and true to the *Vedas*. They are termed *astika*. In contrast, those groups originating in the Indian culture, such as, for example, Buddhism, Jainism, and Charvaka, that either deny or reject the primary authority of the *Vedas,* are characterized as unor-thodox as well as nontheistic. They are collectively referred to as the *nastika* schools. Buddhism and Jainism are also known as the *Shramana* (non-Vedic) schools. While both perspectives have influenced Ayurveda to varying degrees, the *astika darshana* systems remain preeminent. Buddhism, how-ever, continues to be an integral part of the spirit of Ayurveda both in theory and in practice.

The term *darshana* is usually translated as *philosophical system, world-view,* or *religious system.* This vision of reality refers to the content of a particular *darshana.* In fact, *darshana* was originally used to denote the direct, intuitive experience of "seeing" reality as it existed both on the apparent level and at the essential, subtle, and root level. Gods and gurus are said to "give" *darshanas,* and devotees "take" *darshanas.* The *darshanas* were traditionally communicated in an oral fashion from teacher (*guru*) to student or disciple (*chela*). When written down, the body of a *darshana* was considered to fall into one of two categories: *sruti* or *smriti.*

Sruti was understood to be the "heard," oral teachings of the *rishis* or sages who "saw" their content. This revelatory meaning applied whether or not these ideas were transcribed in written form. The *Vedas* and the *Upanishads* are thought to be in the *sruti* class of scriptural documents. *Smriti* (tradition arising from memory and remembrance), whether in written form or not, was understood to be the large body of commentary written about the more primary *sruti* (revelation). The classic epics, *Bhagavad Gita,* the *Ramayana,* the narrative literature of the Puranic period (c. A.D. 320–520), and later *Vedanta* formulations (c. ninth–twelfth century A.D.) may be considered works of *smriti.*

Each of the six major *astika darshana* schools, *Shad Darshanas,* attempts to explain reality by using a particular and differing perspective. Hinduism and Indian philosophy draw their content from one or more of the *darshanas.* Ayurveda incorporates much both from the orthodox *darshanas,* especially *Sankhya,* and also from Buddhism. The great Ayurvedic scholars, Nāgārjuna of the ancient university of Nalanda and Vagbhata of Sind, were also Buddhist priests.

1. **Sankhya** is the *darshana* that provides a more nontheistic creation sequence, which is used to outline the evolution and manifestation of spirit/consciousness into matter. This system is one of the oldest Vedic *darshanas* and most explicitly forms the framework of the Ayurvedic worldview, as will be discussed at length further on. *Sankhya* ideas are found in the *Rig-Veda, Atharva-Veda,* and the *Upanishads.* A central proposition, the *Maha gunas: Rajas* and *Tamas,* relates to the centrality of human suffering and, therefore, can be closely linked to Buddhist thought.

   Sankhya is based on the primacy of consciousness (*Purusha*) as the integral ground or substratum that pervades and maintains the entire universe (*Prakriti*). In Western terms, it can be thought of as a dualistic realism wherein the male *Purusha* and the female *Prakriti* exist in polarity. Due recognition to the proper balance both of maleness and of femaleness and to their dialectical nature is addressed in full measure. Although considered an *astika darshana, Sankhya* does not base its statements entirely on scripture; some have said that it rates *sruti* no higher than reasoning, nor does it recognize a Supreme Divinity higher than *Purusha* and *Prakriti.* Its originator is considered to be Kapila, one of the ancient seers mentioned in the *Rig-Veda.* The figure of

Kapila (c. sixth century B.C.?) remains anonymous, and no details of his life have been recorded. Indian tradition refers to him as the father of philosophy. The main *Sankhya* text is the *Sankhya Karika,* a commentary in verse on *Sankhya* by Ishvara Krishna written about A.D. 200.

2. ***Yoga*** is the *darshana* developed by the Indian sage Patanjali. Classical *Yoga* contains a more theistic base and describes an Eightfold Path characterized by introspection, meditation, self-discipline, and aspects of renunciation and asceticism. These procedures aim toward the gradual liberation of the human spirit from its bondage to the material world, a process of release referred to as *Kaivalya,* and a state of being called *Samadhi* (enlightenment). *Yoga* and *Sankhya* are considered an inseparable pair whose principles pervade Hinduism.

3. ***Nyaya*** *darshana,* the method of thorough investigation, is a monotheistic system that describes a logical approach to apprehending the world by using reason. *Nyaya* emphasizes epistemological methodologies, tools of logic, and inquiry. It uses deductive strategies and syllogistic reasoning. It is a critical realism that holds that logic is a real way to truth and, in turn, to salvation. *Nyaya* has been called *Tarkavidya,* the science of debate, and *Vadavidya,* the science of discussion. This epistemological method is one of logical realism and considers that it is possible to arrive at a valid knowledge of an objective reality, a world that is independent of the mind. Perception (*pratyaksha*), inference (*anumana*), comparison (*upamana*), and testimony (*sabda*) were its epistemological axioms (*pramanas*). *Nyaya* contains a natural theology; its worldview admits both factual material properties, that is, atoms, and immaterial substances such as the consciousness of man. A rather personal God (*Ishvara*) is ardently postulated. *Moksha* or ultimate liberation was believed possible only after bodily death, not in one's lifetime. The founder of *Nyaya* has several appellations: Gotama, Gautama, and Aksapada. He presumably lived between the sixth and third centuries B.C. and authored an important Hindu law book, *Dharma Shastra,* whose 12 volumes discuss creation, transmigration, liberation, and dharmic mandates. He also composed the *Nyaya Sutras,* a fundamental *Nyaya* text.

4. ***Vaisheshika*** *darshana* describes a complex system of categories and classifications of substances, their action potentials, and their properties or attributes. It is an ontological worldview. It is the oldest of the six *darshanas* and tends to be more scientific than philosophical in exposition. It sets forth propositions and uses inductive inference to examine the structure of the material world. *Vaisheshika* is explicitly Vedic in orientation. *Kanada* (c. 600 B.C.), its founder, divides the multiplicity of nature into six categories or mutually exclusive distinct entities. These are considered real essences and are called *padarthas: dravya, guna, karma, samanya, vishesha,* and *samavaya.* Some add a seventh category, *abhava,* which denotes absence or gap.

It proposes nine causative substances under the category of *dravya* as comprising the entire universe: Ether, Air, Fire, Water, Earth, soul (*atman*), mind (*Manas*), time (*kala*), and direction (*dig*). This is called *Dravyaguna Shastra.* Included in these formulations were theories of atoms and primal Elements. Kanada, born in the region of modern Gujarat, India, was the first person to develop a theory of irreducible more amorphous substances, "atoms," variously termed *anu* and *pilu*. Democritus (c. 460 B.C.) in Greece later developed a version of the atomic nature of the world.

In Ayurveda, the primal Elements as irreducible substances that retain an overriding unique identity are termed in Sanskrit the *Mahabhutanis* or *Mahabhutas*. These "great" Elements are five in number (Ether, Air, Fire, Water, and Earth) and constitute the primordial material or gross building blocks or principles of all substances. They may be regarded as the principal states of matter. They play a pivotal role in every aspect of Ayurvedic theory and practice. *Vaisheshika* employs a system of pluralistic realism that is used extensively in Ayurveda in its development of a materia medica, the delineation of the mechanisms by which herbal substances affect the body's functioning, and their effects on the bodily *doshas,* the physiological principles that regulate the body's homeostasis. Ayurveda has incorporated this detailed analytic system into the fabric of almost all of its theoretical principles and its diagnostic assessment techniques.

Kanada is said to have been the abbot of a school for priests and to have written the first version of the *Vaisheshika Sutra* in which he introduced a theory of the atom. *Vaisheshika* and *Nyaya* are viewed as a complementary pair.

5. *Purva-Mimamsa darshana* is called *Mimamsa,* and by some "the old theology." *Purva* means first, initial, or preliminary. It contains elements of the Vedic-based philosophies with an extremely strong emphasis on the discipline, religious ritual, service, and right action that are considered significant Vedic mandates (*vidhi*). *Mimamsa* means exegesis or inquiry, and this school was especially attentive to the language of the *Vedas* and their precise meanings. It espoused the philosophical tenets of realism and pluralism and eschewed what it regarded as idealistic conceptualizations. The idea of God is deemphasized or nonexistent. The role of sacrifice is emphasized, at times, apparently for its own sake in the sense of its being an unquestionable Vedic command. *Apurva* is the concept that denotes the merit (*punya*) or grace that follows obedience to these *vidhi* (ritual injunctions) in one's current lifetime and may give one a better chance for the reward of heaven (*svarga*) after death rather than the ultimate goal of liberation after many lifetimes as implied in the *Moksha* sense. The founder of this school was Jaimini (c. 200 B.C.), about whom little is known.

6. *Uttara-Mimamsa* or **Vedanta** is a more spiritually oriented system that emphasizes the essential spiritual/consciousness base of all reality (*Brahman*), human misperception (*advaita* and *maya*), and ways that the individual and the Ultimate or *Brahman* may become reestablished in their already eternal axiomatic unity. These last discussions regarding Vedic wisdom, *Vedanta,* are believed by many to hold and encapsulate the entire essence of the *Vedas*. They also pull from the larger group of the *Upanishads*. The *Brahma-Sutra,* also called *Vedanta-Sutra,* of *Baradarayana* (c. 400 B.C. to A.D. 200) whom some have identified with *Vyasa,* is a nodal text of *Vedanta*. In it, *Brahman* is the Absolute, quintessential, and only reality. Although there is an emphasis on the impersonal and transcendental aspects of *Brahman, Brahman* as a personal deity is also presented.

Three main branches of *Vedanta* are the following. First, *Advaita-Vedanta* is a nondualistic approach to *Brahman*. The highly renowned sage, Shankara (Sankara), meaning "giver of goodness," born in modern-day Kerala, (A.D. 788–820), established a *darshana* that tends to be nontheistic and monistic. It has the philosophical features of an absolute idealism and has been one of the most influential schools of Hindu thought, *Advaita-Vedanta*. It espouses a "consciousness model" as its irreducible axiomatic base. Shankara, according to some leading authorities, is considered the greatest Vedantin and perhaps the greatest of India's philosophers (Klostermaier, 1994).

Second, the *Vishishadvaiata-Vedanta* of Ramanuja (A.D. 1055–1137) espouses a qualified nondualistic view of *Brahman* and the world. For him, reality is essentially unified but tiered and somewhat differentiated. Ramanuja held that *Brahman* is identical to the personal aspect of divinity termed *Ishvara* and that this is, in fact, Vishnu. This view of *Vedanta* has very pronounced theistic and ritualistic features.

Third, the *Dvaita-Vedanta* of Madhva (A.D. 1199–1278) holds a more dualistic view of the relationship between *Brahman,* the soul, and the world. He is said to have been the most prolific of the great Vedantin scholars with the greatest volume of written works. Like Ramanuja, his *Vedanta* is strongly "religious," yet he holds to the reality of much greater differentiation within the created world. He views *Brahman* as *Ishvara,* who is Vishnu, and stresses that liberation is achieved by self-surrender through active love and ritual worship.

The three *Nastika Darshanas* are Buddhism, Jainism founded by Vardhamana/Mahavira (sixth to fifth century B.C.), and Lokayata of Charvaka (c. 600 B.C.). Buddhism and Jainism, but not Lokayata, have influenced Ayurveda. Jainism is noteworthy for its monumental emphasis on nonviolence (*ahimsa*), reverence for life, and for its overwhelming stress on the need for personal effort and intentional work on the self in order to achieve *Moksha.* Jainism's luminary, the great hero Mahavira, not only is said to have rediscovered the path to *Moksha,* but also to have compassionately demonstrated it to others.

Of the three unorthodox *darshanas,* Buddhism has played an outstanding role in the development of Ayurveda. Its influence is inestimable. The work of the great sage and Ayurvedic physician Nāgārjuna, continues to exert a profound influence in modern times, especially in the field of Ayurvedic iatrochemistry and mineral-based therapeutic preparations. Buddhism and Jainism are also referred to as *Shramanas.* This connotes the path taken by aspirants who strive for the refinement of consciousness, self-realization, and ultimate freedom (*Moksha, Vimukti*) but who do not use the Vedic propositions or rituals as their primary means.

EPISTEMOLOGY

The epistemological perspective that Ayurveda uses comes chiefly from the Vedic observational system termed the *Nyaya darshana* and includes methods, techniques, and means to derive knowledge. In general, it is referred to as *pramana*. *Pramana* denotes both the techniques of measurement used and also the derived data themselves, which may be already formulated, as, for example, propositions from the *Vedas*. The instrument or organ of subjective epistemological experience is termed *Antahkarana*. It denotes the internal instrument of knowledge in contradistinction to the external instrument of the senses. This process comprises sensation, perception, concept formation, and interpretation. The four cognitive faculties subsumed within *Antahkarana* are the following:

1. *Manas.* This is the broad Sanskrit term encompassing the mind as it experiences sensations and perceptions, registers their data input, and then begins the process of identification and conceptualization. It also includes motoric information. It is the active mind that senses, perceives, and coordinates information.

2. *Chitta.* This is usually considered part of the function of *Manas* that specifically acts as a disseminator or transmitter of perception and thinking from *Manas* to the higher cognitive functions within *Ahamkara* and *Buddhi*. It has more of a passive, storage character. *Chitta* is also spelled *citta*.

3. *Ahamkara.* This aspect of mind is considered the differentiated ego or individuality of the person, the self. *Ahamkara* is the specific identity of an individual or of a substance. In the individual, a major function of *Ahamkara* is to evaluate the goodness or badness of an identified experience. *Ahamkara* acts as the stamp of individuality that organizes perceptions with the distinctive interpretative character unique to that individual. The function of *Ahamkara* as the self-identity provides that individual with the experience of relative constancy, perceived sameness, and adaptable continuity over time. Within *Ahamkara* are *Manas* and *Buddhi*.

4. *Buddhi.* This is the most refined aspect of the epistemological process and is termed intellect or intelligence. Its specific connotation suggests that its functioning is most discerning and intrinsically valid having the capacity to accurately interpret experience. The *Buddhi* function decides whether one will act or refrain from acting. This is the aspect of mind closest to the innate wisdom (*prajna*) emanating from pure consciousness. An individual's *Buddhi* is derived from and participates in the universal, cosmic intelligence called *Mahat*. The functions of *Buddhi* transcend mere physiological cognition. *Buddhi* is the link that acts to present elements of *Prakriti* (creation) within the individual (mind, body, internalized aspects of the external environment) to the *Purusha* (pure consciousness). *Buddhi* and *atman* have an anaclitic relationship.

Epistemology or the theory of how one obtains knowledge is termed *pramana*. This connotes both the epistemological means used and the proofs or evidence used to describe aspects of reality. Four techniques for knowing and measuring (*Pramanas*) are described:

1. *Pratyaksha,* direct sensory perception. This involves the straight contact of the five senses (sight, hearing, smell, touch, and taste) with their objects of

perception (*vishaya*). In Ayurveda, *Pratyaksha* is regarded as the preeminent mode of experiencing the material world. It is firsthand experiential sensory evidence. It is considered the premier epistemological method for ascertaining a true perceptual understanding of reality. It is believed to be the most reliable method used to arrive at a proof, a reality-based conclusion, with the reliability of *Sabda* or textual theory considered of secondary and merely supporting value. *Pratyaksha* is understood to support the proper use of the function of *Manas,* the mind. This experience is not merely a simple act of sensory perception, but, in fact, it is the experiencing of perception by living in the five senses with a focus on the perception of sensations. Dwelling within the experience of the five senses and not on their already internalized referents in the form of concepts and preestablished understanding is the sense that *Pratyaksha* conveys.

2. *Anumana,* inference. This involves the inductive process of initial observation and data gathering, such as assessing signs and symptoms, and then the generation of explanatory hypotheses.

3. *Sabda* or *Aptopadesha,* authoritative statement. This "testimony" includes the use of texts, documents, and theories describing relevant material. In ancient times, *Sabda* (sound, hearing) was the primary form of all learning and involved face-to-face contact with a teacher who was recognized as an authoritative figure. This time-honored system was referred to as *guru-sishya parampara,* the transmission of knowledge from generation to generation via an oral tradition. In addition to this more direct instruction, the actual firsthand reports of patients and their families are used as important clinical statements to gather further medical and lifestyle history.

4. *Upamana,* analogy. This *Pramana* or technique for attaining correct knowledge is the method of using abductive reasoning and relying on the best available explanation to be the truest at that time for that situation, that is, for contextual validation.

AYURVEDIC WORLDVIEW

The broad base, the Weltanschauung or worldview, that Ayurveda espouses is essentially unitary and dynamic. The whole of reality is conceived as an integrated coherence with actively interdependent aspects. There is no part of the totality of existence that is functionally separate or disconnected from any other. The dynamic aspect of this is fueled by the constant interaction, in biological life, among the three *doshas, Vata, Pitta,* and *Kapha,* all of which are the three fundamental regulatory principles of the body's psychophysiological functioning. Since these *doshas* have an almost axiomatic role in Ayurveda, synonyms for them are generally not used. *Vata* connotes movement, *Pitta* connotes transformation, and *Kapha* suggests consolidation and inertia. The interplay between and among these principles modulates the interactions of the *gurvadi gunas* or ten pairs of opposite qualities that characterize all created substances. An almost infinite variety of presentations thus becomes possible.

The place of man in greater nature is reflected in the notion of "microcosm within macrocosm" or *pinda-brahmanda*. This suggests an intimate correspondence, if not virtual identity, between the life of the individual and the life of the world around. This cosmic homology is a central tenet of the *Vedas*. Man, in this view, is regarded as a miniature of nature, a world within a world. Man, in effect, is a contraction of Great Nature, *Prakriti*. This connotes that everything existing in the universe is in some way encapsulated within man. Some implications of this include the intimate effect that nature or the environment has on man; for example, the influence of seasonal changes; and the presumption that all aspects of the outer world are, in some way, represented within the individual. Each individual is understood to be a unity composed of body, mind, and consciousness. The Vedic recognition of a spiritual base with an emphasis on consciousness is an important part of the Ayurvedic perspective. Ayurveda, per se, positions the physical body and its functioning both in its balanced and in its unbalanced states as one major focal point. Ayurveda's focus, in fact, is on the complete individual—physical body, mind, and consciousness. Since ordinary attention is most concentrated on the more material aspects of experience, Ayurveda uses the natural focal point of the body as a vehicle to begin its approach toward understanding and treating the total person.

SANSKRIT

Another important consideration in outlining the scope of Ayurveda is an appreciation of the original language, Vedic Sanskrit, in which the ancient texts were composed. Sanskrit is one of the oldest known languages. Legend states that the ancient seers or *rishis* of India developed this system of sound, speech, language, and writing during deep contemplative states. Sanskrit words were believed to reflect and contain the energetic bases of the objects or experiences to which they referred. The oldest Veda, the *Rig-Veda,* was, in fact, a text of chants or hymns. These *mantras,* as they are called, were believed to have a magical power able to effect change.

The pronunciation and correct sounding out of Sanskrit words and *mantras* had been and continues to be an important study within Hinduism. The *Vedangas* (eighth century to fourth century B.C.) or limbs of the *Vedas,* for example, were composed as supplementary texts that covered phonetics, prosody, grammar, etymology, astronomical considerations, and sacrificial rituals. These are within the class of *smriti* (secondarily revealed) literature. Their goal was to ensure an ongoing correct rendition of Sanskrit scripture.

Sanskrit is held to be a sacred language by Hindus, and Ayurveda follows this view. The conceptualizations to which many Sanskrit terms refer are difficult to adequately translate and so are used in their original form in this text. For historical and scholarly purposes, we provide English approximations of some relevant Sanskrit terms (Apte, 1993; Bender, 1967; Fischer-Schreiber, Ehrhard, & Friedrichs, 1994; Staal, 1963). Of note is the language called *Pali.*

It is a derivative of Sanskrit and thought to be the Indian dialect used by the Buddha. Buddhists consider *Pali* a revered language, and many Buddhist scriptural texts are written in this dialect, as well as in Sanskrit.

VEDIC STANDARDS AND VALUES

There are four basic life goals (*purushartha*) or prime values for each individual according to the *Vedas*. The fundamental importance of these and their relevance for Ayurveda is supported by Charaka's mention of them in his description of the origins of Ayurveda. They are the following:

1. *Dharma,* destiny, purpose, duty, obligations, immanent cosmic lawfulness, justice, and righteousness in life. This goal broadly refers to career, vocation, and the conduct of one's life; in addition, it may be understood as one's life's work or mission.

2. *Artha,* possessions. This refers to the necessary material accumulations that one acquires in order to live with a reasonable degree of comfort. Charaka specifically denotes *artha* as being the possessions or objects of the five senses.

3. *Kama,* pleasure. This is the experience that derives from the capacity of desire and relates to the natural propensity of attraction to objects that, it is felt, will satisfy needs, reduce tension, and yield wholesome pleasure or enjoyment.

4. *Moksha,* liberation. This is the central and primary goal under which the other three are subsumed. *Moksha* refers to the gradual process of becoming freed from inordinate desires through the exercise of proper discrimination of a hierarchy of values that regards self-actualization and expanded consciousness as ultimate goals to be actively pursued. *Moksha,* in the Vedic sense, means to regain consciousness of the unity of the individual spirit (*atman*) and the universal Absolute (*Brahman*).

PRINCIPLES OF TREATMENT

The term *upashaya* refers to Ayurveda's two basic principles of treatment:

1. *Samanya,* "like increases like." This principle relates to the interconnectedness of all aspects of the world, as previously mentioned. It connotes universal and pervading essences within particulars. Factors, substances, qualities, or attributes of a specific type exert similar effects on the object to which they are applied. This holds true both for positive and for negative influences. The phenomenon of "like attracts like" is also included in this principle. Homologous constituents in foods and herbs, when consumed, are attracted to and assimilated into their presumed corresponding sites in the body's tissues.

2. *Vishesha,* "opposites balance and so cure each other." This principle relates to the idea of balance and imbalance. It connotes individual differences and

contrasts. The idea of restoring balance through applying qualities opposite to those manifesting in the imbalanced condition is especially related to more material phenomena such as the gross aspects of the physical body, foods, and herbs. Cooling substances like milk or coconut oil, for example, when ingested or applied to the body diminish excess heat and thus treat conditions such as hyperacidity or skin irritation.

UNIVERSAL DESCRIPTIVE QUALITIES IN NATURE: *SAGUNAS*

Ayurveda has constructed a detailed classification system relying heavily on the perceptual five senses; these descriptors are used to identify and characterize the essential properties of virtually all substances. These descriptive attributes or qualities are called the *gurvadi gunas* and consist of ten pairs of opposites. The term *guna* has the connotation of being an assessed physical and chemical property of a substance. All created realities in nature (*Prakriti*) have qualities and attributes and so are considered to be *saguna* or describable. The entire conception of *gunas* denotes the impermanent, ever-changing, interdependent, and constant state of flux that characterizes conditioned reality on all levels—material, psychological, and spiritual. *Gunas* are the ascribed attributes used to delineate the dynamically changing features of a substance using English terms. The ten pairs are the following:

1. *shita/ushna,* cold/hot,
2. *snigdha/ruksha,* wet or oily/dry,
3. *guru/laghu,* heavy/light,
4. *sthula/sukshma,* gross/subtle,
5. *sandra/drava,* dense/liquid,
6. *sthira/chala,* stable or static/mobile,
7. *manda/tikshna,* dull/sharp and penetrating,
8. *mridu/kathina,* soft/hard,
9. *slakshna/khara,* smooth or slimy/rough, and
10. *picchila or avila/sishada,* sticky or cloudy/clear.

The importance and utility of this conceptualization comprises a large part of the Ayurvedic methodology. Foods and herbal substances are understood in this way. The functioning of the body and the interplay of the *doshas* are described in these terms. In addition, virtually any perceptible data can be described using this system. This becomes useful since each attribute carries with it a distinctive set of characteristics, which are both explanatory and suggestive of potential therapeutic actions. These gunic properties have been associated with material substances and also with psychological processes. The close and, perhaps, unfamiliar juxtaposition of physical and material attributes with emotional states, for instance, is a regular part of traditional thinking in Ayurveda. In addition to the customary denotation of each term,

Ayurveda adds further meanings, some of which describe states or conditions, and some of which describe functioning, processes, or trends. Ayurveda places great stress on the value of human perception. The five senses (hearing, touch, sight, taste, and smell) are the basis for contact with the world, data gathering, and for the process of inductive reasoning. The exquisite development of sensory perception is a prerequisite, therefore, for the process of correct conceptualization and deductive reasoning. This again attests to the empirical and experiential method of a naturalistic science rather than a more a priori theoretical operational style. In addition, there is a high regard for the significance of the material world rather than a de-emphasis of it. This valuation of the physical body and the physical world should not be underestimated; it was and continues to be among the dominant values of the *Vedas* and the ancient Vedic view of the meaning of life.

The following is a brief outline of some important aspects associated with the ten pairs of opposite qualities; they are most often referred to using their English designations:

Cold is said to induce contraction, numbness, fear, and insensitivity. *Hima* also connotes cold. The action of stopping flow by cooling (*stambhana*) is thus produced. A reasonable degree of cold, such as is experienced in the cooler seasons, is considered to encourage health by maintaining tissue viability. Cold is an essential aspect of the potency or energy (*virya*) of foods and herbs. *Kapha* and *Vata dosha* are increased; *Pitta dosha* is decreased (KV+, P−). This notation system, applicable to each different attribute, indicates that, when the designated attribute is present, then each of the three *doshas* is either relatively increased (+) or relatively decreased (−). In this particular case, *Kapha* and *Vata* are increased (+), and *Pitta* is decreased (−).

Hot increases digestion and the metabolic fire (*Agni*). It induces expansion, perspiration, inflammation, and anger. Excessive heat as experienced in the hotter seasons is not considered beneficial to health. Heat, like cold, is a prime quality of the potency (*virya*) of food and herbs (KV−, P+, *Agni* +). In addition to the decrease in *Kapha* and *Vata,* there is an increase in *Pitta* and in *Agni,* the digestive fire.

Wet or *oily* is often termed *unctuous*. It induces lubrication, smoothness, and moisture (*kledana*). The emotions of love and compassion are associated with this quality (KP+, V−).

Dry is related to lack of moisture, absorption (*shoshana*), constipation, and anxiety. The quality of dryness is perceived chiefly through sight (KP−, V+).

Heavy is a quality most associated with weight, fullness, richness, and possible difficulty in digestion. Heavy foods contribute to building body tissues (*brimhana*) (K+, VP−).

Light is associated with airiness, buoyancy, less gross substance, being light in weight, easy digestion, and the reduction of body tissues (*langhana*) (K−, VP+, *Agni* +).

Gross has the action of covering (*samvarana*) and is associated with an increase in material structure, coarseness, crudeness, obstruction, and obesity (K+, VP–).

Subtle denotes more immateriality, a pervading action (*vivarana*), the ability to rapidly enter very small spaces, and the capacity to increase emotional states (VP+, K–).

Dense is considered to promote stability, strength, and cohesiveness. Its main action is solidifying (*prasadana*) (K+, VP–).

Liquid or *flowing* has a dissolving or liquefying action (*vilodana*). The quality of compassion is associated with the idea of flowing (KP+, V–).

Stable or *static* creates support and firmness. Stable substances are enduring and strengthening to the body. Their chief action is that of stabilization (*dharana*). Stable is associated with the emotional experience of faith (K+, VP–, *Agni*–).

Mobile promotes movement and restlessness. Its action is stimulating (*prerana*). Mobile when steady, spreading, or creeping (*sara*) is associated with *Pitta;* when erratic (*chala*), mobile is associated with *Vata* (VP+, K–).

Dull creates a blunt quality, is sluggish, marked by slow action, and produces relaxation. It may help to pacify (*shamana*) body elements. Dull is associated with mild, tissue maintaining food substances such as milk and ghee (K+, VP–).

Sharp penetrates with an immediate action on the body associated with purification (*shodhana*) and an increase in the digestive process (K–, VP+).

Soft has a loosening action (*shlathana*) and the tendency to remove hardness from the tissues of the body. This oily, loosening action creates softness, delicacy, relaxation, tenderness, love, and care (KP+, V–).

Hard increases strength, rigidity, and has a hardening action (*dridhikarana*). It is related to selfishness (KV+, P–).

Smooth connotes moisture and lubrication and has a healing action (*ropana*) (KP+, V–).

Rough is perceived by the sense of touch and has characteristics of dry texture, cracks, fissures, and a scraping-away action (*lekhana*) (V+, KP–).

Sticky or *cloudy* is associated with lack of perceptive capacity and with an adhering action (*lepana*) (K+, VP–).

Clear is related to spreading and diversification and has a cleansing action (*kshalana*); clear is also related to translucency and clarity of perception (VP+, K–).

SANKHYA MODEL OF CREATION

The Ayurvedic model of creation is derived from the Vedic system called *Sankhya*. This is a narrative sequence of enumeration that outlines the evolution of the cosmos from the immaterial realm to the material, manifest dimension. There are 24 prime cosmic principles (*tattvas*) that emerge out of a single, unified base.

This model holds that the universe and humans share a common origin; that the individual is a microcosmic unit reflecting the larger macrocosmic universe; and that foundational, primal reality is a single immaterial essence out of which all material forms emerge. Although the 24 prime cosmic principles have an apparently logical, sequential development, they occur simultaneously and so may be coparallel in operation.

AVYAKTA

Pure existence, in its unmanifest state, is called *Avyakta*. Its absolutely transcendental being makes it truly imponderable. Although indescribable and ineffable in essence, the ancient Vedics acknowledged its noumenal reality with the Sanskrit terms *satyam, ritam,* and *brihat. Satyam* implies the essential truth and reality of existence; *ritam,* the deep structure of the universe, connotes a substantive internal and lawful order that is self-perpetuating and self-correcting; and *brihat* refers to the vast and enormous breadth of its being, an infinite eternalness. The two chief components of *Avyakta* are *Purusha* and unmanifested *Prakriti;* they constitute noumenal reality.

Avyakta's eternal emptiness with its connotation of potentiality may be termed *Zephirum,* whose sense is roughly akin to the term "zero." I have intentionally coined this term, *Zephirum,* with its novel and unsaturated connotations to indicate an orientation that suggests the Buddhist notion of *shunyata* or emptiness. Inherent in this is the seeming paradox of attempting to indicate a "position" by using a term that, in itself, denotes no reference points. It includes no dependent dimensions suggestive of a syllogism or duality that could be cognitively or mathematically described. Such a construct, in effect, suggests that excessive attempts to intellectually understand issues that Buddha, himself, regarded as irrelevant to the goal of salvation such as the ontological status of the universe, a soul, an afterlife, and so forth are futile. If anything, these considerations serve as preliminary props that ultimately point to a suggestion with ineffable, perhaps zero, qualities, *Zephirum.* This idea is pointed to in the Chinese concept of *Wu* or *Tao,* the Void. *Tao* is indescribable. However, it is said to have characteristics both of *Wu* as nothingness and of *Yu* as everythingness. *Avyakta* as unmanifest reality and *Vyakta* as the manifest, phenomenal universe constitute the One, the Absolute, the *Brahman.*

PURUSHA

Purusha is the Sanskrit term for the primal immaterial matrix out of which all else emerges. It is indescribable. Language and any descriptions referring to it are mere approximations. This single and absolute reality is understood to be identical with pure consciousness. *Purusha* may be considered the "World Ground" behind and at the heart of the entire universe. It denotes absolute, unconditioned consciousness. It is *Brahman*. It is the primordially uncaused, substantival totality of the real however it is understood. *Purusha* is one, pure, eternal, and changeless. It remains in a state of eternal activation. It is the primordial consciousness that grounds all else and is the witness behind all appearances.

Purusha is regarded as the only being that is not material. It is the only being that is a purely conscious entity. In effect, *Purusha* may be considered the only being that is purely spiritual and thus absolutely immaterial. *Purusha* has been called "Seer," "Witnesser," and "Observer." It is not regarded, however, as having any resemblance to the concept of "mind"; rather, it exists as a field of choiceless, passive awareness. It is associated with the idea of male energy and, although it is outside of creation, it is considered the ground or matrix of all creation.

Purusha is absolutely and always unmanifest; it has no material correlate; it is completely incorporeal and unlimited. From an ontological point of view, the nature of *Purusha* is virtually without descriptive qualities; that is, it is closest to the concept of *nirguna* (having no attributes or qualities). *Purusha,* as pristine consciousness, is regarded as the core of all existence, manifest and unmanifest. This consciousness paradigm is considered to mirror the spiritual basis of all reality. It is entirely spiritual or *karana*.

Purusha is the *Sankhya* term for what in the *Vedanta* is referred to as *Brahman*. When this reality is pointed to as existing within an individual, it has several designations. In Hinduism, it is called the *jiva,* and the *Chaitanya*. In *Vedanta,* it is the *atman*. In Buddhism, it is the Buddha nature, the Buddha-Self, the Buddha *dhatu,* and the *Tathagatagarbha* (Buddha embryo). In Chinese Buddhist traditions, it may be denoted by the term *Dharmakaya*. In general, in English, it is called spirit, and within the individual, the soul.

PRAKRITI

When the primal immaterial matrix, the *Purusha,* spontaneously "moves," a primal emotional state of purified desire or the rudimentary condition of need arises. At that moment, the first material energy, *Prakriti,* comes into being. It is in this sense that *Prakriti* may be understood to be synonymous with both *soma* as matter and *Agni* as energy. *Prakriti* is primordial Nature, creation, and the ground of conditioned consciousness. Its dynamic essence denotes impermanence and a constant state of flux.

Details of this emergence out of *Purusha* are considered unknowable, and it is inferred that this mysterious point of movement initiates creation in a manner roughly akin to, though qualitatively different from, the Western conception of a "big bang," an initial, one-time event, launching the origin of the universe. This is called *Pranava,* the first creation. It manifests as the first soundless, primordial sound, the AUM or OM. It is also called *Udgitha* or the primordial mantra. In the *Atharva-Veda Samhita,* the *Taittiriya Upanishad,* the *Mandukya Upanishad,* and the *Chandogya Upanishad,* the meaningfulness of AUM as a word, a syllable, and a sound is expounded. AUM has been said to incarnate in one instance the entire Vedic *darshana*. It encompasses consciousness as it is experienced in human existence, and as it participates in Absolute consciousness, *Brahman*.

In fact, thousands of years ago, concepts that are now considered modern discoveries were clearly postulated. These ancient ideas include the conception of the *paramanu* as an indivisible subatomic particle, the *anu* or atom, and the coming together of multiple *anus* in forms that today are denoted by the term "molecules."

Prakriti, thus, can be thought of as emerging out of a field of zero point energy. This spontaneous synchronicity, the emergence of auspiciousness (*subha, mangala*), is regarded as the "Divine Mother." This "Blessed Mother" is synonomous with the "Will of God." *Prakriti* denoted as *Shakti* suggests its power, force, and drive.

Prakriti, per se, is unmanifest and constitutes "Ur-Matter" or primordial nature. This primal matter or first substance is a kind of undeveloped energetic matter, also called *Pradhana. Prakriti* is unconscious yet dynamic and is the material that very gradually evolves into all forms of the manifest created world (*pravritti*). *Prakriti* is the first creation, and as such, is the first reality that contains qualities, attributes, or properties (*saguna*) capable of description. *Gunas* condition (*samskara*) existence.

Prakriti contains the potential out of which differentiations, boundaries, and limitations emerge. An ancient Vedic *sutra* (aphoristic verse) reflects *Prakriti's* creative intent: "I am One, I wish to become many." This is related to the Sanskrit idea of *abhasa* and *abhasana,* the process of the one transforming into the many. *Prakriti* is desire in its purist form. It is desire as energy whose singular aim is ineffable expansion through pulsed, cyclic transformations. The evolutionary, bidirectional conception of *Parinamavada* denotes the dynamic flux of the trigunas, *Sattva, Rajas,* and *Tamas,* within *Prakriti* that results in the energies behind creation. In addition, the theoretical construct *Satkaryavada* holds the following: The effect is latent within the cause and requires only a releasing factor to make the effect come about. Cause and effect are seen as the undeveloped and the developed state of the same one entity. This entire process (*parinama*) is *karana* or spiritual in essence.

Different *darshanas* or theoretical schools give varying emphasis and interpretation to the *parinama* construct. *Sankhya* most explicitly maintains that the effect is preexistent in the cause and that karmic actions are real transformations. *Advaita-Vedanta* highlights that all change is essentially only apparent and that the underlying immutable unity is the overriding reality. At the heart of Buddhism is the core idea that cause and effect are both misconceptions, that dependency is illusory, and that the awakened mind ultimately disappears into an unknowable and ineffable ground best characterized as namelessness.

Perhaps, the *Ajativada* (unborn creation; no creation ever happened) concept found in some ultraorthodox forms of Hindu *Advaita-Vedanta* as well as in Buddhism and in Jainism offers an exceedingly worthy counterpoint to the idea of creation as a dynamic doing and undoing process. *Ajativada* views existence as being an eternal now, the eternal unborn having no beginning and no end, no cause and no effect, no origination as production and no devolution as destruction.

In Chinese Taoism, *Prakriti* is akin to the conception of *Tao* as *Tai Yi, Tai Chi,* or the Supreme Ultimate. *Yuan chi* and *Te* are the Taoist terms connoting the *Kundalini* energy of *Prakriti* that produces *wan wu,* the 10,000 things of perception, a concept suggesting the virtually infinite multiplicity that comprises the created universe. *Tzu jan* is the term that connotes the spontaneous activation inherent within *Prakriti*. In philosophical terms, it is the ontological disposition of *Prakriti*. Within human nature, its correlate is *wu wei,* spontaneous, natural, and unmotivated action virtually free of rapacious desire for objects of the senses, both inanimate and animate. *Wu wei* is the aim of the *Tao* and is said to be the purpose of life.

MAHA GUNAS: THE THREE UNIVERSAL ENERGETIC BINDERS WITHIN *PRAKRITI*

The three axiomatic *Maha gunas* (great attributes), the *Trigunas,* that are inherent in *Prakriti* are *Sattva, Rajas,* and *Tamas.* They are in a spiritualized state (*karana*). These *gunas* may be thought of as highly rarefied potentials that impart direction, organization, and create a unique character to that which they imbue. The term *guna* in Sanskrit means that which binds, a fundamental energetic force promoting coherence. The *Maha gunas* are considered sacred and their subtle, yet profound actions are revered. The *gurvadi gunas,* in contrast, are considered coarser and are commonly used to describe features of material substances in everyday use. For example, the *gurvadi guna "laghu"* denotes lightness in weight, whereas the *Maha guna "Sattva"* denotes lightness in terms of the energy of luminosity, radiance, and light as illumination (*prakasha, prakashika, prakshana, prakhya*). The character that the *Maha gunas,* considered "omnisubstances," imparts denotes the degree of subtleness, purity, and the innate trend toward potential consciousness raising that a substance contains. The quality and quantity of *Maha gunas* within an individual's psychological makeup determines the respective psychological *prakruti* or constitution. The *Maha gunas* or *Trigunas* are sacred energies.

Sattva is the purest, most immaterial, and spiritual attribute within the manifest world. It is characterized by degrees of consciousness, intelligence, lightness, purity (*shuddha*), clarity, luminosity (*prakasha*), peace, harmony, equilibrium, and optimal balance. The simple word "goodness" aptly connotes its numinous meaning. *Sattva* denotes the highest level of purity that is unadulterated and thus wholesome. *Rajas* is characterized by dynamic movement, kinetic energy, turbulence, agitation, change, and transformation.

Tamas is the quality of inertia, solidity, dullness, darkness, veiling, coarseness, grossness, resistance, and materiality.

The *Maha gunas* are inextricably bound up with *Prakriti* and remain the most essential and overridingly influential aspects of all of her developed forms. The binding forces and motivational trends at the heart of all creation events emanate from the *Maha gunas*. This is denoted by the concept of *Parinamavada,* the dynamic *Triguna* flux of creation that emanates out of *Prakriti*. When in perfect balance, the *Maha gunas* create a more spiritual or immaterial state in the created object. The usual condition of creation, however, is one of an imbalance of these *Maha gunas*. To the corresponding extent that *Sattva* is *less* prominent, a more material, corporeal, gross, or imperfect state of being exists. When *Rajas* and *Tamas,* therefore, are in ascendance, for example, an individual's life is experienced as more "bound up," rigid, attached to things in a static way, and so is less flexible, creative, and free. Out of these primordial *Maha gunas* come the more materially perceptible *gurvadi gunas* that are the intrinsic properties, qualities, or attributes of substances in the world recognizable by the five senses.

MAHAT: COSMIC, PERVASIVE INTELLIGENCE

At this juncture in the creation sequence, the previous aspects that were noumenal in nature first begin to become manifest and their phenomenality, more material, defining, and specific properties begin to become consolidated. These cosmic principles that make up nature or *Prakriti,* according to the *Sankhya* system, continue to be human centered and so have what may be seen as an anthropomorphic orientation.

The first manifestation, which is considered to have some developed primordial material substance, is called *Mahat* (cosmic intelligence). This is understood to be the innate intelligence within all aspects of the universe. It exists in a spiritualized state (*karana*). This pervasive, universal intelligence is made up of laws and regulatory principles (*ritam* and *dharma*) that determine the course of evolution. *Mahat* is the transitional area between noumenal and phenomenal reality; it has been called the "Divine Mind." Within the individual, *Mahat* is termed the *Buddhi,* the reliable capacity to discriminate truth from falsehood, right from wrong, and reality from delusion and illusion. Intelligence, therefore, in this view, comes into being prior to the grosser forms of matter that only later evolve into existence.

Another important aspect of *Mahat* is its containment of what are called the *Pancha Tattvas* or five root causes, the five prime cosmic forces, that activate and manifest as energy and matter in the universe. They exist on the *karana* or spiritualized level of being. They create four structures: (1) the five sense organs (*jnanendriyas*), (2) the five motor organs (*karmendriyas*), (3) the five *Tanmatras* or irreducible subtle (*sukshma*) energies behind the five Elements, and (4) the Five Great Gross (*sthula*) Elements (*Pancha Mahabhutanis*).

Mahat is regarded as the first organization out of *Prakriti* that is a nodal intelligence having coherence and direction and being capable of imparting the rudimentary template of form. This is the genesis of the *Maha gunas: Sattva, Rajas,* and *Tamas.* The *Pancha Tattvas* within *Mahat,* therefore, are understood to be the spiritualized, *seed precursors* and the spiritual etiological stimuli behind and at the heart of the entire created world.

AHAMKARA: INDIVIDUATION

The next step in the developmental process of *Prakriti* is a giant leap and is what eventually becomes most characteristically individualized in human experience. It is called *Ahamkara.* This is the point at which unity differentiates and splits into individuality and multiplicity. What had been the spiritualized roots now, for the first time, become less fine and are referred to as being *sukshma* or subtle. The English word closest to this concept of human individuality would be *ego. Ahamkara* also connotes individual soul, individual self, and person. It implies a separate and distinct delineation of self from all else, as well as a subjective and unique experiential identity characterized by feelings of separation, isolation, and difference. *Ahamkara* becomes the ego container that makes one thing unique, different, and separate from all else. For human beings, *Ahamkara* becomes the experience of a personal sense of self. It is limited self-awareness. This quality is chiefly applied to human life but is also an aspect of other sentient life, such as exists in the plant and animal world. *Ahamkara* imparts an entity's essential identity that remains constant but which is flexible, changeable, and adaptable via modifications over time.

In Buddhism, *Ahamkara* is the personality, the embodied self, composed of five *skandhas* or ever-changing and impermanent dimensions: (1) physical body, (2) emotional reactions to the five sensory experiences and to *Manas,* (3) perception/conception, (4) conditioned precipitates of perception/conception: habitual and passively reflexive modes of thinking, memory, and behavior, and (5) individualized consciousness with its default dualistically programmed state of cognition: the subject versus object mode of experience and cognition.

Ahamkara, in its connotation of the human psychological ego, imparts to the ego one of its major functions, repression. Repression denotes the mind's continuous pressure to forget. This forgetting is coupled with an intrinsic cognitive default, that of being unable to easily become aware of the unconscious dimensions already existing within the self. Repression is the virtually unyielding pull toward nonconsciousness that the unconscious continuously exerts. The importance of this understanding, of necessity, requires repetition. The significance of this relentless, yet typical, pull toward unconsciousness for self-development is addressed in detail in Chapters 11 and 12.

Through the vehicle of *Ahamkara,* both the five *Tattvas* and the three *Maha gunas* begin to dynamically build the manifest universe. Before and up to the point of *Ahamkara,* the quality of creation has been *karana* or virtu-ally spiritual in its entirety: *causal, seed, magnetic,* or *soul.* From *Ahamkara* onward, the rest of the creation process now becomes more "incarnated" or more materialized: *sukshma* as subtle and energetic, and then *sthula* or gross. There is a trend downward, so to speak, into grosser, more concrete, and tan-gible manifestations of reality.

BIRTH OF THE BIOLOGICAL *DOSHAS*

The *Maha gunas* or *Trigunas* within *Prakriti* interact to precipitate out the "subtle essences" of the psychobiological *doshas.* These *sukshma* essences then become the unspoiled soul ("mental *dosha*") of each material biological *dosha. Prana* is the energetic soul of *Vata dosha, Tejas* is the soul within *Pitta dosha,* and *Ojas* is the subtle essence within *Kapha dosha.* The *Maha gunas* impart psychophysiological properties to the *doshas.*

As *Sattva* interacts with *Rajas* and *Tamas,* the kinetic energy of *Rajas* pre-cipitates out what is to be the vital, energetic essence that pervades all bio-logical life, *Prana.* This *Prana* or life force is virtually identical with what in Traditional Chinese Medicine is called *Qi.* This substantive entity on the verge of formlessless both holds the body, mind, and consciousnesses together and also animates them.

Out of this *Prana* comes the first bioenergetic *dosha, Vata.* Out of *Vata* come the other two *doshas, Pitta* and *Kapha.* This broad level of reality, hav-ing both spiritual as well as more grossly material qualities, is metaphysically termed *sukshma,* the subtle, energetic, or vital level. The older literature has referred to this as the "astral" sphere, especially when alluding to the sheath of *Manas* and that of *Prana.*

The concept of the *doshas* forms a bedrock group of axioms in Ayurveda. *Doshas* have traditionally been called "humors," which implies the histori-cally archaic conceptualization found in ancient Greek, Roman, and *Unani Tibb* (Arab) medical texts. The idea of *dosha,* as a biological and energetic substance, originates in the work of Charaka and then Sushruta, the ancient authors of the original and still fundamental Ayurvedic texts. The Sanskrit word *dosha* literally means spoiling, fault, or darkener. This refers to the *dos-ha*'s inherent capacity to become vitiated or agitated and then disruptive of the current status quo of the *dhatus* (tissues) and the body as a whole. This apparently disruptive action is, in fact, a positive homeostatic mechanism aimed at regulating the health of the body. The connotation of being a dis-rupter suggests the dynamic action that is inherent in the functioning of the *doshas.*

The concept of *dosha* contains two fundamental ideas: (1) its being a bio-energetic substance and (2) its acting as a bioenergetic regulatory physiologi-cal force, process, or principle. The nature of *dosha* is that of a force that resides on the borderline between matter and energy. The biological *doshas* are psychophysiological principles of organization, both structural and functional within the *BioPsychoSpiritual* person.

Since the *doshas* do have material substance, they are, in part, composed of varying amounts of what are called the Five Great Gross Elements (*Pancha Mahabhutanis*) that are the five elemental building blocks of all matter. They are Ether, Air, Fire, Water, and Earth. These "primary pentads," as they are sometimes called, are the very first precipitations of material substance and compose the inorganic elemental building blocks that when ingested and properly digested become part of the internal regulatory principles that make up the biological *doshas*.

Doshas, in general, however, exert their effects in a more functional way in the human body. They are the basic organizing principles that regulate and maintain physical and psychological homeostasis. In effect, they are the intermediaries between the outside world (foods, diet, seasons, daily routine, and life-style) and the inside world of tissues, organ systems, and functioning of the body. These homeostatic regulators act as protective barriers guarding the health and integrity of the body both mental and physical.

The connotation of the *doshas* as faults refers to the fact that the *doshas,* as protective intermediaries, are vulnerable to being disrupted, imbalanced, and temporarily impaired. External and internal (mental) aggressions first assault the *doshas,* which, in effect, try to absorb the stressor and to protect the tissues. This beneficial function provides a cushioning effect. If the assault to the *doshas* is too severe, they then become spoiled. In turn, the vitiated *doshas* further disrupt the body and the mind. This process of spoiling has been traditionally referred to as "vitiation," a customary and standardized term denoting a pathological state. In other words, *doshas* in a state of balance are good; only when the *doshas* become excessively aggravated do they become spoiled and then act as spoilers.

Vata

Vata has been called the biological air humor. *Vata* means wind and suggests movement. Its main characteristic is that of propulsion. *Vata* is responsible for all motion in the body from the cellular to the tissue and musculoskeletal level, for the coordination of the senses, for the equilibrium of the tissues, for the acuity of the senses, and for respiration. The central and peripheral nervous system is under the control of *Vata*. Since it has a primary leadership role, *Vata* has been referred to as the "king *dosha*." In fact, one might also view the nature of *Vata* as being a "servant *dosha*" since it is the only *dosha* that serves the other two by acting as their vehicle and carrier within the paths of their operation. It transports them and itself to peripheral sites in the body. Like *Pitta* and *Kapha dosha, Vata* has a base in the sattvic *Maha guna* (purity), but, unlike the other two *doshas,* it has a significantly larger complement of the rajasic *Maha guna* (turbulence). This rajasic aspect is the basis for *Vata*'s kinetic action. In terms of the ten pairs of descriptive *gunas, Vata* has the following qualities: cold, dry, light, subtle, mobile, sharp, hard, rough, and clear. *Vata* is composed of the Ether (*Akasha*) Element and the Air (*Vayu*) Element.

Pitta

Pitta is known as the biological fire humor. Its etymological derivation is associated with digestion, heating, thermogenesis, and transformation. *Pitta*'s chief action is that of digestion or transformation from the cellular, tissue, and organ levels to the psychological, mental, and emotional spheres. Conversion and thermogenesis are prime activities of *Pitta*. The fundamental Ayurvedic concept of *Agni,* the energy of the digestive fire, is inextricably tied into the activity of its biological container, *Pitta dosha.* The key attributes of *Pitta* are hot, slightly oily, light, subtle, mobile, sharp, penetrating, soft, smooth, clear, flowing, and creeping. *Pitta* is composed of the Fire (*Tejas* or *Agni*) Element and the Water (*Ap, Apas,* or *Jala*) Element. *Pitta* has a strong sattvic base and also contains a significant measure of the rajasic *Maha guna.*

Kapha

Kapha has been called the biological water humor. Its chief characteristic is that of cohesion and binding. The word *Kapha* means phlegm and water flourishing and suggests the quality of connectedness. *Kapha* maintains the stability of the bodily tissues and imparts a quality of protection, which is related to its tendency toward denseness, containment, and materiality. The qualities of *Kapha* include cold, wet, heavy, gross, stable, dull, soft, smooth, cloudy, and dense. *Kapha* is composed of the Water Element (*Ap, Apas,* or *Jala*) and the Earth (*Prithvi*) Element. *Kapha* has a base in the sattvic *Maha guna,* but contains a significant measure of the tamasic *Maha guna* (inertia).

PANCHA TANMATRAS: THE SOUL OF THE FIVE GREAT GROSS ELEMENTS

As we continue our analytic descent in describing the sequence of the origination of the world around us, we come to the beginnings of the five *Tanmatras.* The Sanskrit word "*tanmatra*" means primal, subtle, undeveloped matter. The broader and more universal terms "*Prakriti*" and "*pradhana*" are closely related in meaning to this conception. They all refer to material or substance that is yet to be developed.

The *Tanmatras* are sometimes referred to as the "Subtle Essences." They are the subtle energies that flow out of *Rajas* and *Tamas. Tamas* evolves into the objects of the cognitive senses: sound, touch, form, taste, and odor. They are behind and also generate the manifestations of the next phase in evolution: the Five Great Gross or Material Elements. The *Tanmatras* are the irreducible subtle (*sukshma*) half of the gross Elements. The *Tanmatras* are the food for *Manas.* They nourish the mind. When an individual perceives the world, it is the *Tanmatras* that are within the Elements that compose the world that are grasped and experienced via the flow of *Prana* and then returned into *Manas* via the senses. They are also called *vishishtha (vishaya) gunas* or the five specific qualities that are the *gunas* of the Elements.

The *Tanmatras* incarnate to form the Five Great Gross Elements. Each Element contains all five *Tanmatras,* but has a predominance or primary loading of only one. If one conceives of the *Tanmatras* as being gunic attributes, the sequence and contents of the Elements and their *Tanmatras* are as follows. Ether has *Shabda* (sound) as its primary *Tanmatra.* Air has *Sparsha* (touch) as its primary along with associated *Shabda.* Fire has *Rupa* (color/ form) as its primary along with *Shabda* and *Sparsha.* Water has *Rasa* (taste) as its primary along with *Shabda, Sparsha,* and *Rupa.* Earth has *Gandha* (smell) as its primary along with *Shabda, Sparsha, Rupa,* and *Rasa.*

The *Tanmatras* also have another major meaning. They are the root energies associated with the five sensory organs. The *Tanmatra* of sound (*Shabda*), for example, is the energy whose anatomical field is located in the auditory functioning of the sense organ, the ears. *Tanmatras* are the manner in which each sensory organ experiences itself when it makes contact with the environment as mediated by an anatomical sense organ. In *Sankhya* philosophy, emphasis is on the *Tanmatras* being created first—before the sensory organs that experience the perception of them. Therefore, they have a semi-independent position ontologically in respect to the grosser material world. From a Western philosophical perspective, the *Tanmatras* would denote the *subjective experience* that is mediated by one or a combination of sensory organs. In other words, in conventional Western logic, in contrast to the Ayurvedic idea, the sense organs first must be present; only then can sense experience (*Tanmatras*) emerge in a secondary fashion through the processes of cognition.

The five *Tanmatras* (the underlying subtle energies and objects of perception: sound, touch, sight, taste, and smell), their corollary sense organ, and primary Element correspondences are as follows:

1. *Shabda Tanmatra:* the energy that generates the sensation of *Sound* via the ears; its chief primary Element is Ether.

2. *Sparsha Tanmatra:* the energy that generates the sensation of *Touch* via the skin; its chief primary Element is Air.

3. *Rupa Tanmatra:* the energy that generates the sensation of *Sight* via the eyes; its chief primary Element is Fire.

4. *Rasa Tanmatra:* the energy that generates the sensation of *Taste* via the tongue; its chief primary Element is Water.

5. *Gandha Tanmatra:* the energy that generates the sensation of *Smell* via the nose; its chief primary Element is Earth.

FIVE GREAT GROSS ELEMENTS: *PANCHA MAHABHUTANI*

The Five Great Gross Elements or Primordial Pentads are known as the *Pancha Mahabhutani(s)* or *Pancha Mahabhuta(s)*. They exist on the most material level (*sthula*). All five subtle *Tanmatras,* in varying proportions, come together to produce each one of the five Elements. The *Tanmatras* are the subtle half of the entire Element. In each single Element, moreover, are contained aspects of the other four Elements.

These five Elements, the "primary pentads," are conceptualized as the first and most elemental substances that compose matter. They function as principles of density or states of matter. In addition, as proto-substances, they also carry a strong metaphorical and emblematic connotation that implies their being a representation of physiological functioning when considered from the viewpoint of biological life. In the sense of philosophy, the Five Great Gross Elements are the confluence of concept, word, and the things referred to by the concept and the word.

Varying mixtures of one or more of these Elements compose and are the material "stuff" of all manifest reality, including the mind. Mind in Ayurveda has a distinctly material connotation. This broad conceptual perspective holds that immaterial consciousness manifests materially first in the form of the Five Great Gross Elements. These Elements constitute degrees of density of matter. They represent stages in the manifestation of consciousness as progressive levels of increasing density and materiality (Table 2.1). These inorganic Elements make up the material universe. They contribute to making up the biological *doshas* in living beings. The Elements or primary pentads are the food both for the biological *doshas* and for the biological tissues (*dhatus*). These Elements are the material of the biological *doshas,* the *dhatus,* and the *malas.* In Chinese medicine, the five Elements are termed *wu hsing* or *wu xing*.

The five Elements are as follows:

1. *Akasha,* **Ether.** This is the first Element to precipitate out of the five *Tanmatras.* It holds a unique position among the Elements since it is, in fact, *transitional,* in that it is the only Element that is completely subtle with virtually no material quality. Ether is characterized by the qualities of

Table 2.1 *Pancha Mahabhutanis,* the Five Great Gross Elements

Akasha, Ether
Vayu, Air
Tejas, Fire
Jala, Water
Prithvi, Earth

nonresistance, space, and receptivity. Its attributes include being subtle, soft, and light. The Western concept of vacuum, that is, a volume of space that is essentially empty of matter, roughly correlates with this Ayurvedic idea. The notion of a field such as this is approximated in modern quantum theory by the concept of the so-called Higgs field (1964), which is said to permeate the entire universe. It has never been observed, but there is indirect evidence suggesting its presence, which is required in order to explain the large difference in mass between particles that mediate what are called "weak interactions" (the W and Z bosons) and those that mediate the electromagnetic interactions caused by so-called massless photons.

2. *Vayu* or *Marut,* **Air.** Out of Ether comes the Element Air. Movement and direction characterize it, and its attributes include being light in weight, dry, subtle, cold, and dispersive.

3. *Tejas,* **Fire.** As Air continues to move and cause friction, the Element of Fire emerges. Fire has the manifested qualities of visible light, appearance, and energy. Its qualities include being hot, penetrating, subtle, light, and dry.

4. *Jala,* **Water.** Ancient texts say that Fire causes the densification of consciousness that becomes Water, which has the quality of flowing and allows for a potential cohesion of life. Its qualities include its being fluid, soft, and sticky.

5. *Prithvi,* **Earth.** As Water coagulates, it transforms into Earth, a mass that is dense, stable, and solid. Its qualities include its being gross, stable, heavy, and hard.

PANCHA JNANENDRIYANI: THE FIVE RECEPTIVE ORGANS OF PERCEPTION

The next phase in the cycle of creation is that of the emergence of the five sense organs of perception called the *Pancha Jnanendriyani.* These are the receptive organs of perception and cognition. They are the externally directed instrument of perception in contrast to the *Antahkarana* (*Ahamkara, Buddhi, Manas, and Chitta*), the internally oriented instrument of perception.

The critical importance of these cognitive sense organs, the resting place of the senses, in Ayurveda cannot be emphasized enough. These sensory faculties make possible direct contact with the outside material world. This connotes the importance of the idea of the necessary and valuable experience of contact with the sensory world. The sense of touch, that is, contact and connection, is uniquely intrinsic to every other sense modality. The sense organs flow more out of their anlagen in the five *Tanmatras.* In addition, because of their potential benefit for further human development, they are more imbued with the sattvic *Maha guna.* As mentioned above, the five sense organs are ears (*shrotra*), skin (*tvak*), eyes (*chakshu*), tongue (*jihva*), and nose (*grahana*). Their respective objects are *shabda* (sound), *sparsha* (touch), *rupa* (form), *rasa* (taste), and *gandha* (scent or aroma). Varying amounts and combinations of the Five Great Gross Elements make up each of these objects of the senses.

PANCHA KARMENDRIYANI: THE FIVE EXPRESSIVE ORGANS OF ACTION

On the same conceptual level as the five sense organs, there exist correspondences with the five organs of action, the *Pancha Karmendriyani.* Their more material nature is associated with their emergence from the Five Great Gross Elements, and their more action-oriented functioning is the result of their greater content of the rajasic *Maha guna.*

An outline of the action organs and their correspondences to function, sense organ, and Element are (1) Mouth (*vak*): speech, ear, and Ether; (2) Hands (*pani*): holding, skin, and Air; (3) Feet (*pad*): walking, eyes, and Fire; (4) Urogenital (*upastha*): procreation, tongue, and Water; (5) Anus (*payu*): excretion, nose, and Earth.

MANAS

The *Sankhya* enumeration now describes the distinctively human faculty, mind or *Manas.* While most English translations use the term *mind* to indicate the nature of *Manas, Manas* also refers to the general processes of thinking, mentation, and sequential experience. *Manas* is a major part of the internally oriented instrument of perception. It is understood to be "fed" by impressions (particularly *Tanmatras*) resulting both from the five sensory organs of perception and from the five motor organs of action. These externally oriented instruments of perception and action are sensory and motoric, respectively. These externally directed faculties are termed *indriyas.*

Manas can be conceived of as the "sixth sense" whose objects and contacts act within the intrapsychic or internal mental arena. It has been called "lord" (*natha*) of the five cognitive senses in contrast to *Prana* being the lord of the mind. *Manas* is a unifying and formulating principle that includes the integrated functioning of sensory perception, conceptualization, and some degree of conation or volitional activity. *Manas* has been understood to be a major component of the *Antahkarana,* the inner organ of cognition. In many texts, the *Antahkarana* is described as having four components: (1) *Ahamkara,* (2) *Manas,* (3) *Buddhi,* and (4) *Chitta(m).*

Manas thus connects the individual both to the outside world and, as well, to what is interior, having a degree of apperception, so to speak. *Manas,* in addition, may be roughly equated with the Western psychological concept of ego or personality with particular emphasis on affects/emotions and all the mechanisms of defense, some of which include denial, repression, splitting, devaluation, idealization, dissociation, omnipotence, projection, projective identification, rationalization, reaction formation, suppression, and undoing. The defense mechanism of intellectualization is especially prominent in modern times. These actions of *Manas* along with the normative "spoiling" functions of the *doshas* constitute the ground that makes for human proneness to corruption, fraudulence, and inauthenticity both in body and in mind. The allied concept of the mind's intrinsic cognitive fault, *Prajna-aparadha,* will be discussed at length in Chapter 6.

As each individual person is, to varying degrees, "his or her own person," he or she thus manifests a personal *Ahamkara.* Once born into the world, every experience imprints itself on an individual, thereby modifying and shaping an individual's identity. This conditioning function (*samskara*), so to speak, of *Ahamkara,* is facilitated by *Manas.* Attachment to a personal sense of self is a chief function of *Manas.*

Inherent in the idea of this eco-corporeal connectedness—*Manas* mediating between the senses and their attraction—attachment to the outside world—is the phenomenon of the experience of *desire* (*mara, raga, trishna, iccha, abhinivesha*). *Manas* can be thought of as a functional key, the ticket of admission, to the experiential world. It constitutes the point of contact between inner man and the world. Desire, operative within the functioning of *Manas,* in all its expressions is held to be among the most fundamental driving forces in human nature. The phenomenon of desire denotes both the unconscious and the conscious craving for satisfaction, gratification, and fulfillment of subjectively experienced wishes. The perpetual drive toward wish fulfillment, a pathognomonic feature of man's mind in Eastern traditions, acts both as a motor and as an organizing set of mental impulses that strive to repetitively achieve previously experienced satisfactions.

The problem of "glamour," the uncanny excitement and pull (*upadana*) that the material world has on the mind, is intimately tied in with the functioning of *Manas.* This phenomenon is termed *Vishaya-Shakti,* the power of the world of the senses. The function of *Manas,* by its inherent nature, tends to create a linkage, dependence, or bondage (*bandha*) to the sense objects of the material world. The regulation of desire, then, becomes a central theme in the Ayurvedic system of health, well-being, and self-development. This follows from the premise that Ayurveda seeks to address the needs of the physical dimensions of life, the body and the mind. In the course of achieving and maintaining a healthy physical balance, further harmony is induced within what are considered more spiritual and consciousness-enhancing dimensions. In Ayurveda, a fact, which is never lost sight of, is that of the body being the physical base of consciousness, its material dimension.

The distinctions, then, between different aspects of psychic functioning are as follows. Mental functioning, in general, is structured and regulated by an inner (subjective) organization of functions called the *Antahkarana,* the inner instrument. It has four different aspects: (1) *Ahamkara,* the uniqueness of an individual, (2) *Chitta(m),* the store or memories of passive conditioned consciousness, (3) *Manas,* the active, measuring, and reflexive capacity of the mind to perceive and to be attracted to distinctions, and (4) *Buddhi,* which is an individual's share of sattvic intellect and discrimination very close to the intrinsic intelligence (*Mahat*) within nature, and to the pure consciousness of the *Purusha.*

Manas subjectively differentiates and recognizes experience via mechanisms of comprehending the world in the form of binary polarizations or splits (*vikalpa*). The Sanskrit term *Manas* denotes the broad idea of mind as it experiences desire, needs, and cravings elicited through sensory experience, and possessing the wish for pleasure and gratification. *Chitta(m)* is a term roughly synonymous with *Manas* but containing the idea of having relay capabilities providing stabilized connections to other mental functions. *Chitta(m)* is the storehouse, the memories of conditioned, dualistically experienced consciousness. This also denotes the general concept of the mind as a seat of consciousness with dimensions that are conscious, unconscious, and transcendently conscious or superconscious. *Buddhi* is the inherently intelligent aspect of mind that is most sattvic (pure, conscious, and balanced) and has the power to correctly discriminate that which is good and conducive (*satmya*) to growth, maturation, and development from that which is unwholesome (*asatmya*).

The term *Chit* denotes states of highly purified consciousness. It may be used in the sense of the term *prajna* or wisdom. It suggests pure intelligence, the absolute consciousness of *Purusha* and *Brahman*. This state of being cannot be "known"; it can only be recovered or realized.

HEALTH, BALANCE, PURITY, AND WHOLESOMENESS

The Ayurvedic concept of health is based on the idea of achieving dynamic balance and equilibrium. When the *doshas* are in balance, health ensues. The state of the *doshas* determines the state of all other aspects of the individual—digestion, elimination, prevention of excess *Ama* buildup, tissue integrity, immune resistance to disease, energy level, mental and emotional stability, and optimal overall functioning, to name just a few. Striving for balance is an ongoing task and is fostered and supported by continuing efforts toward maintaining purity (*shuddha*) on all levels of one's being. Optimal *Agni*, the transformational fire that pervades the entire individual and which brings about maximal nutrition in body, mind, and spirit, promotes and accompanies the optimal balance and functioning of the *doshas*. Purity, health, and wholesomeness (*satmya*), therefore, are achieved through prescribed dietary practices, daily and seasonal routines, and healthy lifestyle activities that include active work on the material and spiritual components of the self. In addition to the care of the body and the mind, the cultivation of spirit includes meditative practices and other self-inquiry pursuits. A *BioPsychoSpiritual* worldview is espoused. Refinement and integration of body, mind, and consciousness aligns the individual with the universal, the *atman* or Buddha-Self with the *Purusha*, the *Brahman* of Absolute unity.

Maintenance of the health of the body is not only an end in itself, but also a prerequisite to further development on more subtle levels. This includes the psychological, the subtle-energetic, and the spiritual. This idea rests on several propositions fundamental to Ayurveda. The first is that of the primacy of consciousness and its primordially ordained ontological position. Today, even outside of Ayurveda, the examination of the qualitatively unique significance of consciousness and its critical role in human culture is a generally recognized fact (Block, Flanagan, & Guzeldere, 1997; Cairns-Smith, 1996; Hameroff, Kaszniak, & Scott, 1996; Neumann, 1954; Solso, 1999).

In the Ayurvedic worldview, as consciousness participates in the evolutionary process, it gradually manifests in forms that are denser and have increasingly denser material attributes and expressions, like the physical body. The individual's purpose in life, therefore, is to become aware of the immanence of consciousness at the core of physicality, and to facilitate and enhance the manifestation process of consciousness. Accordingly, man has the innately designed directive to experience to the fullest his material reality accompanied by this realization. The second proposition then advocates the goal of maintaining the optimal health of the body in order to provide an adequate amount of time for a higher quality of life to be achieved.

In the Buddhist tradition, the term *kushala* or wholesomeness connotes those activities of daily living that have high degrees of purity and an absence of inordinate desire, envy, avarice, greed, aggression, hate, and cognitive confusion. Pursuit of wholesomeness, in this sense, is considered to be of great value since it is believed to purify one's *karma,* that is, to contribute to freeing one from the fetters of unresolved conflicts and the bondages that stem from the past. The ultimate aim of this is the achievement of the prime Vedic goal, *Moksha,* that is, liberation into ever more refined states of experiential consciousness (*sakshat kara*).

3

ANATOMY

THE PHYSICAL BODY AND ITS COMPONENTS

Ayurvedic anatomy (*Sharira Rachana*) is a description of the morphological constituents of the individual and an enumeration of the integrated material structures and principles through which the various physiological processes occur. The physical body, in fact, is viewed as the material expression of man's essential core, that is, of consciousness. As was described in the preceding outline of the *Sankhya* creation sequence, the immaterial aspects of reality, particularly the reality of consciousness, are given primacy in terms of origin, value, and significance. The physical body (*sthula sharira*), however, remains the material ballast of man's consciousness and is regarded as the platform upon which all endeavors for well-being must begin.

The basic components of the body are the biological humors (*doshas*), the tissues (*dhatus*), the secondary tissues (*upadhatus*), the tissue membranes (*dhara kalas*), the channels of circulation (*srotas*), the waste products or refuse (*malas*), and the organs. Each of these will be discussed here. The *srotas,* which have more of a physiological function, will be discussed in Chapter 4. The nine orifices or openings of the body have been the source of contemplation in Eastern systems of interpreting the universe and its meaning. They are two eyes, two ears, two nostrils, the mouth, the urethra, and the anus. These openings permit both entry and exit into the environment on multiple levels. Their associations with sensation, sexuality, survival, and adaptation are manifold.

Western scientific perspectives, in contrast to those of Ayurveda, organize the physical body and its functions in a different manner. The two basic categories are the tissues, which are composed of cells that perform a similar function, and the organ systems, which together perform a similar function. Only four tissue groups are recognized: (1) epithelial, which comprises layers of cells covering organ surfaces and the inner lining of the gastrointestinal tract; these serve as protection, for secretion, and for absorption; (2) connective tissue includes extracellular matrices, bone, and blood; (3) muscle tissue; and (4) nervous tissue. There are 11 organ systems enumerated. These include the circulatory, digestive, endocrine, integumentary, lymphatic, muscular, nervous, reproductive, respiratory, skeletal, and urinary.

DOSHAS AND SUBDOSHAS

The concept of the *doshas* is a major focal point in Ayurveda. Ayurvedic evaluation is based on an assessment of the state and interaction of the *doshas* in the body. Health and disease are reflected in the condition of the biological *doshas*. The essence of treatment, as well, is based on efforts to correct vitiations, imbalances, or disruptions in the doshic system. The *doshas* are principally bioenergetic in nature. It is from this angle that they are viewed both theoretically and in formulating treatment plans, especially in respect to diet, herbs, and seasonal considerations. The *doshas* have a subtle half in their makeup: *Prana, Tejas, and Ojas*. These *sukshma* or subtle components denote the psychophysiological dimension of the *doshas*. It is from that angle that the mental, emotional, and spiritual dimensions of the *doshas* are viewed.

As described previously, there are three *doshas: Vata* is the principle of propulsion, *Pitta* is the principle of transformation, and *Kapha* is the principle of consolidation (Table 3.1).

Vata

Vata has been described as having characteristics both of a bioenergetic substance and of a regulatory principle. *Vata* is the *dosha* closest to having

Table 3.1   *Doshas* and their Subdoshas

Vata
1. *Prana Vata*
2. *Udana Vata*
3. *Samana Vata*
4. *Apana Vata*
5. *Vyana Vata*

Pitta
1. *Pachaka Pitta*
2. *Ranjaka Pitta*
3. *Sadhaka Pitta*
4. *Alochaka Pitta*
5. *Bhrajaka Pitta*

Kapha
1. *Kledaka Kapha*
2. *Avalambaka Kapha*
3. *Bodhaka Kapha*
4. *Tarpaka Kapha*
5. *Shleshaka Kapha*

the properties of immateriality, that is, acting as a more amorphous energetic entity. *Vata* has the *gurvadi guna* called *laghu,* which connotes light in weight, rising to the top, airy, and floating. This quality along with *Vata*'s buoyant dispersiveness imparts freshness. Although *Vata* has no form, its presence can be likened to that of the energetic transmissions that travel through the nervous system, or to the motion that accompanies breathing. From an anatomical perspective, the chief seat or "home" of *Vata* is in the large intestine or colon. This specifically refers to the fact that the primary site of accumulation of *Vata,* especially in disease, occurs in the colon. In this sense, the quality of being erratically mobile (*chala*) is attributed to *Vata.* In addition, *Vata*'s influence is also concentrated in such sites as the hips, thighs, ears, trachea, bones, brain, nerves, and skin.

Each of the three principal *doshas* is subdivided into five components. Only one of these five subdoshas controls all the others. It is their master regulator. The subdoshas of *Vata* are termed *Prana, Udana, Samana, Apana,* and *Vyana. Vata* is considered the lead *dosha* since only this *dosha* has the primary function of propulsion that applies to it and to its role in moving and propelling both *Pitta* and *Kapha.* Some have referred to *Vata* as the first equal among the three equally primary *doshas* (Figure 3.1).

Prana Vata pervades the brain, heart, and lungs. Each of the five senses, especially those of hearing and touch, is imbued with the activity of *Prana Vata. Prana* means forward or primary air. It governs and supports respiration, heart rate, and the vegetative and the sensory functions. It is associated with the actions of inhalation, swallowing, sneezing, spitting, and belching. It is the main and directing form of all the other *Vata* subdoshas. It governs intake, input, reception of food, and awareness and introjection of sensory impressions (*Tanmatras*).

There is a high concentration of sattvic *Prana* in the brain. The subtle roots of *Prana,* as the life force, are considered the connecting links to consciousness, especially via its sattvic component, and the cultivation of *Prana* is held in high regard. *Prana Vata* denotes attention. *Prana* in the subject focuses and directs attention via its rajasic component, and, subsequently, an object of attention comes into being (which is the precipitating effect of *Tamas*). The technique of *pranayama* (breath control) is regarded as essential in the pursuit of controlling the movements within the mind and in activating the *kundalini Shakti* (life force power) in self-development techniques such as meditation. *Prana* is absorbed instantly via the air inhaled into the lungs. *Prana* is absorbed in a delayed fashion via the absorption of food and nutrients in the colon.

Udana Vata is concentrated in the throat, chest, lungs, navel, and sinuses. *Udana* means upwardly moving air. It governs exhalation, speech, coughing, vomiting, and belching. It is associated with expiration. Along with speech expression and communication, *Udana* governs memory, remembrance, and will or volition. *Udana* transports material from the inside to the outside. It facilitates output. It aids the upward rising of *Kundalini.*

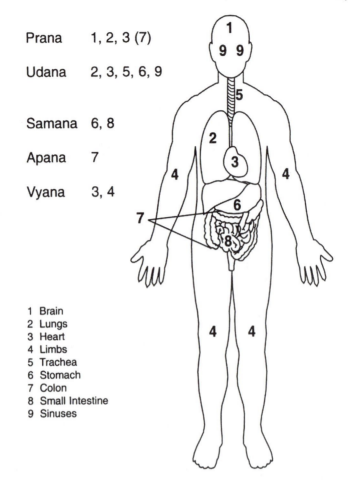

Prana   1, 2, 3 (7)

Udana   2, 3, 5, 6, 9

Samana   6, 8

Apana   7

Vyana   3, 4

1 Brain
2 Lungs
3 Heart
4 Limbs
5 Trachea
6 Stomach
7 Colon
8 Small Intestine
9 Sinuses

Figure 3.1   The five subdoshas of *Vata:* Primary anatomical sites
(Courtesy of illustrator Frank John Ninivaggi, M.D.)

Samana Vata perfuses the whole alimentary tract, especially the small
intestine. It regulates peristalsis. *Samana* means equalizing or balancing air.
It balances the energy of the body and is very closely tied to assimilation, in
general, and specifically to the digestive process. It fans the digestive fire of
Agni. This encompasses the processes of separation, splitting, and discrimination that are preparatory to the assimilation of food in the gastrointestinal
tract, air into the lungs, and sensory experience into the mind. In addition,
Samana Vata is the predominant *Vata* in the internal organs, including the
liver, the spleen, the pancreas, the stomach, and the upper part of the large
intestine. It also contributes to movement in the blood circulatory system
and the nervous system as well as to peristalsis in the gastrointestinal tract.
Samana Vata operates on a psychological level to aid proper discrimination

(*viveka*) and the differential distinction of aspects of reality. It aids discerning understanding; it opposes confusion.

Apana Vata is centered in the colon and controls the other *Vata* subdoshas. It is the master regulator of all the *Vata* subdoshas. It governs and controls them. *Apana* means downward moving air. In addition to absorbing *Prana* from food in the colon, *Apana* is the chief *dosha* directing all elimination. It facilitates discharge. This includes excretion of feces and urine, as well as menstruation, parturition, and sexual discharge. The state of *Apana Vata* is critical in Ayurvedic evaluation since it reflects, to a significant extent, the overall health or disease of the individual.

Vyana Vata is contained in the heart, blood vessels, the skin, bones, muscles, and nerves. *Vyana* means diffusive or pervasive air. The chief actions of *Vyana Vata* are the circulation of blood from the heart to the periphery, the movements of the musculoskeletal system, and the innervation of the sensory organs. It facilitates centrifugal propulsion. The processes of blinking and yawning have been associated with it.

Pitta

Pitta is the biological *dosha* that drives change, conversion, thermogenesis, and transformative processes. It has the quality of a mobile, steady flow (*sara*). Its chief site is in the small intestine. This is the anatomical place in which it will accumulate when it becomes vitiated and excessive. *Pitta* is also found in the liver, the spleen, the stomach, the skin, the eyes, the heart, and parts of the brain (especially the gray matter, the hypothalamus, and the neurotransmitters); it is also present in sweat, sebaceous oil, blood, and, to a small degree, in lymph. Bodily warmth and heat, essential to life, emanate from *Pitta*. *Pitta*'s five subdoshas are *Pachaka, Ranjaka, Sadhaka, Alochaka,* and *Bhrajaka* (Figure 3.2).

Pachaka Pitta, the *Pitta* of digestion, is located mainly in the small intestine and lower stomach and is contained in hydrochloric acid, enzymes, bile, and hormones. It is the master regulator of all *Pitta* subdoshas. It is the main *Pitta* involved in the second or sour phase of primary digestion (*avasthapaka*), and its actions assist in regulating body temperature and fueling the strength of circulation. Its functioning is tied into the operation of *Agni,* the energy of the fundamental digestive fire of the body. This also puts it close to the actions of another digestion-related subdosha, *Samana Vata. Pachaka Pitta* controls and supports all other *Pitta* subdoshas.

Ranjaka Pitta, the *Pitta* that gives color, resides chiefly in the liver, the spleen, bone marrow, the small intestine, the stomach, the blood, bile, and stool. This *Pitta* is mainly associated with secondary digestion, which is referred to as "tissue metabolism," whose site is in the liver (*yakrut*). This *Pitta* contributes to erythropoiesis, the formation of red blood cells, as well as to the formation of every bodily tissue.

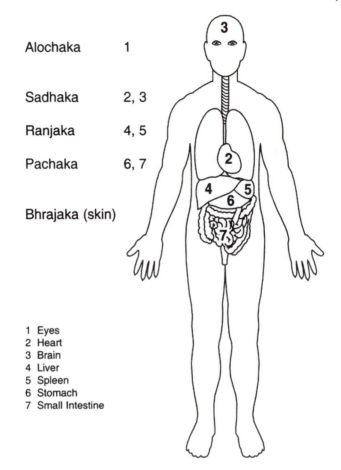

Alochaka   1

Sadhaka   2, 3

Ranjaka   4, 5

Pachaka   6, 7

Bhrajaka (skin)

1 Eyes
2 Heart
3 Brain
4 Liver
5 Spleen
6 Stomach
7 Small Intestine

Figure 3.2   The five subdoshas of *Pitta:* Primary anatomical sites
(Courtesy of illustrator Frank John Ninivaggi, M.D.)

Sadhaka Pitta is located in the heart and the brain. *Sadhaka* means accomplishment, realization, and discernment. It functions through the nervous system (especially in the neurotransmitters) and sensory organs to produce clear thinking, lucidity, penetrating discrimination (*viveka*), understanding of differences, intelligence, recognition, comprehension, memory, courage, and contentment. In this sense, it pulls energy from *Tejas.* Cultivation of this *Pitta* can propel the individual toward realization of the four goals of life according to the *Vedas: dharma, artha, kama,* and *Moksha. Sadhaka Pitta* energizes the acuity of the *Buddhi* aspect of mind. It supports the energy of loving compassion. It is part of the energy that drives spiritual aspirations. On the other hand, many forms of desire and lust are associated with *Sadhaka*'s penetrating power.

Alochaka Pitta is the *Pitta* of the eyes and governs visual perception. In addition, *Alochaka Pitta* contributes to the functioning of all the other sensory organs to some degree.

Bhrajaka Pitta is located in the skin, the sweat, and the sebaceous oils. It is the *Pitta* fire that governs luster (*prabha*) of the skin's complexion (*chaya*), that is, its color, texture, and appearance. It is also related to the temperature of the skin.

Pitta derives its energy from *Agni* and has been given the following characteristics:

1. *Paka* and *pachana:* digestion,
2. *Dahana:* burning and combustion,
3. *Bhinna samghata:* splitting,
4. *Tapana:* producing heat,
5. *Parinamana:* conversion,
6. *Paravritti:* transformation,
7. *Prakashana:* illumination,
8. *Ranjana* and *Varnakara:* imparting color, and
9. *Prabhavakara:* imparting luster.

Kapha

The word *Kapha* means "flourishing of water." *Kapha dosha* is the biological *dosha* of body fluids such as plasma, saliva, mucus, phlegm, cerebrospinal fluid, and synovial fluids. *Kapha* is the most material, dense, gross, and coarse of the three *doshas.* The heavy and dense qualities of *Kapha* give it a richness that engenders form, has a tendency toward solidity of form, and imparts protection from inordinate heat and the wear and tear of everyday functioning. *Kapha* protects the tissues from the unopposed heat that *Pitta* might generate. The five subdoshas of *Kapha* are *Kledaka, Avalambaka, Bodhaka, Tarpaka,* and *Shleshaka* (Figure 3.3).

Kledaka Kapha is located in the stomach. It means the form of water that moistens or humidifies. Its primary action is to liquefy food in the alkaline or sweet phase of the first stage of digestion. In addition, it protects the stomach lining from damage by excess *Pachaka Pitta* and *Agni,* the digestive fire.

Avalambaka Kapha is located in the heart, the lungs, the spine, and the pelvic girdle. It is the form of water that gives support. It resides in mucus and in interstitial and intercellular fluids. In the chest, it provides lubrication for the heart and the lungs and prevents the negative effects of excess friction. It is a central, supportive component for the stability of the vertebral column. *Avalambaka Kapha* is the central *Kapha* and controls all other *Kapha* subdoshas. It is the master regulator of all the *Kapha* subdoshas. Its fundamental significance lies in the fact that it is the force behind the first and primary of the body's tissue (*dhatu*), the plasma (*rasa*). It holds and is a transport

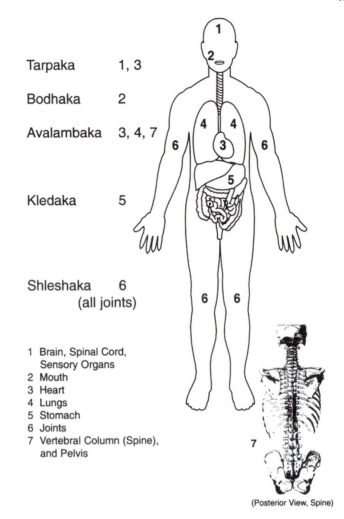

Tarpaka   1, 3

Bodhaka   2

Avalambaka   3, 4, 7

Kledaka   5

Shleshaka   6
               (all joints)

1 Brain, Spinal Cord,
  Sensory Organs
2 Mouth
3 Heart
4 Lungs
5 Stomach
6 Joints
7 Vertebral Column (Spine),
  and Pelvis

(Posterior View, Spine)

Figure 3.3   The five subdoshas of *Kapha:* Primary anatomical sites
(Courtesy of illustrator Frank John Ninivaggi, M.D.)

medium for *Prana,* the life force. In Ayurveda, the plasma is considered the matrix tissue out of which all other tissues are formed. *Avalambaka Kapha* is considered the material medium associated with psychological attachment and detachment, love, and depression. An excess of this *Kapha* is associated with both greed and obesity. In health, it supports the whole self and imparts confidence, zeal, and motivation.

Bodhaka Kapha is located in the tongue, the mouth, and in the saliva. It means that form of water that gives perception. This *Kapha* subdosha has also been called *Rasana Kapha. Bodhaka* is the subdosha related to taste. The Sanskrit word for taste is identical to that for "plasma," the first bodily tissue to be formed and the tissue out of which all other tissues develop. Plasma and taste are both termed *rasa* because of their functional association in Ayurvedic physiology. Taste, a critical faculty in the Ayurvedic scheme, is that sensory guide that not only is a screen to determine the nature and wholesomeness of a substance, but also becomes therapeutic when herbs of differing tastes are used to balance excess *doshas*. Healthy plasma is reflected in a state of healthy, balanced *doshas,* and both are a consequence of the ingestion of the proper tastes being consumed. In this sense, the specific Ayurvedic concept of "taste" is distinct from the meaning of the common word *flavor,* which is nonspecific, general, and more inclusive.

Tarpaka Kapha is located in the brain, nervous system white matter, cerebrospinal fluid, the heart, and in the sinuses. It means that form of water that gives contentment (*tripti*). *Tarpaka Kapha* has also been called *Snehana Kapha. Tarpaka* is associated with emotional stability and peace of mind. Some Ayurvedic sources consider it to be the physical source and container of consciousness. It has been called the *dosha* that nourishes the sense organs of perception (*jnanendriyas*). This *Kapha* is present in muscle tissue. In conjunction with *Prana Vata,* its balanced functioning assuages anxiety and insomnia. In conjunction with *Sadhaka Pitta,* it supports an all-embracing sense of loving compassion.

Shleshaka Kapha is the synovial fluid within the body's joints and articular surfaces. It promotes lubrication and stickiness.

SUBTLE OR ENERGETIC ROOTS OF THE *DOSHAS: PRANA, TEJAS,* AND *OJAS*

The concept of the *doshas,* as has been discussed, is one of the most fundamental working frames of reference in Ayurveda. The *doshas* are bioenergetic both in substance and in functioning. They have psychophysiological properties. The *doshas* tend to be more material in nature and so reside in and make up part of the physical body (*sharira sthula*), and they work through physiological processes. In one sense, the *dhatus* (tissues) provide the coarser form within which the *doshas* provide their functioning.

As the whole of the Ayurvedic worldview is one of dynamic, multidimensional, and integrated functioning, an elaboration of the deeper aspects of the *doshas* reveals their subtle counterparts that reside on the vital or energetic level (*sukshma*). This is the same energetic level upon which the Five *Tanmatras* reside. These subtle roots of the *doshas* are the mental energies underlying the *doshas*. In their most rarefied aspect, this reaches into the spiritual dimensions of consciousness. The subtle roots of the biological *Vata, Pitta,* and *Kapha doshas* are *Prana, Tejas,* and *Ojas,* respectively.

All of them are filled with *Sattva,* the energy of clarity and luminosity. This luminous (*prakashana*) dimension enhances their radiance and spiritual value. The energy of *Rajas* gives them their capacity for movement, and their complement of *Tamas* gives them some substantive presence in the physical body.

The quality and development of an individual's *Kundalini* (spiritual energy and power related to the awakening of consciousness) is correlated with that person's *BioPsychoSpiritual* integration of *Prana, Tejas,* and *Ojas.* The cultivation of consciousness takes place, in particular, through the mediums of *Prana* and of *Tejas.* A correlation with Traditional Chinese Medicine is as follows: *Prana* with *Qi, Tejas* with *Yang,* and *Ojas* with *Yin* and *Jing.* In Hinduism, *Prana* may be associated with *Sat* (Being), *Tejas* with *Chit* (Wisdom), and *Ojas* with *Ananda* (Pure Love, Bliss, and Joy).

Prana: The Life Force

Prana is the subtle root of the coarser, more material subdosha *Prana Vata. Prana* is considered the life force and has been called *Qi* (also spelled *Chi*) in Traditional Chinese Medicine. It is both masculine and feminine in nature. *Prana* is subjectively experienced as the will to live. The significance of *Prana* lies in the fact that it exerts an integrative drive toward a confluence of all aspects within an individual on all levels. It is distributed throughout the entire body, but is especially concentrated in the brain, the heart, and the colon.

The predominant Element associated with *Prana* is Ether; Air also plays a part. The two *Tanmatras* that feed *Prana* are touch (*sparsha*) and sound (*shabda*). The *Maha gunas* that predominate in *Prana* are *Sattva* and *Rajas,* especially *Sattva.* As the life force, *Prana* is indwelling in the individual; *Prana,* however, does require replenishment on a daily basis. The rudiments of what transforms into the vital Pranic substance come into the body through air and through food. Oxygen and food carry *Prana.* Oxygen and blood feed *Prana. Prana* helps to create, circulate, and stabilize the integrity of blood and its channels of circulation. *Pranayama* is the system of intentional and conscious breath regulation and expansion to facilitate the absorption of *Prana* into the lungs and the bloodstream. Eating fresh foods, especially of reasonably high quality, and taking specific herbal substances also increases the body's concentration of *Prana.* The use of essential oils in massage and in aroma therapies feeds this *Prana.* Proper exposure to balanced sounds such as those found in nature, music, mantras, and prayers, for example, feeds *Prana.*

Prana, the subtle essence of *Vata,* makes flow, coordination, and direction possible. This applies to the integrated movements of *Prana, Tejas,* and *Ojas.* It also is responsible for the mind-body coordination. This denotes the proper flow that synchronizes breath, sensory perception, and *Antahkarana* (*Ahamkara, Buddhi, Manas,* and *Chitta*). *Prana* as the life force denotes the power that compels body, mind, and spirit to intimately lean on each other and to function integrally, in simultaneity.

Tejas: The Intelligent Transformative Flame of the Life Force

Tejas is the subtle root of the coarser, more material subdosha *Sadhaka Pitta. Tejas* resides on the *sukshma* (subtle) level of existence just as does *Prana* and part of *Ojas. Tejas,* however, is very close to being a spiritualized (*karana*) subtle essence as is *Prana. Tejas* is considered the flame of life, and its functioning of interactive transformation makes it closely allied to *Agni,* the energy of the overall digestive fire. *Tejas* is associated predominantly with the Fire Element. *Tejas* is fed by the *rupa* (vision) *Tanmatra.* It is associated with the *Sattva* and the *Rajas Maha gunas.*

Whereas the concept of *Agni* emphasizes transformation and digestion in the broadest sense, the concept of *Tejas* puts emphasis on the transformations and digestion of sensory impressions and thoughts—intelligence—on all levels in the person. *Tejas* works through *Sadhaka Pitta* on a spectrum from the cellular, tissue, *srota,* and organ level to the Mind (*Manas*), especially via *Buddhi.*

In Traditional Chinese Medicine, the concept of *Yang* is most closely related to the concept of *Tejas.* In Ayurveda, *Tejas* functions chiefly as the transformative force of penetrating intelligence and discrimination. As such, it is closely connected to the *Buddhi* aspect of cognition. The quality of *Tejas,* as well, is related to the quality of personal self-discipline and self-determination. Its transformative action effects a communicative penetration that reaches all material and subtle aspects within an individual so that they may mutually influence each other. The use of color therapies feeds *Tejas.* Cardamom and saffron taken internally increase *Tejas.*

Tejas denotes a pushing transformation and makes passage between and among all levels of being possible. *Tejas* is the fire behind breaking and cracking blockages. *Tejas* underlies the dynamic, changing, and impermanent dimension within substances.

Ojas: The Bioenergetic Substance of Immunity, Strength, and Vital Energy Reserves

Ojas is the body's vital essence that is manifest by and contained in a particular way in the *Tarpaka Kapha* subdosha. *Ojas* means vigor and strength. It denotes immunity and resistance to developing disease. It is not only an energetic force as is the nature of *Prana* and *Tejas.* It can be considered a substance that is transitional between the physical and the energetic spheres within the body. Some Ayurvedic writers have described *Ojas* as being the nexus substance between consciousness and matter. Unlike *Prana* and *Tejas, Ojas* has more physical or material reality. Some Ayurvedic texts regard *Ojas* as a highly rarefied tissue substance.

Ojas is associated with the Water Element and with the taste (*rasa*) and the smell (*gandha*) *Tanmatras.* In addition to the *Sattva* and the *Rajas Maha gunas,* some degree of *Tamas* is associated with *Ojas.*

In Traditional Chinese Medicine, the Ayurvedic concept of *Ojas* is most closely identified both with that of *Yin* and with that of *Jing* or *Life Essence* whose center is in the kidneys. Enduring immunity, enduring memory, and the quality of peace of mind or contentment (*tripti*) have been considered functions of *Ojas*. A healthy and balanced *Ojas* takes away burning desire. It brings about feelings of confidence and of being securely grounded. This grounding arises from the containment of body, mind, and spirit that *Ojas* provides. *Ojas* is responsible for psychological stability and the strength to endure. It provides resistance to and protection from breakdowns due to emotional conflicts. *Ojas* is regarded as the primary energy reserve of the body. It is the ultimate product of nutrition, digestion, and metabolism.

Ayurveda regards the subtle dimension of the heart (heart *chakra*) to contain several drops of the best *Ojas* (*Para Ojas*). Contemporary Ayurvedic scientists have suggested that the heart area (*hridaya*) may refer to the functioning of the hypothalamic region in the central nervous system. In addition, *Para Ojas* may correlate with the energy of cellular mitochondria, whereas *Apara Ojas* may be associated with cytoplasmic enzymes that contribute to cell death or the process known as apoptosis. These speculations, whatever their frame of reference, suggest an intimate relationship with metabolic (*Agni*) regulation. The major portion of all *Ojas*, however, termed *Apara Ojas*, is distributed throughout the rest of the body (*vyapi*). In Ayurveda, *Ojas* has been likened to a subtle glue or cement that binds body, mind, and spirit into a bounded and contained functional whole.

Ojas has sometimes been referred to as the eighth tissue. It is the subtle essence of *Kapha* and of *shukra* (reproductive tissue). *Ojas* is derived from *shukra* and produces the subtle energetic field around the body called the aura. *Ojas* is increased by sattvic foods such as pure milk, ghee, and rice. Proper and balanced tastes and the aromatic fragrances found in nature, essential oils, and attractive smells (bodily pheromones, for example) feed *Ojas*.

The maintenance of optimal amounts and optimal quality of *Ojas* is an important concept in Ayurveda. Factors responsible for the depletion and the weakening of *Ojas* are similar to those considered important in Western medicine that are responsible for weakened immunity. In Ayurveda, however, special stress is put on the following: anxiety, anger, depression, envy, physical trauma, wasting and emaciating diseases of whatever etiology, excessive fasting, and excessive physical exertion.

There are three stages characterized by various signs and symptoms of *Ojas* depletion. Stage 1 is termed *Ojas vishrama,* the variable displacement of *Ojas* away from its proper sites of healthy functioning. It is precipitated by inefficient *dhatu Agni* (the metabolic and digestive processes of each bodily tissue) such as an abnormally high *Vata* cooling and thus erratically impairing the *Agni* of *Pitta dosha*. Its characteristics are fatigue, laxity of the joints, and general malaise. Stage 2 is termed *Ojas vyapat,* the impairment of *Ojas*. It has many characteristics: heaviness in the body, stiff joints, bodily swellings, drowsiness, and depression. Stage 3 is termed *Ojas kshaya,* the severe depletion of *Ojas.* It is due to abnormally high *dhatu Agni* that is believed to burn and to dry up bodily tissues to an excessive degree. It is an end-stage process characterized by emaciation and wasting of tissues, stupor, delirium, delusional states, and eventual death.

THE SEVEN BODILY TISSUES: *SAPTA DHATUS*

The universe is considered to be constructed with seven planes of existence (*sapta lokas*). The body, in similar fashion, is understood as being composed of seven basic tissue elements (*sapta dhatus*). The Sanskrit word *dhatu* means that which enters into the formation of the body as a whole in order to hold and to support. These seven bodily constituents are composed of all Five Great Gross Elements, but, as in the case of the *doshas,* only one or two Elements predominate in each tissue. The entire body is composed of the seven tissues, and these tissues sustain the organized material structure of the individual. Although both are considered physical substances, the *doshas* take on more of a functional and regulatory role while the tissues provide the integrated physical scaffolding within which the *doshas* operate. There is a definite sequence of tissue production in the body. This spans a range from most gross with the largest mass and least compact quality toward most subtle, having less mass, and a greater degree of compactness (*samhana*). The first tissue and "most gross or material" substance is called the plasma (*rasa*); next is blood (*rakta*), then muscle (*mamsa*), fat (*meda*), bone (*asthi*), marrow and nerve (*majja*), and, last, reproductive (*shukra*). In Ayurvedic tradition, the *Ojas,* being considered the supremely vital, life-sustaining essence, has been sometimes called the "eighth tissue."

Plasma

The term "*rasa*" has two common denotations: plasma and taste. *Rasa* as plasma implies dynamic life-giving circulation throughout the body. *Rasa* as taste connotes the almost instantaneous action of a food or an herb on the *doshas* and on the tissues.

Plasma (*rasa*) is chiefly composed of the Water Element. It constitutes the chyle, lymph, serum, or plasma matrix that bathes all the other bodily tissues. The Ayurvedic concept of *rasa* is, in fact, much broader than the Western medical definition of plasma. *Rasa* is the total water content of the body, which amounts to about 55 percent of body weight and is the most abundant constituent of the body. The Western definition of plasma, on the other hand, is restricted to denote only the intravascular water that contains electrolytes and clotting factors. In the circulatory vessels, this intravascular plasma is the medium in which red blood cells, white blood cells, and platelets are contained. Total body water (TBW) is distributed as follows: intracellular fluid is ⅔ TBW; extracellular fluid is ⅓ TBW. Extracellular water occupies two main body spaces: (1) the intravascular spaces (25 percent) comprised of the blood and lymph in their circulatory vessels and (2) the interstitial spaces (75 percent) containing intercellular fluid (*lashika*) comprised of the areas around cells, blood vessels, and all other tissues. In Ayurveda, however, the concept of *rasa* includes the total body water contained both in the intracellular and in the extracellular body compartments. *Rasa,* therefore, denotes the massive pool of life-sustaining substances permeating all the *dhatus* (tissues) throughout the entire body.

The intimate association between the Ayurvedic concept of taste (*rasa*) and the plasma tissue (*rasa*) has profound implications. This is certainly implied since the Sanskrit term for both is identical. The nutritive and therapeutic value of an ingested substance, for example, food and herbs, is determined by the combination of tastes that it contains and evokes in the body. After these materials are properly digested, they become the first bodily tissue, the *rasa,* which acts as the foundation for all further nutrition and tissue production. *Rasa* is considered the first point at which digested food transforms into the human *Ahamkara* with an individualized, specifically human identity. Plasma has been called the "sap" of the body and, as such, functions to provide nutrition and nourishment for every other component of the body. Generation and maintenance of the physical body has its repeated beginnings and further development at the juncture at which *rasa* is made. All vital nutrients are in solution and are distributed via the plasma. The Sanskrit word *prinana* is used to describe the action of the plasma. *Prinana* connotes fulfillment, fullness, hydration, pleasure, and the expectation of more to come. In the Ayurvedic sense, the *prinana* aspect of *rasa* results from the pleasure that is considered to be the subjective experience resulting from the circulation of *rasa.* The predominant *dosha* contained in plasma is *Kapha,* particularly *Avalambaka Kapha.*

Although all seven tissues are of vital importance, the developmentally first tissue, the plasma, which launches the evolution of the tissue formation chain, is arguably the most important one that determines the health or disease of the body. The plasma, therefore, is the basic nutritive matrix for all bodily substances, and, as well, is the basic matrix out of which all other tissues develop.

Each tissue is considered to have a "membrane" that may be both a material covering and have functional, physiological significance. These holding or embracing tissue membranes or *dhara kalas* are nutritive membranes within and around the tissue and around that tissue's specific channel or circulatory system. These membranes not only seal, hold together, and protect the tissue substance but also filter out wastes in addition to facilitating the absorption and diffusion of nutrients that feed the tissue. Each tissue membrane is the main site of that tissue's particular digestive fire (*dhatu Agni*). The membrane structures associated with the plasma are called *sleshmadhara kala.* *Sleshma* is an ancient synonym for *Kapha* and connotes the virtual identity of plasma and *Kapha.* It is believed that the synovial membranes around joints are specifically related to these plasma-*Kapha* membranes.

Blood

Blood (*rakta*) is chiefly composed of the Fire and Water Elements. It is the particulate matter in the circulatory system, especially the erythrocytes or red blood cells. Its unique status, which makes it essential to life, has prompted Ayurvedic tradition to virtually regard it as the fourth *dosha*. Synonyms for blood are the following: *rudhira, lohitam,* and *shonitam,* all of which indicated red color; other terms include *asruk* (circulation), *asram* (circulation), and *kshatajam* (that which emerges from wounds). A chief function of blood is to carry oxygen and to oxygenate all the other tissues. In addition to this, blood is considered to vitalize and to invigorate through the infusion of *Prana;* in these respects, its functioning is referred to as *jivana* (invigoration). The Sanskrit term for blood, *rakta,* means that which is colored red. This connotes blood's warmth and stimulating capacities. Along with its ability to carry oxygen, blood is the gross fluid that acts to create, hold, and carry the *Prana* or vital energy. Blood and hemopoiesis are closely identified with *Ranjaka Pitta.* Blood thus functions to oxygenate the tissues, to contribute to the production and circulation of *Prana,* and to induce a sense of invigoration, ardor, and passion. In intimate contiguity to this, *Prana* is the motor that drives blood. The role of nitric oxide in vasodilation and blood flow correlates with this and is yet to be explored in Ayurveda and Western science.

The membranes associated with the blood are called *pittadhara kala*. This connotes the intimate connection between the blood and *Pitta,* its origin. In Ayurveda, the *pittadhara kala* are considered to have their anatomical sites not only in the endothelial lining of the blood vessels but also in the membranes of the gastrointestinal tract, especially the small intestine. The *dhatu Agni* (tissue fire of digestion) of *Ranjaka Pitta,* situated in the liver (but also in the spleen and bone marrow), is the primary site of the secondary metabolism or general tissue metabolism, which occurs after the primary digestive processes occur in the stomach and in the small intestine.

Muscle

Muscle (*mamsa*) is composed chiefly of the Earth Element with some additional Water and Fire Elements. Muscle imparts strength and has the function of plastering or binding (*lepana*). The connotation of the root of the term *mamsa* suggests the function of holding firm. The membrane that holds muscle tissue is called *mamsadhara kala*. It is usually associated with the anatomical structures of the deep fascia.

Fat

Fat (*meda*) is composed chiefly of the Water Element. Its function is that of lubrication (*snehana*). The term for fat, *meda,* denotes that which is oily.

This tissue has been traditionally associated with the melodious functioning of the voice, and also with the emotion of loving affection. The membranes that are associated with fat are called *medodhara kala*. These are anatomically associated with the greater and lesser omentum, sheaths of fascia in the abdominal area anterior to the lower parts of the stomach and to the transverse colon.

Bone

Bone (*asthi*) is composed of the two Elements: Earth and Air. Its function is support (*dharana*). The Sanskrit term for bone, *asthi,* means to stand or to endure. Bone is the physical container of the *Vata dosha,* particularly *Vyana Vata* and *Apana Vata*. The membranes that contain and nourish it are called the *purishadhara kala*. These periosteal membranes, according to Ayurveda, are intimately associated with the mucous membranes of the large intestine or colon. Any *Vata* imbalance, normally having its seat of perturbation centered in the colon, therefore, will ultimately affect the skeletal system (*asthi dhatu*) in some manner. Although this association appears unusual, it is a traditional Ayurvedic concept and has great therapeutic significance, particularly demonstrated by the efficacy of therapeutic enemas used in the treatment of bone disorders.

Marrow and Nerve Tissue

Marrow and nerve (*majja*) is composed of the Water Element. In Ayurveda, the function of marrow is to produce fullness and contentment (*purana*). The meaning of marrow derives from the root *maj,* which denotes sinking. This is understood to suggest that which is sunk and encased in bone. This encompasses both bone marrow and the entire central and peripheral nervous system. All the *Vatas* circulate through the marrow and nervous system or *majja*. The membrane that holds the marrow and nerves is referred to as *majjadhara kala* (marrow and nerve nutritive membrane).

Reproductive Tissue

Reproductive tissue (*shukra*), both male and female, is composed of the Water Element. It is considered to be the essence derived from all the tissues, especially the marrow and nerve tissues. Its multiple functions include producing progeny, giving strength, producing energy, and fostering stamina. The Sanskrit word for reproductive tissue, *shukra,* means seed and luminous. It also refers to the planet Venus. The membranes that hold reproductive fluids are called *shukradhara kala* (reproductive tissue nutritive membranes).

SEQUENCE OF TISSUE DEVELOPMENT AND OF TISSUE NUTRITION THEORIES

In the developmental origin and production of the bodily tissues, the first tissue to be formed is believed to be the plasma. When food (*ahara*) is taken into the mouth, it is considered "unhomologous." In Ayurveda, this means that its individual identity (*Ahamkara*) as nonhuman continues to be retained until it is properly digested. Since this is experienced by the body as foreign at first, it is not fully utilizable. In the process of digestion in the stomach and small intestine, the "raw" unhomologous material begins to be transformed (digested and absorbed) into useful nutrition. At this point, this "pre-plasma" is called *ahara rasa,* the still unhomologous nutritive substance. Once the *ahara rasa* enters the liver and is further digested by the appropriate transformative processes, it then becomes a homologous chylelike fluid and is called *rasa* proper or plasma. Through a series of ongoing and dynamic processes, this assimilable plasma is used for nutrition and also is used for the process of transformation into the other tissues in a sequential manner. Plasma transforms into blood, blood into muscle, muscle into fat, fat into bone, bone into marrow, and marrow into semen.

This direct, transformative sequence of tissue formation (*Ksheera Dadhi*) is a dynamic process that produces ongoing stable tissue (*sthayi dhatu*), unstable tissue (*asthayi dhatu*), gross waste products (*sthula mala*), subtle waste products (*kleda*), and secondary tissues (*upadhatus*).

There are, however, two other theories of the mechanism of the nutrition and formation of tissue. The first is called *Kedara Kula* and refers in an analogous fashion to the mechanisms seen in the channel irrigation method used on farms. Nutrients travel through the blood vessels and larger circulatory system to nourish and produce tissues. The second is called *Kale Kapota* and refers to the "land and pigeon" selectivity mechanism wherein each tissue extracts the specific nutrients it needs from the plasma so that it may grow and develop.

The time sequences for tissue productions vary. Plasma is developed daily and transforms into blood in about 5 days. The full transformation of plasma into reproductive fluid is believed to occur in about 35 days.

BODILY WASTE PRODUCTS (*SHARIRA MALAS*) DERIVED FROM FOOD

The body produces three main gross waste products (*sharira malas*) from the intake of food after all digestion is completed: urine (*mutra*), feces (*purisha*), and sweat (*sveda*). These are considered functionally important although ultimately they are the discardable end products of ingested food. Each *mala* has a dual role, that is, one of initial support to the body and when spent, it has the role of an excrement. Urine is derived from the intake of water and from the metabolic fluid wastes. The function of urine is considered to be the carrying away of wastewater (*kleda vahanam*). The basic portion of urine is first in the colon and then extracted into the circulation to go through the channels (*srotas*) so that *kleda* or wastes may be collected and carried away to the kidneys for excretion. Sweat is believed to be an end product derived originally from the intake of air. Its main function is considered to be the process (*kleda vidhruti*) of separating waste from nutritive material. Sweat brings *kleda* wastes to the skin, not only to dispel them, but also for the purposes of moisturizing and oiling the skin. Feces are originally derived from the food or *ahara* intake. In addition to its obvious function of ridding the body of excrement, Ayurveda highlights the dual supportive roles of the feces. First, the feces are considered to have a primary role called *avasthamabhana;* this refers to the function of supporting the structure and tone of the colon and the entire pelvic area. Second, the feces are believed to support the *Agni* or digestive fire and contribute to the body's normal temperature regulation. After these functions have occurred over a time, the feces are eliminated.

SECONDARY TISSUES OR *UPADHATUS*

As the seven primary tissues (*dhatus*) are produced, they also produce accessory or secondary tissues (*upadhatus*). The primary tissues maintain the functioning of the secondary and supplementary tissues. *Rasa* produces *sthanya* (breast milk) and *raja* or *artava* (menstrual fluid). *Rakta* produces *sira* (blood vessels) and *kandara* (tendons). *Mamsa* produces *vasa* (muscle fat), *tvacha* (skin), and *snayus* (ligaments). *Meda* produces omentum sheaths around fat, small tendons, and small bony joints. *Asthi* produces *danta* (teeth). *Majja* produces *dushika* (sclerotic fluid of the eyes). *Shukra* produces *Ojas,* the bodily fluid associated with immune functions.

GROSS WASTE PRODUCTS DERIVED FROM TISSUE METABOLISM (*DHATU MALAS*)

The gross waste products of the tissues (*dhatu malas*) are considered significant by-products necessary for the health of the body. Along with the formation of these tissue gross by-products, a small amount of subtle tissue wastes called *kleda* are also produced. *Kleda* constitutes an amorphous mixture of waste materials that have moist and evaporative properties but no other coarser correlates in the body that can be measured in appreciable amounts.

The gross waste products of tissues (*dhatu malas*) produced from their respective primary tissues (*dhatus*) are as follows. Plasma is considered to be originally derived from *Kapha*. In the process of its multiple transformative stages, plasma yields *Kapha dosha* as one of its primary tissue by-products. Blood is believed to be originally derived from *Pitta*. Like plasma, in its multiple transformative processes, blood yields *Pitta dosha* as one of its primary tissue by-products. Muscle is originally derived from *Kapha*. Its by-products are called *khamalas* and are described as being the waste material found in the cavities of the body's outer surfaces: ears and nose, for example. Fat is originally derived from *Kapha* and has sweat as its major gross tissue waste product. Bone is originally derived from *Vata dosha*. Its two main gross tissue by-products are *nakha* (nails) and *kesha* (hair).

Marrow and nerve tissues are originally derived from *Kapha* and produce the by-product associated with the glaze or fluids of the eyes. Reproductive fluids are derived from *Kapha* and are believed to yield the by-products smegma as well as facial, axillary, and pubic hair.

Thus, after the ingestion of food, its unassimilated and postdigestive end products or gross waste products (*sharira malas*) are excreted from the body in the form of sweat, urine, and feces. Proper digestion and assimilation, therefore, ultimately produce primary tissues (*dhatus*), secondary tissues (*upadhatus*), gross tissue wastes (*dhatus malas*), very subtle tissue wastes (*kleda*), and excretory gross wastes (*sharira malas*).

GROSS ANATOMY

In Ayurveda, the detailed gross (*sthula*) anatomy of the body is virtually similar to that described in Western medicine. The morphological and functional Ayurvedic perspective, however, is different and reflects the centrality of the *doshas* as they function both in health and in disease. There are several versions of a body structure concept. The two most common are the following.

1. Head, Trunk, and Branches View. The body in this view is composed of three main sections. They are (a) *shira,* the head-neck portion; (b) *koshta,* the trunk portion; and (c) *shakha,* the branches portion. The head and neck part contains both solid tissue and hollow organs. The trunk portion contains the gastrointestinal tract and most of the organs (*ashaya*) that have hollow interiors. The branches include the four limbs and are composed of the highest proportion of solid tissue such as muscle and bone.

2. Hollow Organs and Compact Tissue View. The body here also consists of three groupings. They are (a) *koshta* that includes the gastrointestinal tract, the plasma, and some hollow organs; (b) *shakha* that includes the four limbs, the blood, the muscles, and fat tissue; and (c) *marmas* or *madhyama* that includes the head-brain, the heart, the kidneys, the urinary bladder, and bone, nerve-marrow, and reproductive tissue. The *madhyama* are considered the most important group of vital organs and tissues.

MARMA POINTS

Marma points, of which there are about 107, are significant areas on the surface of the body that are sensitive and responsive to injury and to therapeutic pressure. The first reference to these points is found in the *Atharva-Veda,* an ancient Vedic text containing some medical content. The later medical text *Sushruta Samhita* more fully expands on their locations and therapeutic use. Ayurvedic sources speculate on the possibility of these larger area *Marma* points being the progenitors of the smaller area acupuncture points used in Traditional Chinese Medicine. At this time, there is no material evidence to substantiate this speculation, other than Ayurvedic oral tradition. The antiquity of the Indian *Marma* concept is believed to extend back to a very ancient Ayurvedic medical text, the *Suchi Veda,* as yet undiscovered.

Marma areas are defined as the anatomical site on or near the surface of the body where muscle, blood vessel, bones, tendons, ligaments, and joints meet. There are three major ways of classifying *Marma:* (1) by their region or area on the body, (2) by the tissues and structures of which they are predominantly composed, and (3) by the signs they produce when they are injured. By careful massage, especially with specific essential oils, *Marma* stimulation is believed to regulate the functioning of the *doshas* and the physiologic processes in the body.

The three great *Marmas* (*Mahamarmas*) are (1) *Hridaya Marma* located over the heart area, (2) *Shira Marma* located on the head area, and (3) *Basti Marma* located over the lower abdominal area.

THE ORGANS OF THE BODY

In Ayurveda, the tissues (*dhatus*) of the body are a central focus of attention in determining health and imbalance as well as in assessing and formulating therapeutic interventions. The body's organs (*ashaya*), important as they are, take on a secondary role. This apparent de-emphasis of the organs may, in fact, be due to the Ayurvedic conception of *dosha-dhatu* (humortissue) structure and functioning, which implicitly includes the actions of the organs, although this is not made explicit in the Ayurvedic literature or in clinical practice. Each organ, however, is correlated with its important tissue, channel, subdosha, and allied substance such as its waste product and its relevance to *Ojas,* the physical substance associated with immunity, vigor, and strength. The major organs and their correlation to the *doshas* and tissues will be outlined here.

The functioning of the gastrointestinal tract is pivotal in Ayurveda. The organs directly related to it, therefore, are of primary importance. The stomach is considered a *Kapha* organ in which the *Kledaka Kapha* is prominent. The sweet phase of primary digestion occurs here. The small intestine is the site of *Pachaka Pitta,* which is intimately allied with the central *Agni* or digestive fire and is called the *Jatharagni.* The sour phase of primary digestion occurs here. The colon is the major site of *Apana Vata* and the site of the pungent phase of primary digestion.

The nature and the understanding of the pancreas (*kloman*) and the spleen are important and take on a different significance, for example, from that in Traditional Chinese Medicine. The pancreas has also been referred to by the term *agnisaya*. In Ayurveda the spleen is considered a *Pitta* organ with a preponderance of *Ranjaka Pitta* similar to the status of *Pitta* in the liver. The spleen is understood to be involved with the production and the destruction of blood components. In contrast, the pancreas is thought of as a *Kapha* organ with a preponderance of *Kledaka Kapha*. As such, it is involved in the processes of primary digestion with an emphasis on water and blood sugar regulation. For example, according to Ayurveda, the imbalances produced by diabetes and hypoglycemia, and also the clinical phenomena of nonpitting edema, are related to impairments of the pancreas. In addition, primary metabolic processes are impaired; *Pachaka Pitta* is excessively high while *dhatu Agni* is low. In the Chinese medical system, by contrast, the important concept of "damp spleen" refers more to what Ayurveda considers pancreatic disorders, although the term *pancreas* is not used in the Chinese description.

The brain is considered a central organ that houses three significant subdoshas. *Prana Vata* has its primary site in the brain. *Sadhaka Pitta* and *Tarpaka Kapha* share prominence here as well. These are vital subdoshas and have profound psychological and consciousness-related impacts. They contribute to the experience of sacredness, awe, and reverence. The heart contains *Sadhaka Pitta, Avalambaka Kapha,* and both *Prana* and *Udana Vata.* The liver and gallbladder are imbued with *Ranjaka Pitta.* The kidneys have a predominance of *Apana Vata.* The reproductive organs of the female contain *Kapha* in the breast tissue and *Pitta* in the uterus, ovaries, and Fallopian tubes. The male gonads contain *Kapha.*

Specific organs contribute, in part, to the regulation of the tissues and their functioning. This takes on clinical significance in disease because a diseased tissue's governing organs are believed to be also impaired and, in part, etiologically responsible for their tissue's dysfunction. Therapeutic intervention, therefore, may be directed to the governing organs. The plasma is considered to be governed by the heart and the lungs. The heart, the liver, and the spleen govern the blood. The liver, the spleen, and the pancreas govern the muscle. The pancreas and the kidneys govern fat. The colon and the kidneys govern bone. The colon is believed to be responsible for the direct nourishment of bone through the functioning of the *purishadhara kala* or colon membrane. The brain and the colon govern the marrow. The gonads and the kidney govern the reproductive fluids. This close tie of tissues with their controlling organs again demonstrates the almost inseparable interrelatedness of the body according to Ayurveda.

BIOPSYCHOSPIRITUAL STRUCTURAL AND FUNCTIONAL ORGANIZATION

The Ayurvedic model of the individual is an integrative one. This conception acknowledges and describes a structural and functional interpenetration of dynamic components that includes physical, psychological, and spiritual-consciousness dimensions. *BioPsychoSpiritual* mankind denotes men and women viewed in all their infinite complexity and dynamisms (Table 3.2).

Table 3.2   The *BioPsychoSpiritual* Model

Man and woman: each is one indivisible person who participates both in a material and in a spiritual nature. Self-development denotes the consciously intentional path from a state of less integration, that is, splitting among the various dimensions of the self, toward the realization of self-integration within the larger context of reality.

The Person consists of three dimensions:
  Physical Body: eco-corporeal
  Subtle Energetic Mental Body: eco-psychological
  Spiritual/Consciousness

The *BioPsychoSpiritual* model is a systems approach toward an under-standing of the interrelatedness of the individual, not only within but also as an integral part of the wider universe. The microcosmic interplay of body, mind, and spirit is innervated and given meaning through its participation in the extended environmental systems of which it is a key player. The individual exists both for himself and herself and also for the interpersonal and social worlds that comprise family, society, and cultural group. This concep-tion again attests to the dynamic understanding of issues related to the con-struct of "the one and the many" that may be formulated on any level of consideration of the individuals that collectively comprise humanity.

Ayurveda, as has been alluded to previously, emerged out of the ancient *Vedas* and was influenced by the work of Patanjali, the propounder of the Yoga system. The following description derives from both these traditions; its import rests in the comprehensive picture of man's multifaceted constitution that it presents.

The human body (*sharira*), the person, may be understood as having three major aspects that range from the gross, coarse, and most material (*sthula*) level of being, through a more rarefied, subtle, or energetic level (*sukshma*), to the most immaterial, spiritual, causal, or seed-origination sphere (*karana*). An individual is considered to be one person with three bodies. Within the trinity of each of these three fundamental domains, there exist differing gra-dations or organizational nodes called *koshas* (sheaths) in which aspects of the five Elements, the *doshas,* the subtle, energetic roots of the *doshas,* and the *Maha gunas* (*Sattva, Rajas,* and *Tamas*) operate. The core at the center of these five sheaths or coverings is called *atman,* the individual spirit or con-sciousness. *Atman* is considered to be *Brahman,* the universal Absolute, as it exists in the individual. Every individual person has a share both in a physical and in a spiritual nature.

The first aspect is the gross or physical body (*sharira sthula*) made up of coarse matter that has perceptible mass and is most tangible. On this level, the Five Great Gross Elements (Ether, Air, Fire, Water, and Earth) predomi-nate and create the unique physical morphology of that specific individual. These link an individual with the ecological material environment. This *eco-corporeality* creates the dynamic resonance between man and nature.

The three biological *doshas, Vata-Pitta-Kapha* (VPK), constitute the physio-logical aspect of the five Elements and act as the body's functional and regu-latory principles. This physical sheath is called the *Annamaya Kosha*. It has been referred to as the outermost, that is, the most material, layer or dimen-sion of the individual. This material sheath of *dhatus* is considered relatively coarse and crude in comparison to the composition, structure, and fineness of the other dimensions that constitute the individual.

The second aspect is the subtle or energetic body (*sharira sukshma, linga sharira*) made up of more immaterial yet vital substances that function as the psychological, mental, and emotional spheres. It is here that the subtle forces of *Prana, Tejas,* and *Ojas* are situated. Two sheaths are organized at this level: (1) *Pranamaya Kosha,* the breath sheath: this houses the activity of *Prana* and the breath, the basic life forces. This has been referred to as the "body of energy," the etheric body, and has been considered to have a special relation to what are called the five organs of motor action, the *kar-mendriyas. Pranayama* or breath exercises prevent the sensory and nervous disturbances that may develop and situate themselves here. (2) *Manomaya Kosha* is the emotional-mental sheath. This is the site of *Manas* (mind). *Prana, Tejas,* and *Ojas* are also active here. This sheath has been considered to have a special relation to the organs of the five senses, the *jnanendriyas.* Breathing and the mind form a delicately interrelated entity. The *eco-psychological* resonance between man and nature is epitomized in the breath-ing in and out of sensory impressions into the mind and the manner in which these shape experience. The practice of *mantras* and of music therapy may help to manage anxiety and thought disorders. Yoga meditations contribute to preventing various forms of mental decline.

The third aspect is the spiritual or causal-seed body (*sharira karana*) con-stituting the most immaterial level of the human being. The *Maha gunas, Sattva, Rajas,* and *Tamas,* are most active here. It is with this arena that the quality of one's consciousness, self-realization, and awareness resides. Two sheaths are found at this most rarefied plane: (1) *Vijnanomaya Kosha,* the intelligence-wisdom-*Buddhi* sheath. *Buddhi* is the infallible intelligence that is able to discern truth from falsehood; and (2) *Anandamaya Kosha,* the bliss or joy sheath that is considered closest to the spiritual core (*atman*) of the individual.

The Yoga concept of Patanjali regards the five sheaths as surrounding, but not touching, the primary spiritual core called *atman.* Yoga systems aim at re-leasing (*Moksha*) the *atman* from its fetters to these sheaths and to the material world. Ayurveda tends to regard the multidimensional concept of man in a more integral, perhaps less segregated fashion, with consciousness pervading and supporting the entire unity. Cultivation of consciousness in all its manifestations, material and nonmaterial, is a Vedic precept. *Moksha* or liberation, in this sense, is regarded as freedom from the mistaken belief that man and nature, in themselves and in relation to each other, are split and divided. The Vedic concept of *Moksha* denotes attaining the realization of personal wholeness within a unified field that is consciousness based. The physical body, therefore, is considered, in fact, to be more than a mere vessel or container of the spirit; it is the material dimension of spirit. Spirit, indivisible from matter, is an acknowledged real presence. In Ayurveda, the physical body, rather than being considered as a prison, is understood to be the medium within which consciousness unfolds. The root of the Sanskrit word *budh* means to regain consciousness. It is this consciousness of unity within apparent diversity that constitutes the Vedic view. Self-development leading to *Moksha* refines consciousness and brings it toward the ultimate ideal of the unblemished, equipoised witnessing (*sakshin*) of the play (*lila*) of creation in the world (*Prakriti*).

CONCEPT OF OM/AUM

OM or AUM is a term used to denote a symbol (Figure 3.4) and a sacred syllable or sound (*Pranava, udgitha*). It is a central entity in Hinduism and also has prominence in Buddhism. OM is believed to be more than a mere word; it is the tangible expression of spirit in the way the mind can perceive it. When recited, it is said that this humlike sound helps the meditator to cross the ocean of existence and reach the shore of purer consciousness.

The OM may be understood, in *eco-psychological* terms, to display the mind and its situated states (*avastha*) of consciousness: consciously awake, preconscious, and unconscious in relation to *Maya* and *Brahman*. The bottom

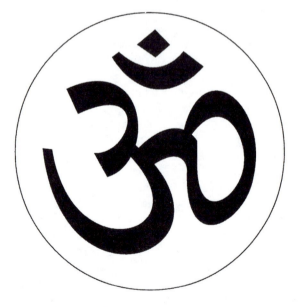

Figure 3.4   OM/AUM: Sacred Hindu symbol of form and sound
(Courtesy of illustrator Frank John Ninivaggi, M.D.)

curve in Figure 3.4 symbolizes the domain of conscious awareness and wakefulness (*jagrat*). The mind typically grounds itself here and ordinarily believes that the material body and the cognitive processes of reason and logic that are used to know itself and the environment constitute the (entire) truth of what is real. The right curve, which may be depicted as open or closed, symbolizes the preconscious arena (*svapna*) that plays a major part in the production of the dream state within sleep. The uppermost attached curve symbolizes the ordinarily inaccessible, dynamic unconscious (*sushupti*) that houses the raw fabric of human existence such as the life instincts, the death instinct, and unconscious phantasies, all of which drive root motivations and desire. The topmost smaller, unattached semicircle with its shallow side facing up is used to depict *Maya*.

Maya connotes the illusion that reality is a series of unrelated parts. It is the power (*shakti*) of *Brahman* that inexplicably veils human vision so that only single aspects of the integrity of existence can be grasped. *Maya* deceives when the world of appearances is taken to be immutable rather than impermanent and that this agglomeration constitutes the only reality. *Maya* is both the inability to see the truth and also the ability to see the world in a delusional manner. The topmost dot represents *turiya,* "the fourth way." It is the superconscious state of illumination (*sakshin*) that is transcendental to the three states of wakeful consciousness, preconsciousness, and the unconscious. This awareness maintains an identity with *Brahman. Brahman* is the Absolute, consciousness in itself, and the ground within which and out of which everything arises.

CONCEPT OF *CHAKRAS*

Chakras (energy wheels) are subtle energy structures or nodes organized at different sites along the spinal cord. These focal points function to selectively bind *Ahamkara* into self-identification with the physical body of an individual through each of the five Elements. The energy of these *chakras* is termed *Kundalini,* which implies snake- and serpentlike power. Tantra Yoga or Kundalini Yoga holds this paradigm in high esteem. The *Kundalini* is likened to a female energy that, when awakened by proper techniques and practices, rises from the base of the vertebral column, traverses the *chakras,* and then culminates in the ultimate, *Sahasrara,* the seat of Shiva; this is often referred to as the seventh or crown *chakra.* The mating of the female energy with the male complement, the *Purusha,* brings forth the enlightenment termed *Samadhi.*

The Hindu culture abounds with anthropomorphic tales whose value lies in reframing highly abstract psychological and spiritual propositions into concrete and experience-near narratives. An illustration of this is in the wedding story of Shiva. At first, presenting himself in ash and grotesque costume to his prospective wife, *Parvati,* and to her mother, he ultimately transformed himself into *Sundaramurti,* the embodiment of all masculine beauty on earth.

This marital union is termed *Kalyana Sundaram,* the beauty which grants unshakable welfare and auspiciousness. Shiva's epithet is *Shankara,* one who grants welfare and peace. The mating of the *Purusha* (Shiva) with *Shakti/Kundalini/Parvati* is the ultimate ideal.

Although they are not considered to have physical substance, the *chakras* are located in the region of major nerve plexuses and exist with them but on the subtle or vital plane along a subtle distribution channel (*nadi*) called the *sushumna.* The chakras are part of the *majja dhatu* nerve tissue and are related to the endocrine glands. *Hita* denotes the distribution channels that branch off *nadi.* The specific action of the *chakras* involves the concentration, organization, and regulation of an individual's vital life force, *Prana,* also called *Kundalini Shakti.* In this sense, the *chakras* are functional entities that exert an energetic and subtle physiological role. This conceptualization, used in Ayurveda, comes from the work of Patanjali and remains a significant part of the Yoga system. The Pranic life force is considered to contain the currents of consciousness. It is used in a practical way in the course of the process of meditation as a preparatory stage in which attention is withdrawn from the sensory arena and refocused on the more subtle level of the *chakras* in order to activate their specific functioning. When each *chakra* is energized in this manner, its main Pranic life force is intensified. As each of the seven *chakras* activates in this way, a progression begins from the lowest *chakra,* the *Muladhara,* up to the highest *chakra,* the *Sahasrara.* During the course of this process, the quality of one's consciousness is believed to change, clarify, intensify, and broaden.

The *Muladhara Chakra* is considered the root center and the main foundation or support for the *chakras* above. This spatial positioning refers both to physical and to anatomical locations, and, as well, to the degree of subtleness and the qualitative relationship to consciousness that the *chakra* holds. This *chakra* is located in the region of the anal and perineal area and is related to the sacral and coccygeal plexus. It is correlated with the male and female gonads. Its related *Marma* point is called *Guda,* and its primary Element is Earth.

The *Svadhisthana Chakra* is considered the sex center. It is located near the genitals and related to the hypogastric, lumbar plexus. It is correlated with the adrenal glands and the prostate. Its related *Marma* point is *Kukundara,* and its primary Element is Water.

The *Manipura Chakra* is located near the navel and is related to the solar and celiac plexuses. It is correlated with the pancreas. Its related *Marma* points are *Nabhi* and *Bruhati,* and its major Element is Fire.

The *Anahata Chakra* is located near the heart and is related to the cardiac plexus. It is correlated with the thymus gland. Its related *Marma* points are the *Hridaya* and the *Amsaphalaka;* its major Element is Air. This center has been referred to as the "lotus of the heart," and the place within which the experience of the OM/AUM may be heard.

The *Vishuddha Chakra* is located near the throat and the group of nerve plexuses includes the cervical, the carotid, and the pulmonary. It is correlated with the thyroid and the parathyroid glands. Its related *Marma* is the *Nila Manya,* and its primary Element is Ether.

The *Ajna Chakra* is located between the eyes and is related to the cavernous plexus, the optic chiasma, and the thalamic-hypothalamic-limbic-pituitary system. It is correlated with the pituitary gland. Its related *Marma* is the *Sthapani*. This *chakra* has been called the "third eye" because of its intimate connection with the meditative process, insight, and the development of refined levels of conscious awareness. The third eye depicted in images of Shiva correlates with *Ajna. Ahamkara,* mind, and brain merge at this point. *Ojas* arises and gives containment to these. *Ajna* is depicted as two flower petals with a central OM.

The *Sahasrara* has been called the crown *chakra* and occupies the area near and above the top of the head. It has been correlated with the pineal gland. Its significance goes beyond the ordinary concept of the six *chakras*. Its activation is associated with the highest degree of the refinement of consciousness. This state of consciousness is called *Samadhi*. At *Sahasrara,* the microcosm of an individual's share of *Prana* interfaces with "the thousand-petal lotus," a concept that connotes one's individual flow of *Prana* participating in the macrocosm's infinite flow of *Prana*.

4

PHYSIOLOGY AND DIGESTION

Ayurvedic physiology (*sharira krija*) focuses on the functioning, processes, and mechanisms of the bodily structures. In this chapter, the systems of channels of circulation (*srotas*) that pervade the entire physical body, the concept of *Agni,* and the processes of digestion operative from the cellular through the tissue, organ, and channel system levels are discussed.

In Ayurveda, the concept of *Agni* and digestion is a fundamental cornerstone both in theory and in clinical understanding. The digestive process is extremely complicated and rather difficult to convey to Western thinkers. A great deal of effort has been given to delineate all the major and minor facets that surround digestion in a manner that scientifically reflects the enormity of these macrodigestive and microdigestive processes. It is hoped that this will illuminate rather than impede an understanding of this crucial topic.

SROTAS: THE CHANNELS OF A SPECIFIC SYSTEM'S CIRCULATION

The Ayurvedic concept of *srotas* refers to a complex interconnected system of communicating networks that perfuse all bodily substances. Each one of the major relatively discrete tissue, physiological, and mental systems has its own organization of *srotas.*

The term *srotas* derives from the Sanskrit root *sru* meaning "to flow." The *srotas* are considered tubular canals of circulation in and through which nutrients, *dhatus* (tissues), and *malas* (wastes) are produced, distributed, and eliminated. Each cell, moreover, contains innumerable *sukshma srotas,* which are its communicative channels and pores. The concept of circulation in Ayurveda is not restricted only to the flow of blood and plasma throughout the body, but is extended to include substances such as the *doshas,* nutrients, waste products, and even tissue elements. These *srotas* aid in the production and transport of nutrients and waste materials both to and between cells, the *dhatus,* and the organs.

Srotas, therefore, are involved in the formation, destruction, and conduction of *doshas, dhatus,* and *malas.* The *srotas* and the *dhatu dhara kalas* (tissue-embracing membranes) are functionally and structurally related. Each *srotas* has a root organ that is considered its point of origination as well as its regulatory and controlling center. Any disturbance in an organ is reflected in a disturbance in the functioning of its *srotas*. Some Ayurvedic texts use the term *srotamsi* when referring to the plural of *srotas,* although current convention is to use the term *srotas* when referring to the channel system in either the single or plural sense (Table 4.1). In a more restrictive sense, the generic concept of *srotas* may be delimited by more particular but, admittedly, loosely defined terms such as *rohini* (arteries), *nila* or *sira* (veins), *keshika* (capillaries), *gauri* (lymphatic vessels), *dhamani* (arteries, motor nerves), and *aruna* (sympathetic nerves). Charaka has given a special distinction in this regard when he speaks of *dhamanis* as being pulsatile, *srotamsi* as oozing and semipermeable, and *siras* as maintaining continuous flow. In this sense, *dhamanis* may be correlated to arteries, *srotamsi* to capillaries, and *siras* to veins.

Optimal flow through these channel systems reflects optimal health. Disturbed flow may result from multiple causes some of which are hereditary, congenital, and traumatic deformities, and the structural and functional deformities caused by vitiations. Disturbed flow (*sroto dushti*), associated with illness, may take the following forms:

1. Excessive flow (*atipravrutti*): this is usually caused by conditions that increase *Vata*.
2. Deficient flow (*sanga*): this is usually caused by conditions that increase *Kapha*.
3. Blocked, knotted up, or obstructed flow (*srotorhodha*): this is usually caused by conditions of increased *Kapha*, *Ama* (toxins), or waste product buildup. *Sroto dushti* (*srotas vitiation*) occurs and is followed by *srotorhodha*.

Table 4.1   *Srotas,* the Major Channel Systems

Pranavaha Srotas, the respiratory system
Udakavaha Srotas, the water metabolism system
Annavaha Srotas, the digestive system
Rasavaha Srotas, the plasma circulatory system
Raktavaha Srotas, the blood circulatory system
Mamsavaha Srotas, the channels of circulation for muscle tissue
Medhovaha Srotas, the channels of circulation for adipose tissue
Asthivaha Srotas, the channels of circulation for bone
Majjavaha Srotas, the channels of circulation for nerve
Shukravaha Srotas, the channels of circulation for reproductive tissue
Artavavaha Srotas, the channels of circulation for the menstrual system
Stanyavaha Srotas, the channels of circulation of the lactation system
Svedavaha Srotas, the channels of circulation for sweat
Mutravaha Srotas, the channels of circulation for urine
Purishavaha Srotas, the channels of circulation of the excretory system

4. Diverted flow out of the proper channel (*vimarga gamana*): this is caused by blockages or spasms. This is a serious condition that may damage the channel itself and may damage the surrounding tissue. *Vimarga gamana* may produce a structural deformity of the channel (*kervaigunya*) that may become a fundamental factor in establishing a future disease process.

5. Abnormal direction of the flow within the channel (*pratiloma*): this may result from a blockage or from a reversal of the direction of *Vata* in the channel. Any dilation, abnormal growth, or swelling of a *srota* such as in the case of cancer may be called *sira granthi*.

There are five main classes of *srotas* containing a total of about 16 primary channels, each categorized by its particular functioning. The principal classes are (1) intake of nutrients, (2) nutrition of tissues, (3) elimination of wastes, (4) mental and emotional functioning, and (5) sexual and reproductive functioning. Each class has particular subdivisions, and while only 16 are primarily delineated, the actual number of channels is virtually innumerable since they pervade all areas of the entire body and consist of an intricate latticework of main and subsidiary branches.

Intake of Nutrients

Pranavaha Srotas is roughly equated with the respiratory system. The organs that constitute its origin, regulation, and control are the heart and the lungs, the colon, and the brain. The functioning of this channel is intimately connected to the *Pranamaya Kosha* or breath sheath of the individual that exists on the *Pranic* or subtle level. Oxygen and *Prana* are carried in this *srotas*.

Annavaha Srotas, also called *Maha Srotas,* is equated with the functioning of the gastrointestinal tract. The areas that constitute its origin, regulation, and control are the stomach and the left side of the body. The *Maha Srotas* is one of the most important channel systems since it is the primary pathway for nutrition from the outside and its condition depends on the daily intake of proper foods and their proper assimilation. Food is carried in this channel.

Ambuvaha Srotas, also called *Udakavaha Srotas,* is the channel system that regulates the water metabolism in the body. There is no direct correspondence in the Western conception of physiology other than the functioning of organs such as the pancreas, the colon, and the kidneys. The origin and regulating areas of this *srotas* are the hard and soft palates in the mouth and the pancreas. Water and fluids are carried in this channel.

Nutrition of Tissues

Rasavaha Srotas is the system of vessels that carry the plasma and lymph. The areas where it originates and that regulate its functioning are the heart and the blood vessels. The liver, the spleen, and bone marrow are also involved. This is considered an especially important *srotas* since it provides the foundation for the internal pool that is the matrix of nutrients for the entire body. Chyle, lymph, and plasma are carried in this channel. *Raktavaha Srotas* is the circulatory system, the system of vessels that carry blood. Its organs of origination and control are the liver and the spleen. *Mamsavaha Srotas* is the system of channels that pervade the muscles. Its origin is considered to be in the skin and the ligaments, which control it. The factors associated with muscle tissue structure and physiology are carried in this channel. *Medavaha Srotas* is the system of channels that pervade the adipose or fat tissues. Its origin and regulation is situated in the kidneys (including the adrenal glands) and the abdominal omentum. The components necessary for fat tissue are carried in this channel. *Asthivaha Srotas* is the system of channels that perfuse the osseous or bone tissues. Its origin is considered to be in adipose tissue and the pelvic bones of the hip. The components necessary for bone tissue are carried here. *Majjavaha Srotas* is the system of channels that supply the marrow and nervous system, including the cerebrospinal fluid. Its origin and control sites are in the bones and in joints, and the materials related to bone marrow, cerebrospinal fluid, and nervous tissue.

Elimination of Wastes

Svedavaha Srotas is the channel system that is the vehicle for the movement of sweat and the sebaceous fluids. Its origin is adipose tissue, skin, and hair follicles. *Mutravaha Srotas* is the channel system that transports urine. Its origin is the kidneys and the urinary bladder. *Purishavaha Srotas* or *Varcovaha Srotas* is the channel system that carries the feces. Its origin is the colon and the rectum.

Mental Functioning

Manovaha Srotas is the channel system that is correlated to mentation, thinking as well as mood and emotions. Its material origin is considered to be in nerve tissue. The "mental" aspect of this system is termed *Manas* (mind) and is connected to the *Majjavaha Srotas* and the *Shukravaha Srotas* in a special way. Mental experience, per se, is considered to be more closely tied in with the *Manomaya Kosha* or mental sheath that exists on the subtle energetic level of the individual's total makeup.

Sexual and Reproductive Functioning

Shukravaha Srotas is the group of channels that constitute the reproductive system in the male and in the female. Its origin in the male is the testes; in the female, its origin is in the uterus and ovaries. Reproductive fluids are carried in this channel. Some texts differentiate the *Shukravaha Srotas* as being the male reproductive system in contrast to the *Artavavaha Srotas,* considered the female reproductive system, and place the female *srotas* in its own class. *Artavavaha Srotas* or *Rajavaha Srotas* is the system of channels that are involved in menstruation and, in part, some reproductive functions and sexual secretory products. Its origin is the uterus. *Stanyavaha Srotas* is the channel system relating to lactation and to carrying breast milk. Its origin is the uterus.

THE DIGESTIVE PROCESS

Digestion: East and West

In Western medicine, the digestive system is considered the domain of processes that occur chiefly within the gastrointestinal (GI) tract. By contrast, in Ayurveda, digestion is considered a whole body process within and outside of the GI tract. Digestion always takes into account not only foods in the conventional sense, but also herbal substances, which are considered to have medicinal effects. It occurs not only within the gastrointestinal tract but extends to processes as they cross into the circulation (absorption) and into every tissue, tissue system, cell membrane, intracellular substance, and across and within the nucleus of the cell (assimilation). The concept of digestion is also applied to the nutrition of mental faculties; the mind is fed by experience. Nutrition is made possible by the entire spectrum of digestive processes as viewed by Ayurveda: GI primary digestion, absorption across the GI tract, and assimilation into tissues, cells, and also into the mind. Ultimately, the spirit and the quality of consciousness are affected.

Digestion, Pharmacokinetics, and Pharmacodynamics: A Short Course in Western Pharmacology

In Western physiology and pharmacology, digestion denotes the preparatory processing of food substances (proteins, fats, and carbohydrates) when taken into the mouth and, in final phases, acted upon in the colon. The processing (metabolism) of drugs (pharmacokinetics and pharmacodynamics) is viewed in a qualitatively different manner (Hardman & Limbird, 2001). A drug is defined as any substance (natural, semisynthetic, or purely chemical in origin) that in very small quantities can be used to modify a chemical process or physiological processes in the body. Ordinarily, drugs are thought of as medicines to cure diseases, or as psychoactive substances that alter brain and mental functioning. The word "drug" is etymologically derived from the Dutch/Low German word "droog," which means "dry," since in the past, most drugs were, in fact, dried plant parts.

Digestion of foods begins in the mouth with saliva and amylase enzymes digesting starch. In the stomach, the enzymatic digestion of proteins is initiated and foodstuffs are reduced to liquid form. The liver, considered the center of metabolic activity in the body, provides bile salts to the small intestine to digest and to facilitate the absorption of fats. The pancreas, an endocrine and exocrine organ, provides digestive enzymes to the small intestine to digest fats, carbohydrates, and protein. The final stages of chemical enzymatic digestion occur in the small intestine where the initially large macromolecules of protein, fats, and starch have been digested into the micromolecules of amino acids, fatty acids, and glucose in order to expedite the transport and absorption of these nutrients into the circulation. Cutting-edge research in endocrinology and digestive processes has only recently discovered the critical role of the "gut hormone," incretin. As soon as food reaches the stomach, incretin is secreted by the small intestine. It has manifold effects on the systemic regulation of blood glucose. In the pancreas, it activates beta-cells to produce insulin and alpha-cells to decrease glucagon production; in the stomach, it modulates glucose absorption; in the liver, glucagon from the pancreas slows down the production of glucose from stored liver glycogen; and in the brain, incretin acts to regulate appetite. Endogenous incretin is very short-lived, lasting less than two minutes. Synthetic incretins are now available for diabetic management. Intravenous incretins such as exendin-4 mimic natural incretin in the body; oral incretins act as enhancers of endogenous incretin. In the colon, water is absorbed, bacterial fermentation takes place, and feces are formed.

The question of how long ingested foods remain in the GI tract is unsettled. It is generally accepted, however, that 50 percent of stomach contents are emptied between 2.5 and 3 hours; total emptying of the stomach occurs between 4 to 5 hours; 50 percent emptying of the small intestine occurs between 2.5 to 3 hours; and transit through the colon is accomplished between 30 to 40 hours.

Drugs are handled differently from foods. They are not digested. Drugs participate in pharmacokinetic and pharmacodynamic operations in order to be processed, exert their effects, and then to be metabolized and eliminated.

Pharmacokinetics denotes the regulation of the manner in which the whole body acts on a drug from its ingestion through to its elimination or excretion. There are four major phases of pharmacokinetics. First, *absorption,* the transport of the active drug moiety from the GI system, essentially the small intestine, takes place. Second, *distribution* of the drug through the portal vein into the liver occurs. Here, a process of initial metabolism takes place, which is called "the first-pass effect." A great deal of the drug substance is inactivated and then eliminated at this stage. In this presystemic elimination phase, a significant amount of ingested drug is extracted from the available blood pool. Whatever active drug remains is then carried away from the liver by hepatic veins into the inferior vena cava. The inferior vena cava is a large vein that carries deoxygenated blood from this area and from the lower body to the right atrium of the heart to be oxygenated. From here, the drug goes into the general, systemic intravascular circulation, the bloodstream.

The essential feature of the distribution phase is the transfer of the drug from intravascular to extravascular compartments in the body. The target site might be localized to the brain, heart, or some other organ. Multiple sites pervading the entire body may also attract the drug. At this point, the drug binds to plasma and to tissue proteins. This occurs in interstitial and intracellular areas. When bindings occur, the response of cell receptors occurs. On an empirical level, one sees the clinical response. The effects a drug produces are called the process of pharmacodynamics.

Pharmacodynamics denotes the regulatory process governing the therapeutic effects of a drug, the mechanisms that produce a drug's effects. It is the pharmacologic response at the active target site, the cell receptor. This receptor is usually a cellular or tissue protein, as, for example, hormones, growth factors, neurotransmitters, nucleic acids, and proteins. Changes in the rate of neurotransmitter synthesis, increases, and decreases occur. Issues such as dose response curve, therapeutic index, drug tolerance, drug dependence, and drug withdrawal are pharmacodynamically determined. Receptor proteins at target sites may be highly specific to only one organ (for example, brain or heart), or they may be widespread and generalized over the entire body.

Although most drugs act through receptor-binding mechanisms, other processes play into drug responsiveness within the body. Some of the more important ones are the following: cellular membrane disruption, chemical reactivity, interaction with enzyme proteins, interaction with structural proteins, interaction with carrier proteins, and interaction with ion channels.

In order to inactivate a drug, the third phase of pharmacokinetics occurs. It is called *metabolism*. After a drug has exerted its effect on cell receptors, it is returned to the liver. Drug metabolism, biotransformation, and inactivation occur within the liver. The metabolism of most drugs occurs primarily in the liver but also to some extent in the small intestine. Drug-metabolizing enzymes catalyze demethylation, dealkylization, and oxidation of nitrogen, sulfur, and carbon atoms. Although metabolism usually inactivates a drug, it may have the opposite effect at times. Drug metabolism is considered to occur in two phases: an oxidative change, and conjugation of a drug or drug metabolite to form a more water-soluble compound that can be readily excreted by the kidneys. Phase-one drug metabolism is catalyzed by the hepatic cytochrome P450 (CYP) isoenzymes. Inhibition of drug metabolism by the interaction of two drugs, or a drug and an herb, can elevate levels of the parent drug, prolong its pharmacological effects, and possibly cause untoward or toxic effects.

The final phase of the pharmacokinetic processing of a drug is called *elimination*. At this point, the drug has been chemically altered so that it may be excreted in the urine through the kidneys.

This brief and simplified overview of standard Western conceptions of food digestion and drug pharmacology, in fact, merely approximates an understanding of a highly complex series of biochemical and physiological processes. After absorption out of the GI tract occurs, the pharmacokinetic processes of drug disposition (distribution, metabolism, and elimination) proceed almost in simultaneity. Within these multifaceted processes, the pharmacodynamic actions of the drug occur to cause cell receptor changes and empirically observable clinical responses.

AGNI: THE ENERGY OF THE DIGESTIVE AND METABOLIC FIRE

In Ayurveda, digestion and the concept of *Agni* are virtually identical. *Agni* and digestive processes, therefore, are discussed at this juncture since they can be considered fundamental physiological activities within the body. Further aspects of digestion will be addressed in Chapter 8 on nutrition. It is to be remembered that in Ayurveda, the broad concept of digestion of substances refers not only to proteins, fats, and carbohydrates, but also to botanicals, plant substances, herbs, and mineral preparations (*bhasmas*).

The concept of *Agni* is central in Ayurveda. It is the energy of transformation having divine attributes. References to it are found in the ancient Vedic texts, especially *Rig-Veda* and *Atharva-Veda*. In the latter, *Agni* is described as a destroyer of demons and diseases; in addition, it is seen as the body's capacity to replenish the muscle tissue that has been destroyed by external factors. *Agni* is viewed as the power of transformation and as the mediator between the macrocosm (*Brahmanda*) and man (*Pinda*). *Agni* is characterized by various qualities: upward mobility, fragrance, heat, dryness, and lightness. The feature of upward mobility in *Agni* is considered its prime attribute.

Agni, ontologically positioned on the subtle, ethereal, or energetic plane, is situated in the whole body but especially in the functional aspects of the biological *Pitta dosha. Agni,* which is *sukshma,* works through the medium of *Pitta,* which is *sthula* (gross). Whereas *Agni* as a subtle force controls all metabolic processes in the body, it is regarded as the digestive fire itself, and as such is traditionally understood as a dry and upwardly flowing energy (*urdhva gamitva*). The *Pitta* in the body is regarded as a coarser or more material substance that acts chiefly as the container of *Agni,* and as such is more liquid and able to flow in all directions. This digestive *Pitta* is usually understood as the functioning of the subdosha, *Pachaka Pitta,* the *Pitta* of the small intestine. *Ranjaka Pitta* is the *Agni* of tissue metabolism. *Alochaka Pitta* facilitates visual perception. *Bhrajaka Pitta* maintains the skin's color and temperature.

Sadhaka Pitta in the brain and in the heart acts to facilitate comprehension, lucidity, understanding, knowledge, memory, and emotion. Desire, envy, and confusion as well as loving feelings rise from *Sadhaka Pitta.*

The body *Agni* is called *deha Agni*. It is also called *kaya Agni* when the body is viewed in its dynamic, metabolic, and transformative dimension. *Agni* has the following associations:

1. *Ayu:* life,
2. *Varna:* the skin's complexion—color, texture, and appearance,
3. *Bala:* physical strength,
4. *Utsaha:* dynamism,
5. *Upchaya:* physical build,

6. *Prabha:* the body's luster,
7. *Ojas:* the body's vitality,
8. *Swastha:* health, and
9. *Prana:* the Pranic energy of the breath.

Although the entire concept of *Agni* is highly complex and nuanced with a variety of far-reaching subtleties, a short reference and correlation to Western physiological concepts is apt at this juncture. *Agni* as the process of digestion implies a multitude of conversion processes. Chief among these is the conversion of oxygen to energy, and the conversion of ingested substances to energy. Perhaps, the principal site in the body for both these transformations resides within the mitochondria. These are small organelles ranging from one per cell to millions per cell. The inner membranes of the mitochondria are sites of electron transport and cellular or aerobic respiration. Most of the oxygen taken in through the lungs finds its way here and is thus converted into cellular and bodily energy. Within the mitochondrial matrix inside the inner membrane are found complex molecular systems, chief of which is the citrate cycle. It is here that assimilated nutrient foods convert into energy in the form of ATP, adenosine 5 triphosphate. In addition to its significance as the powerhouse of the cell and the healthy maintenance of energy levels, the mitochondria are also involved with the process of aging. Cutting-edge research in psychiatric neuroscience is beginning to postulate a link between mitochondrial impairments and mental illness (Gardner & Boles, 2005). Mitochondrial defects are, in part, produced by intracellular nucleic acid damage caused by free radicals and oxidative stress. These degrade overall cellular function and are directly related to the aging process. Such oxidative stresses along with chronic and subclinical states of inflammation have been implicated with dysfunction of the endothelial lining of all blood vessels within tissues and associated with many disease conditions. As will be addressed throughout this book, Ayurvedic interventions target oxidative stress, free radical formation, inflammatory processes, and *Ama* (toxin) production.

The impact of stress, therefore, on intracellular and tissue functioning has received and is currently receiving renewed attention in Western medicine. The neuroscience research alluded to in the Introduction suggests that the psychological experience of stress correlates with a variety of measurable hormonal (e.g., cortisol) and endothelial cell membrane changes. These changes impact brain structures such as the hippocampus and amygdala and so affect learning, memory, and emotional regulation. The physiological status of the body, for example, that of glucose regulation (Metabolic Syndrome, pre-diabetes, and hypoglycemia) is also directly affected. Hence, the rationale for Ayurveda's close attention to *Agni* and all its ramifications can be seen as undeniably pragmatic. Its real-life applications as described in Chapters 8, 9, 10, and 11 are timely.

DIGESTION AND THE THREE PRINCIPAL *AGNIS*

Agni is most intimately identified with the entire energetic processes of digestion, absorption, transport into the circulation, and cellular and tissue assimilation. *Agni* is present and active in the body from the cellular level to the more complex levels of tissues, organs, and organ systems. This concept of *Agni* and digestion extends to include transformations and processing that also occur in the psychological domains of thinking and feeling. *Agni,* therefore, is the active principle of transformation that operates on all five sheaths that make up each individual in his or her entirety: (1) *Annamaya Kosha,* the physical sheath; (2) *Pranamaya Kosha,* the breath sheath; (3) *Manomaya Kosha,* the mental-emotional sheath; (4) *Vijnanomaya Kosha,* the wisdom-intelligence sheath; and (5) *Anandamaya Kosha,* the bliss sheath. The optimal functioning of *Agni* is directly related to the optimal quality of one's life on all levels: physical, psychological, subtle, and consciousness.

Charaka describes 13 forms of *Agni:* 1 *Jathatagni,* 5 *Bhutagnis,* and 7 *Dhatuagnis.* Sushruta describes 10 forms of *Agni:* 5 subdoshas of *Pitta,* and 5 *Bhutagnis.* Vagbhata describes 23 forms of *Agni:* 5 subdoshas of *Pitta,* 5 *Bhutagnis,* 7 *Dhatuagnis,* 3 *dosha-Agnis,* and 3 *mala-Agnis.*

The description and functioning of the principal digestive *Agnis* is threefold:

1. **Jatharagni,** the primary digestive metabolic fire that occurs in the gastrointestinal tract; *Jatharagni* has two parts: (a) *Avasthapaka* and (b) *Vipaka;*

2. **Bhutagni,** which includes the digestive transformations that are related to the processing of the five Elements in the liver; and

3. **Dhatuagni** (secondary digestion or tissue metabolism), which includes the digestive and metabolic processes within the *dhatus* or tissues and in the liver.

The processing of nutrition is one of *Agni*'s central functional roles. This has two important components: (1) handling the six primary tastes (*rasa*) that Ayurveda identifies within any ingested substance and (2) facilitating the tissue assimilation into the body of each of the five primary Elements within a food or herb. An extensive discussion of *rasa* as "taste" in the Ayurvedic view will be found in Chapter 8. Two ordinary procedures for optimizing *Agni* on all levels are drinking plain hot water on a regular basis and fasting periodically.

JATHARAGNI AND PRIMARY DIGESTION: AN OVERVIEW

Jatharagni is the primary or central digestive fire located in the lower part of the stomach (*amashaya*) and in the small intestine (*grahani*). There is only one *Jatharagni,* and it is closely allied to *Pachaka Pitta.* Foods and medicines that enter the mouth elicit a specific energy (*virya*) that is released by and operates through the *Jatharagni*. Food (*anna*) that enters the mouth becomes partially processed into one uniform suspension that when completely digested by *Jatharagni* (yet unassimilated) becomes known as *ahara rasa*. This is a complex suspension of nutrients that is the penultimate end product of digested food. It can be equated in many ways to the Western physiologic concept of digestive "chyle," which is the turbid white or pale yellow fluid taken up by the lacteals from the intestine during digestion and is carried by the lymphatic system via the thoracic duct into the circulation. This first phase of the primary macrodigestive process in the gastrointestinal tract is *Avasthapaka,* also termed *Prapaka*. It is the initial or preparatory processing of food. Food and *ahara rasa* are processed by *Jatharagni*.

Ahara rasa is composed of unhomologous, biologically unavailable nutrients. It is transported by hepatic veins out of the gastrointestinal tract and into the liver. When processed by the *Bhutagnis* of the liver, it becomes homologous, biologically available, and assimilable to the human body, mind, and consciousness. At that point, chyle is a precursor to all ultimate tissue formation. This precursor or *poshaka* is called *asthayi dhatu*. When this pool of initial *asthayi dhatu* nutrients is acted upon by *Dhatuagnis* (digestive tissue fires), it then becomes the stable (*sthayi*) fundamental and essential (*poshya*) cell and tissue nutrient called *rasa dhatu*. The word "rasa" is derived from the verb "*sara,*" which means to move or to flow steadily. The concept of *rasa* connotes continuous circulation and is fundamental in Ayurveda.

Rasa dhatu (mature plasma tissue) is formed simultaneously with *asthayi rakta dhatu* (immature blood tissue). This occurs in the liver and also in the spleen and in bone marrow. The *asthayi rakta dhatu* (immature blood tissue) is converted into *sthayi rakta dhatu* (mature blood tissue) by *rakta dhatuagni* (blood tissue digestive fire) within the *Raktadhara kala* (blood tissue holding membrane) about ten days after the formation of mature *rasa*. The *Raktadhara kala* is intimately related to the endothelial lining of blood vessels. After this fully formed blood passes through the heart for oxygenation, it then goes into the general, systemic circulation and flows through the entire body to supply nutrients, oxygen, and *prana*. This process is also part of the successive formation of the body's seven fundamental tissues.

The second part of primary digestion, the final microdigestive effect of the digestive process, is termed *Vipaka,* the postdigestive effect. It is also termed *Isthapaka*. In *Vipaka,* nutrients are assimilated into cells and tissues. Between part one of primary digestion, *Avasthapaka,* and part two, *Vipaka,* there are two other major digestive processes: first, *Bhutagni,* which is the microdigestive *bhavana* (processing) of the Five Great Gross Elements that occurs inside the liver, and second, *Dhatuagni,* which is called "secondary digestion" or tissue metabolism. *Bhutagni* is intimately allied with primary digestion in time, space, and functional integrity. *Dhatuagni,* although occurring continuously, is more allied with both *Vipaka* and processes that occur after primary digestion as a whole. All digestion occurs simultaneously and in parallel. For academic purposes, a linear schematic of four sequential phases is described as follows.

THE FOUR MAJOR PHASES OF DIGESTION

I. *Avasthapaka:* Macrodigestion inside the Gastrointestinal Tract, Part One of Primary Digestion

Avasthapaka is the only macrodigestive process that occurs inside the gastrointestinal tract.

Avasthapaka has three subphases: (1) *Kapha* or the sweet phase, (2) *Pitta* or the sour phase, and (3) *Vata* or the pungent phase.

The *Kapha* or sweet phase begins in the mouth under the influence of the *Bodhaka Kapha*. It is dominated by the Sweet taste. As food descends into the esophagus and reaches the stomach, the alkaline and heavier secretions of the *Kledaka Kapha* continue the frothification and "humidifying" digestive action. In the stomach, the Earth and the Water Elements are digested and absorbed.

The *Pitta* or sour phase begins after about 90 minutes in the lower part of the stomach and in the small intestine by the action of the *Pachaka Pitta*. The Sour taste predominates. The *Pittas* of the liver and pancreas heavily contribute to this digestive phase. In this main digestive stage, the Fire Element is digested and absorbed.

The *Vata* or pungent phase begins about four hours after the initial ingestion of food and takes place in the large intestine. This is dominated by a Pungent taste caused by the action of the *Apana subdosha* of *Vata*. The Air and Ether Elements are considered to be digested and absorbed here. Waste materials are also processed in this phase. The undigested portion of the Earth Element is discarded as feces. In addition to the usable portion of water and minerals that are absorbed, indigestible portions are also reabsorbed and traverse the body to collect other wastes (*kleda*) in the journey to the kidneys for ultimate excretion. The purest aspects of the Air Element that contain *Prana* are absorbed into the body; unusable Air is expelled.

II. *Bhutagni:* Microdigestive *bhavana* (Processing) of Primary Elements inside the Liver

Bhutagni refers to the five Elemental digestive/metabolic fires that reside in the liver. Each of the Five Great Gross Elements has its own particular transformative *Agni*. They are closely related to the activity of *Ranjaka Pitta of the liver*. Both correlate with liver enzymes. After the *ahara rasa* is produced from the *Avasthapaka* process of primary digestion, it travels to the liver for a critical transformation. The *ahara rasa* is considered a nonhomologous or nonhuman *Ahamkara* collection of "food" with the five primary Elements in an initially raw, unassimilable state. It is regarded as unprocessed (*asamskara*). The primary function of the *Bhutagnis* is to transmute the unhomologous primary pentads into the homologous or "humanized" Elements that are in a form (materially, energetically, and spiritually) that may become part of the human *rasa* or plasma. The *Bhutagnis,* therefore, function like a humanizing *Ahamkara* stamp to transform materials, such as foods and herbs, which have their own nonhuman identity, into the *rasa* that is qualitatively human and, thus, capable of being optimally utilized.

This qualitative transformation is essential for the entire digestive/metabolic/assimilative process, especially for the assimilative processes of *Vipaka,* to continue in the balanced and healthy production of the tissues. The *Bhutagnis,* therefore, create homologous primary Elements that are part of the unstable precursors (*asthayi dhatus*) of the tissues. Later on, in the secondary processes of digestion or tissue metabolism after each tissue *Agni* (*dhatu Agni*) acts upon its precursor, then a stable, formed, and mature tissue is produced, the *sthayi dhatu.*

The *Bhutagnis* also play another critical role in providing the five sensory organs with their respective primary Element in order to enhance their structural integrity and to promote their healthy functioning. If *Ahamkara* fails to properly stamp the Elements within the dietary inputs with its individualized and human identity, then these raw inputs remain raw and are not absorbed as nutrients. They become toxic and are referred to as *Ama.* This has critical significance for health and disease. The more *Ama* produced, the more difficult it is for the individual's innate *Ahamkara* and intuitive sense to discriminate what further materials in the environment would be best to take in. The faulty functioning of *Manas* thus prevails and wrong choices are made. This further increases *Ama* and leads to a vicious cycle until some corrective action is taken to dispel the accumulated toxins and restore *Ahamkara* to a more balanced state enabling the individual to make healthier choices for his or her particular constitutional needs.

III. *Vipaka:* The Postdigestive Effect, The Second Part of Primary Digestion

The conception of *Vipaka,* the postdigestive effect of food, is unique to Ayurveda. *Vipaka* refers to the delayed and whole body, systemic effect exerted by each of the six tastes (Sweet, Sour, Salty, Bitter, Pungent, and Astringent) of a food or an herb. *Vipaka* denotes the actual assimilation of nutrients into cells and tissues. It is a kind of microdigestive process, the last phase of primary digestion, which contrasts with and complements the macrodigestive actions that take place in *Avasthapaka.*

Vipaka has two sites of action. First, it occurs in the colon; and second, it occurs at the tissue and at the cellular level of assimilation. *Vipaka* is the dynamic action, the point of contact, wherein *Agni* sparks the unique assimilative transformation of nutrients into the tissue cells. This is the juncture at which what was previously the "not self" transmutes to become the human *Ahamkara,* a profound identification with and humanization of the outside world to become one with man.

Vipaka has a long-term effect on the *doshas*. Since the effects of *Vipaka* occur and are generalized throughout the entire body, there is no one specific site of action. The end results of *Vipaka,* however, are more circumscribed than those of *Avasthapaka.* Whereas in early primary digestion, each of the six primary tastes of food produces a different digestive effect matching each of the six tastes, in *Vipaka* only three resulting tastes with metabolic effects are produced. This viewpoint, generally held today, was first described by Charaka (c. 700 B.C.) in his ancient medical treatise *Charaka Samhita.* The three *Vipakas* are (1) Sweet, which promotes *Kapha;* (2) Sour, which promotes *Pitta;* and (3) Pungent, which promotes *Vata.* Their effects relate to the *doshas.* A short time thereafter, Sushruta (c. 600 B.C.), in his medical text *Sushruta Samhita,* described the *Vipaka* concept but emphasized only two nutritive taste end results: (1) *brimhana,* the building up of tissue substance and (2) *langhana,* the catabolic breakdown of bodily substance. Their effects relate to the tissues.

The sweet *Vipaka* results when either the Sweet or Salty taste (*rasa*) has been ingested. This results in an increase of saliva and the alkaline secretions of the stomach. The primary metabolic effect is one of cellular nutrition and the building up of the body's tissues. Nutritive aspects of *Kapha* are primarily increased. Ayurvedic tonic foods and herbs most often have a sweet *Vipaka.* In addition, the elimination of waste products from the colon is enhanced.

The sour *Vipaka* results when the Sour taste has been ingested. This increases acid and bile secretions in the stomach. Although not as highly nutritious as in the sweet phase, the sour phase produces some nutrition for all the body's tissues, especially the plasma, with the exception of the reproductive tissue. Since *Pitta* is stimulated, metabolic processes are enhanced. Nutritive *Kapha* for cells and tissues is chiefly produced. The elimination of waste products from the colon is also enhanced.

The pungent *Vipaka* results when the Bitter, Astringent, and Pungent tastes are ingested. This *Vipaka* is not considered to be useful for either nutrition or for elimination. *Vata* may be increased, at times, and *Kapha* may be reduced. In other words, catabolic processes are enhanced. The therapeutic actions of medicinal herbs, however, can be enhanced. This knowledge of foods and herbs that have a pungent *Vipaka* becomes useful in recommending proper dietary regimes and in selecting therapeutically efficacious herbal remedies.

IV. *Dhatuagni:* Secondary Digestion, or Tissue Metabolism, or Microdigestion inside Each Tissue

Dhatuagni is tissue metabolism and digestion. *Dhatuagni* is also referred to as the *tissue fire, tissue metabolism* of the *srotas,* and as *secondary digestion.* Tissue metabolism is a microdigestion. It occurs within the *dhara kala* (the containing, nutritive, and metabolic membrane), specific for each particular tissue *srotas* or tissue channel system. All *Dhatuagnis* must be in balance to prevent excessive tissue breakdown and to ensure proper tissue buildup. A supporting primary site for *Dhatuagni,* in addition to tissue sites in the *srotas* and in the specific *dhara kala* membranes, is within the liver, especially through the medium of *Ranjaka Pitta.* This important metabolic site correlates heavily with the endothelial lining of blood vessels.

The term "digestion" in Western medicine properly denotes only those primary breakdown processes during the course of nutrition that occur solely within the gastrointestinal tract. They are preparatory to the absorption and the transport of nutrients across the gut into blood and plasma. In Ayurveda, by contrast, the term "digestion" is broadened to denote a dual concept: first, digestion inside the gastrointestinal tract (*Avasthapaka and Vipaka*) and second, digestion outside the gastrointestinal tract. The latter includes *Bhutagni* transformations in the liver, *Dhatuagni* (liver and tissue-based) assimilations, and tissue-based *Vipaka* assimilations into the cells and the tissues.

Dhatuagni transforms the homologous, though unstable, tissue precursors (*asthayi dhatus*) into the stable, formed, and mature tissues (*sthayi dhatus*). Thus, *poshaka* precursors by means of *Dhatuagnis* become the matured, fully nourished *poshya* tissues. *Dhatuagni* follows and also accompanies *Vipaka* processes of assimilation.

There are seven *Dhatuagnis* that produce their respective tissue elements (*dhatus*) and their respective waste products (*dhatus malas* and *kleda*). They are (1) *rasadhatuagni,* (2) *raktadhatuagni,* (3) *mamsadhatuagni,* (4) *medadhatuagni,* (5) *asthidhatuagni,* (6) *majjadhatuagni,* and (7) *shukradhatuagni.*

The seven *Dhatuagnis* activate after and work in conjunction with *Vipaka.* Tissue formation is a cascade process that begins with the formation of *rasa* (plasma) and ends with the formation of *shukra* (reproductive tissue) and *Ojas.*

THE FIVE ELEMENTS AND THE RESPECTIVE TISSUES THEY NOURISH

The five Elements are conceptually regarded both as material building blocks and as representing physiological functions. This dual aspect is reflected in their contribution to the makeup of the bodily tissues, and to overall bodily structure and functioning. The Elements provide the scaffolding for the physical, anatomical *prakruti.*

1. The Earth Element is the primary material that is the basis for the body's nutrition and bulk. The protein of the body in the form of muscle is fed by the Earth Element. In principle, all bodily substances, for example, *doshas, dhatus,* and *malas,* and so forth, must contain some portion of the Earth Element.

2. The Water Element contributes to plasma, blood, reproductive fluids, muscle, nerve, and fat tissue.

3. The Fire Element contributes to the digestive enzymes, hydrochloric acid, and hemoglobin. Muscle and fat tissue contain some Fire Element.

4. The Air Element contributes to the buildup of bone and nerves.
5. The Ether Element contributes to the nutrition of the five senses and to the mind.

The reproductive tissue in both males and females contains all five Elements.

AMA: METABOLIC TOXIN

A fundamental concept in Ayurveda is that of *Ama. Ama* is a broad conception that generally refers to metabolic toxins or impurities that participate in disease and cause overall unhealthy conditions. The word *Ama* is derived from the Sanskrit root *am,* which means to harm, damage, and weaken.

Along with the optimal production of the end products of digestion that contribute to the overall health and nutrition of the body, there is usually a simultaneous and ongoing buildup of *Ama. Ama* results from less than optimal digestion, biotransformation, and detoxification processes, and this is the *usual* rather than the exceptional case even in essentially healthy individuals. *Ama* may form at several junctures in the span of the entire digestive and assimilative process. If the *Jatharagni* operating in the GI tract during primary digestion is weak, *Ama* may be produced within the GI tract. It may remain there and it may also travel outside the GI tract into tissues. In the liver, if the *Bhutagnis* are weakened, *Ama* may form. If in the secondary metabolism of the tissues, the *Dhatuagnis* are weak, then *Ama* may form. If *Pilu Agni* (cell *Agni*) is weak, *Ama* may be produced. If *Pithara Agni* (digestive fire of the nuclear membrane of the cell) is disturbed, then *Ama* may form. *Pithara* may be likened to the large complexes of *pilus,* that is, molecules developing as a result of combinations of *anus* or *pilus* by the transformative action of *Agni.*

Improper eating habits, poor food choices, seasonal and lifestyle factors, aging, and *dosha* vitiations all contribute to impairments of the digestive process and to the production of *Ama,* which constitutes an array of metabolic impurities. *Ama* is considered a metabolic toxin since it, in part, represents the incomplete or undigested portion of food that becomes nonassimilable yet materially present in the gastrointestinal tract. Vitiated *doshas,* particularly *Vata,* instigate *Ama* and propel (*prakupita*) it into the circulation and into the tissues. *Ama* becomes mixed in with *doshas.* Such states of contaminated *doshas* are termed *sama dosha. Ama* becomes mixed in with tissues and also can obstruct *srotas* or channels of circulation on many levels.

Ama acts as a toxic, virtually "foreign" mass within the tissues. From a Western perspective, unstable metabolic end products (reactive oxygen species, free radicals, and so forth) resulting from biotransformations of exogenous nutrients and toxins and endogenous sources (mitochondria, peroxisomes, lipoxygenases, NADPH oxidase, the cytochrome systems, and cellular wastes) contribute heavily to *Ama* production and subsequently to impaired physiological function. Such oxidative stress, inflammatory responses, and cytokine formation contribute heavily to the endothelial dysfunction of the cardiovascular system's lining throughout the entire body. Endothelial cell dysfunction is associated with a variety of disease states such as impaired glucose regulation, impaired vasodilation and vasoconstriction, hypertension, atherosclerosis, inflammatory conditions, blood-clotting abnormalities, and impaired angiogenesis. It has been suggested that the amyloid bodies found in pathological conditions such as Alzheimer's disease are products of *Ama*. *Ama* has a propensity to seek out and then deposit itself in weakened and devitalized body tissues (*kervaigunya*). This becomes the ground for future disease processes. In Ayurveda, herbal substances commonly used in cooking as well as available in supplement form have been shown to reduce inflammatory responses; these include *tulsi* (holy basil), *haridra* (turmeric), *sunthi* (ginger), and *shallaki* (Boswellia serrata). The central factor, however, that determines whether *Ama* will be produced is the healthy or impaired state of *Agni,* the digestive fire, on every level.

FOUR CONDITIONS OF THE BODY'S *AGNI*

An individual's *Agni,* transformative energy, is a function of his or her individual baseline constitution or body/mind type (*prakruti*). *Agni* may become disturbed intermittently as a result of daily and seasonal intervening factors as has been previously mentioned, for example, diet, life-style, weather, and so forth. Four functional conditions of the *Agni* are recognized: (1) *Sama Agni,* balanced *Agni;* (2) *Tikshna Agni,* high *Agni;* (3) *Mandagni,* low *Agni;* and (4) *Vishama Agni,* variable, irregular *Agni.*

The Ayurvedic system strives to achieve and maintain *Sama Agni.* The condition of impaired *Agni,* however, is the more usual finding. *Mandagni,* a state of hypometabolic functioning, is commonly found in individuals with *Kapha* predominance, constitutional types characterized by a large frame, tendency toward overweight, consistent appetite, good endurance, and an overall tendency toward stability and possible lethargy. *Tikshna Agni,* a state of hypermetabolic functioning, is found in *Pitta* predominant persons. These individuals have medium frames, average body weight, strong appetites, compelling drive, and competitive and directive personality styles. *Vishama Agni* is seen in those who tend toward the *Vata* constitution characterized by irregularity and unevenness both in physical and in psychological areas but adept at spontaneity and creativity.

Any impairment of *Agni,* whether it is related to high, low, or variable *Agni* energy levels, causes *dosha* vitiation and disturbance. It may be said that impaired *Agni* (typically *Mandagni*) acts as the ultimate piece of a complemental series of causative factors to spoil the *doshas,* and spoiled *doshas,* in turn, act to impair *Agni. Agni* and the *doshas* have a dynamic, reciprocal interaction, which can be beneficial or detrimental.

Some discriminative contrasts differentiate *Agni* from *Pitta*. *Agni* flows upward, is dry, and is fragrant. *Agni* resides on the *sukshma* level of existence. *Pitta* flows downward, is damp, slightly oily, liquid, and can be malodorous. *Pitta* resides on the *sthula* level of existence. *Pitta dosha* is the biological container for *Agni,* which is energy.

Finally, it would not be an overstatement to say that *Agni,* in truth, is more than just the digestive/metabolic fire. *Tejas* is the subtle (*sukshma*), energetic, and more consciousness-based force of fire from which the biological (*sthula*) *dosha, Pitta,* arises. *Agni,* in some sense, can be considered to be the actual *flame of life* although the ontological and ultimate nature of *Agni* is so vast and numinous that it defies any academic classification. *Agni,* in essence, denotes transformation, conversion, transmutation, and change. In the history of Hinduism and in Ayurveda, *Agni* and power, almost approaching divine proportions, have been equated.

Agni can be thought of as the energy of the physiologic fire that keeps the body warm and in a constant state of active metabolic transformation. *Agni* not only controls the body's temperature; it is the body's temperature. Akin to the concept of *virya,* the energetic potency of substances whose root is the *Jatharagni, Agni* maintains the optimal, functional heating of the entire body. This includes proper temperature regulation in order to limit the inordinate proliferation of *krimi,* the ancient Sanskrit term referring to bacteria, viruses, fungi, parasites, and other infectious organisms. In its more concrete forms, *Agni* energizes and exerts its actions through the five subdoshas of *Pitta.* The ingestion of food ignites *Agni,* and this, in turn, activates the workings of *Pitta,* especially in the processes of digestion, absorption, metabolism, transformation, and assimilation.

5

PRAKRUTI AND VIKRUTI

PRAKRUTI: CONSTITUTIONAL TYPE

The Ayurvedic conceptualization of individualized constitutional types or *prakruti* is a cornerstone of basic theory and practical application (Svoboda, 1989). An individual may be understood to have three specific constitutional dimensions: (1) physiological (*dosha*) makeup, (2) physical body (the Elements), and (3) psychological character, the mind (the *Maha gunas*). Their unified pattern, the relationship of all these together, constitutes the individual's baseline *prakruti*. The pattern of their imbalance and disharmony is called the *vikruti*.

The term *prakruti* is identical with the term *Prakriti;* both mean first creation. To differentiate their pragmatic use in the Ayurvedic system, they are here spelled differently. *Prakriti* is the metaphysical concept that refers to the primordial, first, and continual stirrings within the Absolute, the *Purusha,* that initiate the beginnings of all the rest of the created world.

The word *prakruti* specifically refers to the unique psychobiological (anatomical, physiological, and psychological) constitution of a specific individual person. The individual *prakruti* is expressed on several levels. The first is through the anatomical body, which is the expression of the particular arrangements of the Five Great Gross Elements. The second is through the body's physiological functioning, which is an expression of the genetic code and the manner in which the *doshas* operate. The third level is through the mind, which reflects the quality and influence of one's share of the *Maha gunas, Sattva, Rajas,* and *Tamas.* An individual's *prakruti* determines how the varieties of matter that structure the body, the energies that regulate its functioning, and the mind are handled. The *prakruti* reflects an inborn baseline metabolic pattern, the strength, weakness, and trends that the genetic equipment as it interacts with the environment produces. *Prakruti* is intimately allied with *Agni,* the core template determining an individual's baseline metabolic code and capacity for transformations on physical, energetic, and mental levels.

In a psychological sense, understanding of the self, so to speak, is equated with an understanding of one's *prakruti.* To maintain overall mental and physical health, one must know one's *prakruti*. Knowing which *doshas* predominate within the constitution, for example, permits one to select an array of proper life choices (*pathya*) that includes compatible foods, lifestyle activities, exercise, and a career that will not aggravate or unduly increase naturally dominant bodily *doshas*. The usual guidelines suggest incorporating things with opposite doshic qualities, therefore maintaining balance of the *doshas* and of the *prakruti*. In addition, knowing which of the Five Great Gross Elements and knowing one's measure of the *Maha gunas* aids in self-understanding.

Ayurveda firmly adheres to the proposition that each person, though sharing common human characteristics, is essentially a unique creation, a "first creation." The use of the concept *prakruti,* therefore, is a fractal dimension of the concept of *Prakriti;* it connotes the property of complex self-similarity and implies the understanding that all of reality operates ontologically as series of dynamic, cyclic repetitions. The individual *prakruti* is as significant as the cosmic *Prakriti;* both are first creations, yet on different scales in time and space. The concept of normality, in this view, sets the individual as his own standard. An individual is considered normal to the extent that his *prakruti* is functioning in a balanced and optimal manner according to its own unique, inherent configuration.

Individual, baseline *prakruti* is established at conception and during the gestation process. Four main factors contribute to it: (1) *shukra beej,* the paternal genes; (2) *artav beej,* the maternal genes; (3) *ksheta* and *garbhashaya,* the state of the mother's womb and her plasma nutrition (*ambu*); and (4) *ritu* or *rutu,* the season of the year. Some Ayurvedic schools of thought differentiate the unalterable *prakruti* established at birth (*janma prakruti*) from the developed and later stabilized *prakruti* (*deha prakruti*) found in adulthood.

The genetic contributions of the parents contain varying amounts and combinations of the influence of the three *doshas, Vata, Pitta,* and *Kapha* (VPK), as well as definite proportions both of the primary Elements (Ether, Air, Fire, Water, and Earth) and of the *Maha gunas* (*Sattva, Rajas,* and *Tamas*). Each individual has certain inborn proportions of these. They constitute the "normal" given baseline of *Vata, Pitta, Kapha,* Elements, and *Maha gunas.* Only when this overall baseline becomes imbalanced does the *vikruti* (temporally imbalanced constitution for the specific individual) state of the constitution arise.

An individual's *prakruti* is tridimensional: *doshas,* Elements, and *Maha gunas.* However, ordinarily only the doshic (VPK) aspect is emphasized since a major goal of Ayurvedic treatment is balancing the *doshas.* When the *prakruti* of an individual is set, it then has a relatively stable arrangement of the VPK principles. This established composition of the doshic principles is one part of an individual's *prakruti,* which determines that individual's particular physiologic mechanisms for energy regulation.

For example, although everyone has *Vata, Pitta,* and *Kapha,* some may have a predominance of the *Vata* (propulsion) principle and only very small amounts of the *Pitta* (transformation) and *Kapha* (consolidation) doshic principles. This *prakruti,* therefore, would be called a *Vata prakruti.* If there were a predominance of *Pitta* and *Kapha* with a very small amount of *Vata,* then that *prakruti* would be called a *Pitta/Kapha prakruti.*

Although each person has some of all three *doshas* in the *prakruti,* usually one or two *doshas* predominate. The *prakruti* combination, while relatively constant, will undergo the natural cyclic changes of relative increase and relative decrease of component *doshas* depending on diet, life-style, stress, season, and intercurrent illness. The actual possible combinations are numerous. It would not be an exaggeration to state that, in fact, there are as many individual *prakrutis* as there are individuals. In general, however, seven basic types of doshic *prakrutis* are commonly found. They are (1) *Vata,* (2) *Pitta,* (3) *Kapha,* (4) *Vata/Pitta,* (5) *Pitta/Kapha,* (6) *Vata/Kapha,* and (7) *Vata/ Pitta/Kapha.*

The concept of *prakruti* has both morphological and functional implications. Since *prakruti* denotes one's body type and constitution, the physical appearance, structure, and innate metabolic tendencies that are produced contribute in characteristic ways to the instinctive responses elicited in an individual by all varieties of external and internal stimuli. The *prakruti* determines, in part, an individual's attraction to sensory inputs, food, ideas, and so forth. In addition, *prakruti* shapes how these are taken in and processed both physically and psychologically. The *prakruti* has been called one's "first nature." This connotes the given and reflexive response of an individual to the environment. It may periodically produce negative disturbances over the course of time since growth, maturation, and development change with varying environmental situations. In Ayurveda, these are recognized and addressed. An Ayurvedic understanding of *prakruti,* which includes a correct recognition of real needs and how to address them, produces what has been called one's "second nature." This second nature may be thought of as one's intelligently developed capacity to manage the more undisciplined and reflexive inclinations of one's first nature.

In Ayurveda, the individual is considered to have an innate faculty for correct discrimination, the *Buddhi* aspect. This is supported by the *Sattva Maha guna* and by adequate *Tejas.* The body (*sthula sharira*), in fact, tends toward responding to life events in this innately programmed correct manner. The errors, mistakes, and impairments in judgment, however, that usually prevail, are a function of *Manas* or mind. Mind, in this sense, refers to the more undisciplined and indiscriminately pleasure-seeking human proclivity. This reflects excess *Tamas Maha guna.* The system of Ayurveda assists in educating one to be cognizant of these physical and mental influences. Taming the mind and developing the powers of intelligent discrimination follow from this. One's *prakruti* or constitutional predilection, therefore, does not absolutely predetermine preferences and subsequent doshic balances or imbalances. *Prakruti* sets a psychophysiological tone that can be modulated by the experiential interactions between itself and the environment. Although one's *prakruti* has innate proclivities, the ability to selectively choose different options such as foods or lifestyle habits permits one to experience considerable flexibility in daily living.

CONSTITUTIONAL CHARACTERISTICS

I. *Dosha Prakruti:* Physiological and Metabolic *Prakruti*

Prakruti is made up of varying mixes of *Vata, Pitta,* and *Kapha,* and one's unique *prakruti* reflects the varying functional qualities inherent in that constitutional doshic type. Keen attention to this doshic *prakruti* is the central and leading consideration that runs through all of Ayurveda.

Since all *prakruti* types contain some degree of all three *doshas,* and since the doshic predominance may not contain every one of that *dosha*'s characteristic attributes (*gurvadi gunas*), there is a gradation of and a nuanced tone to each individual's *prakruti* expression. Overall *prakruti* has three basic domains of expression: (1) physical, (2) physiological, and (3) psychological, which all together add to the almost infinite variety of individual *prakruti* expressions. *Dosha prakruti,* the physiological dimension, will be discussed here; and it will also include aspects of its inextricable physical and psychological dimensions. With this in mind, a general outline of the seven basic *dosha prakruti* conformations is examined.

Vata-*Predominant* Prakruti

Vata prakruti has the basic attributes of *Vata dosha:* cold, dry, light, subtle, mobile and erratic, sharp and quick, hard, rough, and clear. Excess *Vata* causes constriction (*sanchoc*) and spasm both mentally and physically. The physical characteristics associated with those having *Vata* predominance are tendencies toward thin bodies, small frames, protuberant and cracking joints, crooked or uneven teeth, small eyes, cold limbs, and dry skin. The variable and irregular metabolism characteristic of *Vata* types contributes to this. Sleep may be light and of brief duration. Physical activity is irregular and may run in spurts of excess versus little activity. There may be restlessness and low stamina. The quality of the voice may be breathy and its strength weak. *Vata* types are usually very talkative. There is difficulty falling and staying asleep. Appetite and digestion is irregular, as well, and there is a tendency toward constipation. There is a preference for warmer climates and an aversion toward cold. Body odor and sweating are minimal. Women may have irregular menstrual cycles. Sex drive and libido are said to be characterized by much imagination, intermittent excesses, and lower than average fertility. In contrast to the other doshic types, there is a significantly greater susceptibility to disease, and life span is believed to be relatively shorter. Disease manifestations tend to include pain, arthritis, neurological problems, and proneness to mental disorders.

The cognitive characteristics of *Vata* include exceptional alertness and quick, active mental functioning. New ideas are quickly grasped, but just as quickly forgotten.

The psychological characteristics of the *Vata* constitution include creativity, freshness, and enthusiasm. *Vata* types may be emotionally sensitive, high strung, changeable, fidgety, impulsive, and restless. They may have tendencies toward anxiety and fear (*bhaya*). Many new activities are launched, but since concentration is usually mobile and difficult to sustain, they often fail to complete an endeavor. Finally, there is a tendency toward ambivalence and indecisiveness.

Pitta-*Predominant* Prakruti

Pitta prakruti has attributes characteristic of *Pitta dosha:* hot, slightly oily, light, subtle, mobile and steady, sharp and penetrating, soft, smooth, clear, flowing, and insidiously creeping. The physical characteristics of *Pitta prakruti* include moderate body build, fair or reddish and warm complexion (*chaya*), thin and sparse hair, and a tendency toward having skin moles and freckles. Appetite is usually strong and digestion is good. There may be problems with gastric hyperacidity. Bowel movements are regular but may be loose; at times, *Pitta*'s heat may produce constipation. Sleep is sound and of medium duration. There is a tendency toward sweating and more pronounced body odor. There is an aversion to warm and humid weather and a preference for the cold. Sexual desire is moderate and its gratification is able to be modulated; fertility is average. Life span is believed to be moderate. Disease proneness includes manifestations of inflammatory conditions, fevers, hyperacidity, hypertension, and liver and blood problems.

The cognitive characteristics of *Pitta* include a sharp, penetrating intellectual faculty with little ambivalence. *Pitta* types tend to be well organized, methodical, and managerial in style.

The psychological characteristics of *Pitta* types include bold, focused, courageous, and intense outlooks with strong leadership qualities. There is a tendency toward competitiveness and critical judgment. Emotionally, *Pitta* types may be demanding, irritable, temperamental, and seek dominance in relationships and groups.

Kapha-*Predominant* Prakruti

Kapha prakruti has properties of the *Kapha dosha:* cold, damp, heavy, coarse, compact, dull, soft, smooth, sticky, and dense. Physical characteristics include solid, heavy body build, good musculature, a tendency toward overweight and subcutaneous fat, soft and oily skin, thick, dark, wavy hair, large soft eyes, and large uniform pearly white teeth. Appetite is hearty, digestion is slow, and elimination is regular. Although there is a pronounced tendency toward lethargy and laziness, physical stamina is excellent, as is general health. There is a tendency to sleep a great deal; sleep is heavy and deep. There is an aversion for cool, damp climates. *Kapha prakruti* experiences steady sexual desire, which is typically very strong. Sustained sexual arousal is easily achieved. Fertility is usually excellent. Life span is believed to be very long. Disease proneness includes manifestations of respiratory disorders, edema, hypercholesterolemias, obesity, and tumors.

Cognitive characteristics reflect a slowness to learn but very good long-term memory. Intellectual pursuits are not especially sought since learning requires effort and repetition, which is not characteristic of the *Kapha* style.

The emotional characteristics of *Kapha prakruti* include a calm, tranquil, and steady mode. There is a great deal of patience, perseverance, and compassion. They tend to be generous, affectionate, loving, forgiving, conservative, and loyal. Speech is clear and unhurried; the voice is deep and melodious. In excess, *Kapha* types tend toward possessiveness, attachment, greed, depression, and lethargy.

Vata/Pitta Prakruti

Vata/Pitta prakruti shares characteristics of both of its *doshas*. Build may be slightly more muscular than that of the sinewy *Vata* persons. They may be gregarious, friendly, and talkative. Digestion is good with more of a quality of regularity. The possible *Vata* motivated tendency toward addiction may express itself as self-medicating with prescribed or illicit drugs; this may be enhanced by the *Pitta* tendency toward wishing to intensify experiences. There is an energetic and more focused quality to their daily activities.

Pitta/Kapha Prakruti

This *prakruti* favorably combines the penetrating sharpness of the *Pitta* with the stability and evenness of the *Kapha dosha*. Body build is more muscular and solid. Energy level is high and sustainable. There may be a tendency, however, to unwarranted overconfidence.

Vata/Kapha Prakruti

The *Vata/Kapha* may be quick and efficient as well as steady and determined in a more regular fashion. There may be some impairment of digestion because of a predominance of the cold attribute common to both *Vata* and *Kapha,* as well as a marked intolerance of cold climates.

Vata/Pitta/Kapha Prakruti

This triple *dosha* type is termed the *sama prakruti*. When in balance, this *prakruti* has the optimal characteristics of all three *doshas*. This constitutional type, however, is not common.

FINER DISTINCTIONS OF *PRAKRUTI*

The basic conceptualization of *prakruti,* however apparently simple, is not, in fact, simplistic. There are finer degrees of differentiation that take into account aspects of the individual across the metaphysical-physical spectrum.

II. Physical *Prakruti* and the Five Elements

Prakruti as described so far has taken into consideration the doshic composition that reflects specific physiologic tendencies. The structural and morphological constitution of the physical body by comparison can be understood in a more detailed fashion from the perspective of the *Pancha Mahabhutanis,* the Five Great Gross Elements (Ether, Air, Fire, Water, and Earth).

The Ayurvedic conceptualization of the Elements, it is to be remembered, goes beyond a denotation of their merely being groupings of material atoms. It includes their additional transcendent operations consisting of a host of implicit innate trends that impart characteristic and enduring form, content, and functional traits to the substances that they compose. The Five Great Gross Elements (*Mahabhutanis*) can be conceived of as a set of "emblems" with which all things in the created universe are composed and organized into patterns, which can be perceived.

Each individual has a predominance of one or more of the primary pentads, the Five Great Gross Elements. Each one of the pentadic Elements is associated with distinctive characteristics that are more apparent on the physical, material level, although these Elements also impart psychological characteristics as well. It is to be remembered that the individual *doshas,* themselves, are combinations of specific primary Elements. The operation of the *doshas* is determined, in part, by their share of the Elements they contain. *Vata* is composed of a predominance of Ether and Air, *Pitta* has a predominance of Fire and Water, and *Kapha* has a predominance of Water and the Earth Element.

1. *Akasha,* or the Ether Element, is associated with large, spacious, and grand characteristics. Very large physical features such as excessively large ears or bone structure, for instance, suggest a predominance of Ether in the body. Large, external body openings such as the ears, the eyes, and the nostrils are characteristic of the Ether Element. Those who have a predominance of Ether have internal organs that are well differentiated; their internal body spaces, the thoracic and abdominal cavities, for example, may be large. The intercellular spaces may occupy more area. This greater spatial configuration contributes to an increased potential for movement and change. Hearing and sound sensitivities are associated with Ether and so are more prominent as is the strength of the speech faculty. Weak areas in the makeup of the body include a tendency for dilatation potentially manifesting in cardiac (congestive heart failure) and in lung problems (emphysema). Tinnitus of the ears may also be present. Psychological qualities that are expansive, highly

intuitive, and reflect high values and moral standards are also characteristic, especially since the sattvic *Maha guna* is predominant. *Sattva* is the innate tendency in *Prakriti,* creation in all its manifestations, toward purity, balance, coherence, intelligence, and spirituality.

2. *Vayu,* or the Air Element, is associated with a great deal of mobility, dynamism, and amorphousness. Physical appearance manifests complexions that are light, pink, dry, and rough. The skin may be thin and show prominent blood vessels, tendons, and joints. There is a characteristic popping sound to the joints commonly referred to as "cracking of the joints." Those with a pre-dominance of the Air Element may be excessively active and may become easily exhausted. Their sleep is light. In addition to being easily distractible, potential weaknesses include susceptibility to the cold, various neuromuscu-lar disorders, neuralgia, arthritis, and a tendency to constipation. *Prana* and *Vayu* are intimately related and produce a well-developed sense of touch and a talent for healing. The rajasic *guna* is active in this Element. *Rajas* is the *Maha guna* within *Prakriti* that is associated with turbulence, stimulation, and activity.

3. *Tejas* or *Agni,* the Fire Element, is associated with transformation, change, conversion, and visual perception. Intensity and penetration are asso-ciated with a predominance of this Element. Those with a *Tejas* predomi-nance appear bright, light, and may have complexions with a pinkish hue. They do not tolerate heat well and have light but sound sleep. They are highly intelligent, organized, managerial, competitive, somewhat impatient, and strive for success and achievement. When ill, they suffer from inflammatory conditions, hyperacidity, ulcers, hypertension, and are prone to hematologi-cal disorders. Their sense of sight is particularly acute. *Sattva* and *Rajas* are the *Maha gunas* that predominate.

4. *Ap* or *Jala,* the Water Element, is characterized by features that are liquid, flowing, and capable of taking on multiple forms without losing iden-tity. Those with a Water Element predominance appear to have light and fair complexions with bodies that are soft, smooth, somewhat "chubby," and cool to the touch. Their hair is soft and wavy; they appear well nourished and "moist." They are particularly affectionate and loving, and their sexual drive is strong. The sensory faculty of taste may be acutely developed. When out of balance, they are prone to congestive disorders such as colds, sinus difficul-ties, and asthma. They may develop edema and diabetic conditions. *Rajas* and *Tamas* are dominant. *Tamas* is the *Maha guna* associated with inertia, cohesion, density, and materiality.

5. *Prithvi,* the Earth Element, is a solid, dense, rigid, and relatively inert substance. This manifests in a physical appearance that is "earthy" with large, heavy muscular and bone development. The complexion may tend to be swarthy, darkish in tone. Although their general demeanor is slow and some-what lethargic, they tend to be calm and stable. They have a need for more than an average amount of sleep. Those with a dominant Earth Element tend to be forgiving and capable of deep and lasting attachments. With such a

strong complement of the most material Element, there is a susceptibility to tumors of bone and muscle. The olfactory sense may be particularly well developed. These persons are more tamasic in nature. *Tamas* is dominant.

III. Psychological *Prakruti* and the *Maha Gunas*

The predominance of the quality of one or more of the three *Maha gunas* or *Trigunas* (*Sattva, Rajas,* and *Tamas*) at the time of birth contributes to the psychological constitution of an individual. The cultivation of consciousness later on in life heavily contributes to one's psychology and the dominance of one or more of the *Maha gunas*. The *Maha gunas* can never exist singly in nature; they are always present in differing admixtures, and this gives infinite variety to the substances they imbue. Nuances of temperament and overall character style are virtually unlimited and defy adequate classification. A general description of the key attributes of various subdivisions of the major three doshic constitutions will be given, however, in order to suggest an approximate understanding of the Ayurvedic notion of some psychological *prakruti* types. Sattvic (pure) qualities are primary and foster movement toward increased consciousness. Rajasic (turbulence) and tamasic (dulling) qualities, significant, necessary, and modulating as they are, tend to be less consciousness enhancing.

Vata *Psychological* Prakruti

The sattvic complement provides a positive energy with features that include harmony, equilibrium, adaptability, strong healing qualities, quick comprehension, and a general sense of cheerfulness, happiness, and freshness. This is the mental domain closest to pure consciousness. The subtle essence of *Vata* is *Prana*. When the *Maha guna Sattva* is cultivated, *Prana,* the life force, expands in a leading manner. It imparts a life-enhancing energy that optimizes healthy will power and psychological directedness. The subtle essence of *Pitta,* which is *Tejas,* and that of *Kapha,* which is *Ojas,* also grow in dominance.

The rajasic component, although providing the driving force of enthusiasm, fresh creation, and novelty, may create, at times of imbalance, a disturbing overall dynamic that includes features of anxiety, insecurity, agitation, volatility, explosiveness, impulsivity, inattention, indecisiveness, mania, loquaciousness, oppositional behavior, irresponsibility, and insomnia.

The tamasic *Maha guna,* in states of imbalance, may tend to produce *fear,* depression, dishonesty, boredom, and proneness to drug addiction, sexual perversion, and other mental disturbances.

Pitta *Psychological* Prakruti

The sattvic complement creates discriminating intelligence (*prajna*), clarity of consciousness, lucidity, sound judgment, harmony, courage, organizational proficiency, self-discipline, will power, and leadership. Loving attitudes and empathy also arise from sattvic *Pitta*. When the *Maha guna Sattva* is cultivated, the subtle essence of *Pitta,* which is *Tejas,* gains exceptional prominence. *Tejas* brings with it penetrating intelligence, luminosity, and keen powers of discrimination. The subtle essence of *Vata,* which is *Prana,* and that of *Kapha,* which is *Ojas,* also intensify.

The rajasic *Maha guna* can introduce turbulence, competitiveness, ambitious and dominating tendencies, manipulation, irritability, defiance, inordinate anger, *envy,* pride, narcissism, and lustful desire. The insidiously creeping quality of *Pitta* manifests as secretive undermining of the productive efforts of others. This is envy.

Likewise, in a state of imbalance, the tamasic component may elicit hate, violence, destructiveness, and a proneness to criminal activities. When unopposed by *Sattva, Tamas* plus *Rajas* brings confusion.

Kapha *Psychological* Prakruti

The sattvic *guna* creates a quality of harmony, calm, serenity, peace of mind, compassion (*karuna*), empathy, devotion, nurturance, loving, devotion, the ability to forgive, stability, and strength. When the *Maha guna Sattva* is cultivated, the subtle essence of *Kapha,* which is *Ojas,* strengthens. *Ojas* imparts confidence, mental equanimity, peace of mind, and secure groundedness. The subtle essence of *Vata,* which is *Prana,* and that of *Pitta,* which is *Tejas,* also are enhanced.

The rajasic component may enhance the qualities of inordinate attachment, materialism, greed, greedy lustfulness, and jealousy.

The tamasic component can produce inordinate coarseness, lethargy, sloth, dull comprehension, apathy, boredom, procrastination, and severe depression.

ANCIENT AYURVEDIC CLASSIFICATION OF PSYCHOLOGICAL *PRAKRUTI*

Ancient Ayurvedic texts describe seven psychological types of sattvic *prakruti,* six rajasic types, and three tamasic types. These have been based, in part, on cultural, archetypal, religious, and mythological figures. This sort of typing is not commonly done in initial assessments nowadays. A very brief description, which is of historical interest, however, is as follows.

1. Sattvic *prakruti* types: All sattvic persons possess strong features of intelligence, purity, clarity, and balance. *Brahma prakruti* demonstrates characteristics of purity, sincerity, respect, and profound intelligence. *Mahendra prakruti,* modeled after the figure Indra, shows bold leadership, courage, bravery, power, obedience, and devotion. *Varuna prakruti* has strong faculties for integration, regulation, tolerance, patience, pleasing language, prefers cold, and is associated with water. *Kaubera prakruti* is

skilled at accumulating wealth and implementing ideas. *Gandharva prakruti* appreciates beauty, dance, and fine fragrances. *Yama prakruti* is fearless (*abhaya*), pure, a person of action, observant of propriety of timely action, and shows mental equanimity. *Asra prakruti,* in the spirit of the *rishis,* demonstrates balanced, steady intellectual and spiritual development; it reflects responsible, faithful, and disciplined behavior for self and for the welfare of the social group.

2. Rajasic *prakruti* types: All rajasic *prakruti* types possess strong desire, drive, ambition, and envy. *Asura prakruti* is solitary, somewhat hedonistic, and intimidating. *Sarpa prakruti* is intelligent but may be deceitful and deceptive. *Sakuna prakruti* shows volatility, anger, and overindulgence in eating and sexual behavior. *Raksasa prakruti* shows very strong anger and envy, irreligiously, and arrogance. *Paisaca prakruti* is bold, daring, amorous, and lacking in shame. *Praita prakruti* is selfish, greedy, lazy, irritable, and quite miserable because of inordinate envy, jealousy, and greed.

3. Tamasic *prakruti* types: All tamasic *prakruti* types share an unintelligent base, dullness, lethargy, and tendencies toward overindulgence. *Pasava prakruti* is very dull, sluggish, unable to follow directions, and overindulgent in sleep and sexual activity. *Matysa prakruti* is unwise, cowardly, interpersonally aggressive, unstable, and said to be fond of water. *Vanaspatya prakruti* shows vegetative traits such as being sessile and lacking in attention to the prescribed Vedic goals of *dharma* (responsibility and virtue), *artha* (working for food, clothing, and shelter), *kama* (healthy enjoyment), and *Moksha* (the freedom of self-actualization).

OVERALL ASSESSMENT OF *PRAKRUTI*

The evaluation of an individual's *prakruti* constitutes the first step in the Ayurvedic assessment process. *Prakruti* is generally regarded as an estimation of the doshic constitution that regulates metabolic functioning. A more comprehensive analysis yields a spectrum of highly individualized constitutional types that is comprehensive and includes anatomical, physiological, and psychological subgroupings. The constitution of the physical body has a predominance of one or more of the primary Elements. This imparts the special qualities characteristic of that Elemental predominance. The constitution reflecting the physiological functioning is determined by *dosha* predominance. This, too, has at its base an underlying dominance of the features of the Elements unique to those respective predominant *doshas.* Through pulse diagnosis, to be discussed later, one may ascertain a subdosha predominance, as well, that would give more specificity to the overall *prakruti* assessment. Finally, there is a significant psychological dimension to the *prakruti.* The dominance and quality of the *Maha gunas* determine these psychological trends.

Ayurveda recognizes the individuality of each person. A comprehensive analysis of *prakruti* reveals the detailed specificity of the constitution. One finds variations in body type and psychological type, for example, *Kapha dosha prakruti* with *Manas* having a rajasic and tamasic quality. A person like this, for example, would have a sturdy, well-nourished body, and a mind that was driven at times and lethargic at others. The *prakruti* conception, therefore, should be understood as indicating an operational form that acts as a template or blueprint to process data that come in from the changing environments and subjective states that each individual experiences. The influence of the environment and the intentions and actions of an individual in joint fashion cause learning, insight, and change to occur. The cultivation of consciousness requires active and intentional work in order for change to develop over time. This makes for a virtually infinite number of constitutional types and possible responses and eliminates the idea of a set and rigidly predetermined system.

SATTVIC ENHANCEMENT

A basic principle in Ayurveda is to foster the development of sattvic (pure) qualities and to regulate the balance of rajasic (turbulent) and tamasic (dulling) tendencies. The *BioPsychoSpiritual* perspective takes into consideration *prakruti* on all levels: physical, physiological, mental, and spiritual. *Sattva* and spirituality, the refinement of consciousness, go together hand-in-hand.

Sattvic attributes include enhanced, refined consciousness, intelligence, compassion, purity, balance, integration, mental and emotional equanimity, trustfulness, and the inclination toward a healthy life-style. To the extent that a simple word might approximate, yet possibly oversimplify, the profound meaning of *Sattva,* the term *goodness* is suggested. Rajasic trends, especially when negative, include the inordinate experience of desire, lust, concupiscence, anger, and cynicism. Tamasic qualities, when devoid of sattvic modulation, tend toward inertia, concreteness, avarice, depression, fear, ignorance, and violence. Sattvic enhancement reinforces one's *BioPsychoSpiritual* integration.

VIKRUTI

Prakruti refers to the specific Elemental, doshic, and *Maha guna* pattern that makes up an individual's normal, baseline body type or constitution. When the baseline *prakruti* reflects the healthy, normal functioning of each of its component *doshas* alone and in their combined state along with proper Elemental status and *Maha gunas,* this condition of balance is the condition of health (*swastha*). When the overall *prakruti* becomes disturbed, especially when the *doshas* qualitatively vitiate, accumulate in excess, decline and become deficient, or interact among themselves negatively, the *prakruti,* now, is referred to as *vikruti,* the imbalanced state of an individual's constitution. This pattern of disharmony and imbalance (*vyadhi*) is the subject of Ayurvedic diagnosis and treatment.

The *vikruti* condition is common and reflects the rapidly changing state of the *doshas*. These imbalances can result from diet, life-style, stress, age, and the seasonal shifts. They may be temporary and last for a few days or weeks or accumulate over the seasons and last for years. Doshic imbalances ordinarily accompany imbalances in the Elemental and *Maha guna* dimensions of overall *prakruti*. An important aim of Ayurveda is to evaluate the basic *prakruti*, assess the current imbalanced state, the *vikruti*, and restore optimal functioning to each *dosha* and proper balance to the overall functioning of the *doshas* individually and as they interact in combination. The Ayurvedic view of health and disease, health maintenance, disease prophylaxis, and treatment addresses these issues.

6

HEALTH AND THE DISEASE PROCESS. I

HEALTH AND DISEASE CONCEPTS

The concept of health and well-being (*swastha*) in Ayurveda grounds itself in the idea of fostering the balanced and normal functioning of the *doshas,* that is, restoring the *prakruti* to equilibrium when states of constitutional imbalance (*vikruti*) occur. The optimal functioning of each *dosha* in the body creates a homeostatic condition that is conducive to overall health and well-being. Ayurveda views health as a comprehensive state of physical, mental, and spiritual balance that includes the optimal quality, quantity, and functioning of the *doshas, dhatus* (tissues), *srotas* (channels), *malas* (waste products), *Agni* (digestive fire), and *Ojas* (immune system).

Disease is viewed as a state of imbalance (*vyadhi*) of component dimensions on all physical, mental, and spiritual levels that when integrated make up the entire person. Within an individual, disease takes hold when the *Agni* becomes impaired. Multiple factors both within and outside the person contribute to impaired *Agni*. *Agni* is the fire of conversion, digestion, and change within every aspect of an individual.

Subsequently, imbalances in the *doshas* produce further impairments in the functioning of the *Agni,* the channels, the tissues and organs, waste products, and the immune system. Terms for disease are *roga* and *amaya*. The commonly used term *roga* denotes that which causes pain and is derived from the Sanskrit root *ruj* meaning to pain.

The word *duhkha* denotes suffering and usually accompanies descriptions of ill health and disease. It represents a fundamental Buddhist and highly significant Ayurvedic assumption. Man and woman's existence in the created world appears to be inextricably bound to fluctuating cycles both of pleasure and of unpleasure. The negative pole of these encompasses a broad experiential range from unpleasure, discomfort, unpleasantness, discontent, and unhappiness to pain, suffering, sorrow, and misery. Hence, the concepts of disease and *duhkha* reflect a disharmony in the integrity of the person as a *BioPsychoSpiritual* being.

The antonym of *duhkha* is *sukha,* which translates as happiness, favorableness, or pleasantness. It is said that Charaka, the renowned Ayurvedic luminary, described disease as the condition in which "ease" is lost. The sense of this is understandable since the root *kha* suggests a space (similar to the notion of Ether or *Akasha*) within the body, and *su* suggests a positive or favorable state, a condition of ease. The term *sukha* implies that bodily spaces such as the channels are in a positive or favorable condition.

The concept of health in Ayurveda also implies the condition of wholeness. This conceptualization has several connotations such as included in the term *samhita* that means integrated compendium, and in the term *advaita* meaning nonduality. Since the medical practice of Ayurveda, as its name implies, derives from the ancient tradition of the *Vedas,* a significant metaphysical dimension of the health concept is fundamental and complements its biological denotation.

The heart of the Ayurvedic concept of health contains the idea that the quality of one's consciousness should reflect wholeness, clarity, coherence, and integration. Consciousness here denotes the most intimate experience of awareness. It goes beyond a merely neurological description of alertness, orientation, and the cognitive capacity to concentrate. The definition of disease in the Ayurvedic view would suggest that any condition of impaired consciousness connotes a state of imbalance and some degree of disease, unhappiness, dysphoria, malaise, yearning, and a desire for the satisfaction of unfulfilled needs. This perspective demonstrates the intrinsic spiritual foundation of Ayurvedic thought. Although Ayurveda in theory and in practice places emphasis on the physical dimensions of man, a core spiritual underpinning, consciousness based, remains its central ballast.

THE THREE UNIVERSAL CAUSES OF ALL DISEASE

Ayurveda describes three common overriding causes that contribute to all disease. They are (1) *Prajna-aparadha,* (2) *Kala-Parinama,* and (3) *Asat-myendriyartha Samyoga.*

Prajna-aparadha

Prajna-aparadha is a concept that is variously translated as *the mistake of the intellect, volitional transgression,* or *an error in wisdom;* it is the loss of the memory of oneness. This default cognitive blindness is perpetuated, in part, by coercive habit/habituation over time, for example, repeating the same stereotyped thinking and behaviors in a reflexive, automatic manner without pause, introspection, and contemplative reflection.

Man's manifestation in the material world of flesh and blood constitutes his potential for rediscovering intrinsic unity within diversity by means of efforts toward repair, restoration, and the development of ever-greater expansions of consciousness. This is the meaning of *Moksha* (liberation) and *samadhi* (enlightenment). *Prajna-aparadha* is the universal human condition marked by a pervasive neglect or forgetting of the aforementioned interconnectedness of the essential unity of spirit and matter. With the original state of all being considered to be one of pure consciousness, birth into the world makes us oblivious of our origins. Most are distracted by the belief that only the conventionally discernible, material aspects of experience exist and, therefore, must constitute reality in its entirety. The assumption that man is, in fact, an integral composite of matter and spirit in an enormous, almost ineffable, universe of matter and spirit is the underpinning for positing the underlying cause of this cognitive distortion.

In the Ayurvedic view, material realities are not understood as being false or even as being "bad." *Prajna-aparadha* maintains an everyday amnesia whose consequences result in forgetting the integrated field of existence, of consciousness at the heart of matter. Ordinary cognition influenced by *Manas* (mind) experiences life as *Viparita-Bhavana,* that is, with the erroneous conviction that the visible world of appearances alone is the only reality. This given condition is explained by the influence of *Manas* on *Buddhi* (the discriminating intellect). Intrinsic to the nature of *Manas* is a dulling of *Buddhi*'s clarity. The epistemological term in Sanskrit for this misinterpretation is called *avidya* and is roughly translated as ignorance. The delusional understanding of reality that results from this becomes formalized in the Sanskrit term *Maya,* meaning the world as ordinarily experienced is a grand illusion.

The fundamental significance of *Prajna-aparadha* lies in the fact that the presence of *Manas* tends to produce an incorrect mind-set. This is the source of the perversions of desire that repetitively seek pleasure in an almost reflexive fashion. The upshot of this is the ordinary tendency to make wrong and unwholesome choices. In this view, wrong choices are ultimately caused by the puissant influence of *Prajna-aparadha* on the operation of *Manas.* The functioning of *Manas* is virtually synonymous with that of "desire" (*mara, raga, trishna, and iccha*) in almost every sense.

The natural, reflexive tendency of *Manas* is to divert attention to extremes. These focal extremes are points near the ends of the spectrum of indulgence and renunciation. *Manas* is always tempted to seek opposites. In fact, the middle path is suicide for *Manas. Manas* desiring life avoids the middle.

What must be clearly understood, if not stressed, is that *Manas,* per se, is not intrinsically bad or evil. *Manas* can be considered man's calling card, ticket of admission, and key to unlocking entry into the manifest world as ordinarily experienced. In this sense, *Manas* is neutral; it functions as an instrument that provides ample access to a world that can be experienced in perceptual, sensuous, and sensual ways. It provides information and opportunities that an individual is free to process in an unlimited number of ways.

If choices and behaviors that are more wholesome (*satmya*) continually discipline and healthfully shape *Manas,* then the functioning of *Buddhi,* the reality intellect, will be empowered, especially in the physical body (*sthula sharira*). This, in turn, will foster more wholesome, safe, and reality-based psychological choices (*pathya*) that are conducive to health. In this way, listening to the body and addressing its needs yields health; the mind or *Manas,* however, may continue to perpetuate ignorance, hedonistic choice, and thus disease.

Prajna-aparadha is responsible for impairments in the functioning of three important psychological faculties: (1) *dhi,* (2) *dhruti,* and (3) *smruti.* *Dhi* (wisdom) is the capacity of the *Buddhi* intellect to comprehend the intrinsic laws of nature (*ritam*) and to cognize that which is real from that which is unreal, illusory, and delusional. *Dhruti* (or *Dhriti*) (patience, steadfast directedness of will) is the courage to avoid that which is harmful; it implies impulse control and willpower. *Smruti* or *smriti* (memory) is the capacity to recall or to be mindful of on a continuous basis the activities proper and conducive to health.

Kala-Parinama

Kala-Parinama refers to the transformations produced by the passage of time. It connotes the evolution and involution of states of order and disorder. This change over time refers to the activity of the *doshas.* When the normal level of a *dosha* is increased, this elevation is potentially unhealthful for the functioning of that *dosha.* When a *dosha* is decreased, this suggests less than optimal physiological functioning. Only in the condition of excess, elevated *doshas* and increased doshic functioning does a tendency toward significant imbalance and disease occur. This encompasses changes that may occur in three ways: (1) over the course of the life cycle, (2) during the course of the day, and (3) during the course of the seasonal shifts of the year.

Doshas *and the Life Cycle*

According to Ayurveda, the life cycle is divided into three epochs each having a general *doshic* predominance that acts as an underpinning to the other influences that affect the *doshic* balance. The period of childhood (*bala*), from birth to adolescence, is the time when *Kapha* (consolidation) predominates. Childhood *Kapha* dominance is associated with the normal processes of growth and the rapid development of the tissues and body structure. *Kapha* imbalances and diseases tend to be respiratory and manifest as colds and as asthma, for example. The period of adolescence (*madhya*) through midlife is considered the epoch of *Pitta* (transformation) predominance. This is the time for refining intellectual and vocational abilities. Displays of natural competitiveness are seen in sports activities, educational training, and vocational pursuits. *Pitta*-predominant diseases include inflammatory conditions such as acne, hyperacidity, ulcer, and irritable bowel syndrome, to name just a few. The period of beginning older age (*vriddha*), roughly from about 55 years onward, is the era in which *Vata* (propulsion) predominates. The influence of *Vata* tends to show itself in a broader experiential range of awareness, the "wisdom of older age," and in difficulties such as insomnia, constipation, and arthritis. These age-dependent three different doshic predominances parallel the timing of the maturational, developmental, and hormonal changes that accompany puberty and later menopause and the male climacteric. The three life cycle divisions and their chronological age correlations, however, are to be understood in a broad sense and suggest only approximations. Individual variations are so common that they take precedence in determining, for instance, the specific age of onset of the older years.

Normal Physiological Diurnal Fluctuations of the Doshas

In the course of 24 hours, the three *doshas* regularly cycle, and one will predominate over the others. *Kapha* predominates from 6 A.M. to 11 A.M.; *Pitta* predominates from 11 A.M. to 2 P.M.; *Vata* predominates from 2 P.M. to 6 P.M. At this point, the cycle begins again. *Kapha* predominates from 6 P.M. to 11 P.M., then *Pitta* from 11 P.M. to 2 A.M., and last, *Vata* from 2 A.M. to 6 A.M.

During this normal diurnal cycling, the specific attributes of the *dosha* that predominates hold sway and influence the overall functioning of the body. For example, the early morning *Kapha* predominance is associated with phlegm, water, and other waste product elimination. *Pitta* predominance around noon is associated with increased appetite and normally increased digestive capacity. Ayurveda considers noontime as the best time to have the largest meal of the day.

Normal Seasonal Fluctuations of the Doshas

The normal cyclical rise and fall of the bodily *doshas* that is produced by the effect of seasonal changes is a gradual process. The *doshas* are contained in all biological life, and this includes the plant world in addition to man and the animals. Varying seasonal conditions act as specific stimuli that elicit *doshic* reactions in the body. Since man and nature are linked in significantly identificatory ways, both respond accordingly. When qualities and attributes in nature that are *dosha* specific begin to predominate, they elicit a rise in the corresponding *dosha* within man. As one or more of an individual's baseline *doshas* increase, the baseline *prakruti* becomes temporarily imbalanced. If it returns back to its normal baseline in a reasonable amount of time, health is maintained. If its pattern remains imbalanced, the disease process begins. The seasonal variations in *dosha* predominance have three phases:

1. *Sanchaya,* Accumulation. This phase is one of very gradual accumulation or increase.
2. *Prakopa,* Aggravation or Provocation. During this phase, the particular *dosha* is at an almost maximally increased level. *Prakopa* is excessive vitiation.
3. *Prashama,* Alleviation or Pacification. This phase occurs when the previously elevated *dosha* decreases and returns to a more balanced level.

In the United States, there are four seasons: fall, winter, spring, and summer. *Vata* is related to fall and early winter, which is cold and dry. *Kapha* is related to mid- and late winter and to early spring, which is cold and damp. *Pitta* is related to early spring and summer, which is damp and hot. *Vata* begins its gradual accumulation in the summer and reaches its peak intensity of aggravation in the fall and early winter. In the late winter and spring, when the dry and cold weather becomes more clement, *Vata* is alleviated, the process of a *dosha*'s return to levels that are more physiologically normal for the body. *Pitta* begins its gradual accumulation in the late winter and spring and reaches its peak intensity in the summer. Summer is the season, therefore, when *Pitta* is provoked and aggravated. When the extreme heat of summer begins to subside as the fall season ensues, increased *Pitta* declines to levels that are more normal, a process referred to as alleviation. *Kapha* gradually accumulates in the fall and early winter and reaches peak intensity in the late winter and spring. It becomes pacified and alleviated with its normal decline in intensity in the summer.

Asatmyendriyartha Samyoga

The distinctly Ayurvedic concept of *Asatmyendriyartha Samyoga* can be translated as the unwholesome contact of the sense organs with their sense objects (*vishaya*). The "objects of the senses" ordinarily denotes perceptions both of parts (qualities) and also of complete (whole) sensory objects. This conception has typically been understood to connote sensory perception referring to the inanimate world. An important, if not even more primary, psychological extension includes the mind's intellectual conceptions of and emotional links to the animate world of uniquely significant human objects. These "object relations," as they have been called in psychodynamic psychology, are sexual in the widest sense since human desire by definition instinctively seeks an object for pleasurable satisfaction. In this sense, sexual denotes attraction whose goal is attachment with reproducing this linking experience and even more novel experiences as an inextricable motivating force. The mind (*Manas*), therefore, is sexual by nature; hence, an important value resides in purifying sexuality and in refining the mind. Relations (*samyoga*) to other human beings, moreover, constitute overriding psychodynamic meaningfulness. They influence all aspects of the self's relationship to itself and to everything else. Love, hate, envy, greed, and jealousy, for example, are forged in this way. The functioning of the sense organs has great significance since it is the central nexus (yoga, *yukti*) between the individual and the outside world. The five sense organs, ears, skin, eyes, tongue, and nose, are called the *jnanendriyas,* the organs that ingest the objects of sensory perception, the sense objects.

When the contact of a sense organ and its object is proper or wholesome (*satmya*), the subtle half of the corresponding primary great Element grasped at that contact point is absorbed. These quanta of energy, the *sukshma*

Tanmatras, then go on to feed the more immaterial sheaths (*koshas*) just as actual food and water feeds the physical sheath of the body with the primary Elements. The sense organs, therefore, are the physical vehicles through which the mind (*Manas*) and the discriminating intellect (*Buddhi*), in fact, effect the absorption of the *Tanmatras,* the subtle Essences, from experience of the outside world into the internal energetic dimensions of the individual. This energetic feeding, so to speak, not only replenishes the individual's own store of *Tanmatras.* The subsequently enhanced *Tanmatras* then go on to produce further vitalization of the body's own primary Elements that, in turn, continue to nourish and replenish the bodily *doshas, dhatus* (tissues), and so forth.

Balanced and proper contact (*sama* yoga) of the outside with the inside of the individual produces the condition of equilibrium (*samya*). Disequilibrium (*vaisamya*) may be due either to increases (*vruddhi*) or to decreases (*kashaya*).

Improper contact of the sense organs with their objects, therefore, is significant since it results in diminished nutritional input on the most subtle, vital psychospiritual levels, with consequential impairment of the interconnected system that affects nutrition on the material tissue level. It is beyond the scope of the present work to adequately discuss the "problem of electricity." Electricity was discovered about 250 years ago, and the electric light bulb was invented about 125 years later. Both these cultural introductions have had monumental effects that can be understood as having positive and negative features. A great deal of experiential impairment is correlated with electricity in its protean uses. Some outstanding aspects of this will be discussed.

Improper contact may take three distinct forms: (1) excessive contact (*atiyoga*); (2) negligible or deficient contact (*ayoga*); and (3) unnatural, perverted, or wrong contact (*mithya yoga*).

1. Ear: the sense organ for hearing. Perhaps second to vision in its multiple roles of facilitating survival and adaptation is the complex function of hearing. The inner ear acts as the sensorineural receptor organ of the auditory system. It converts an acoustic waveform ("sound") into an electrochemical stimulus that can be transmitted to the central nervous system. As this sensory transduction process occurs, the inner ear via the stereocilia hairs of the cochlear analyzes a sound signal in terms of frequency, intensity, and temporal properties. The acoustic nerves transmit this information to the brain for further complex interpretation.

Sound intensity is measured in decibels (dB). Conversational speech typically measures 60 dB. Sounds at or exceeding 75–90 dB are considered potentially damaging to delicate inner ear structures if very close and prolonged contact is made. Excessive contact consists of listening to harsh sounds, sounds with inordinately high frequencies, or repetitive discordant sounds. Noise pollution, for example, city traffic (80 dB), motorcycles at high speeds, power tools, and loud machinery (for example, lawn mowers: 90–100 dB; riveters and pneumatic chippers: 120 dB) represent an array of sounds that may be excessive over a extended period. Prolonged exposure to sound that exceeds 100 dB is harmful. Decibel levels of about 110 to 120 include chain saws, snowmobiles, and very loud music as found in rock concerts or even aerobic class environments. Firearms, guns, and cannon fire measure about 130 dB. Sounds above 110 dB, considered dangerous by the National Institute on Deafness and Other Communication Disorders, include those produced by firearms, fireworks, jet engines, and also excessively loud concerts and loud music club situations. Negligible contact consists of listening to sounds restricted to only narrow ranges of frequencies or sensory deprivation of sound input altogether. The concept of negligible contact has been referred to as "insufficient or feeble" contact. Another form of improper contact is defined as exposure to sounds that are irritating and that may be unnatural, such as a sonic boom made by an aircraft or a nuclear explosion, for example. Some Ayurvedic texts refer to this class of improper sensory contact as "perverted."

2. Skin: the sense organ for tactile sensation. Excessive contact may come from exposure to very rough objects, objects that are of extreme temperatures, or from conditions that are unfavorable over time such as damp or cold climates. Excessive exposure to wind, particularly from electric fans, is very *Vata* provoking. Excessive exposure to the cold air produced by air conditioning will lower *Agni* and its functions within *Pitta*. Negligible contact results from the absence of adequate massage. Ayurveda holds that this may constitute a significant impairment, especially for the *Vata dosha,* over the long term. Other wrong contacts involve exposure to irritants (to skin and upon inhalation) such as tobacco smoke, toxic chemicals, and potential carcinogens such as the lead in paint and possibly the ink in some older printing materials, for example.

3. Eye: the sense organ for vision. Excessive contact includes viewing inordinately bright objects, scenes of excessive or violent activity, and exposure to scenes with repetitive, unnatural, and artificial action and themes. Some examples of these include excessive viewing or staring at the sun, explosions, volcanoes, television, the cinema, computer screens, and so forth. Negligible contact results from remaining in very dark or dim places for prolonged periods. Other forms of wrong contact include viewing objects too closely or from too far a distance. The Ayurvedic literature also describes other examples of improper visual contact by citing the following: viewing frightening animals such as tigers and lions; hideously damaged objects; a solar eclipse; and natural disasters such as destructive floods, earthquakes, and so forth. The modern world also provides examples of improper or perverted visual contact as, for instance, in exposure to inordinate violence, sexuality, and artificial and natural disasters that are seen in television shows, the news media, and the cinema. The current psychiatric disorder termed Posttraumatic Stress Disorder can be linked to these.

4. Tongue: sense organ for taste. Excessive contact includes excessive intake of food and drink. Negligible contact refers to eating a disproportionately small quantity and poor quality of food. It also includes the failure to experience through taste the proper complement of the Ayurvedically required nutritional tastes that are necessary for the optimal functioning of the *doshas* in one's *prakruti*. Perverted taste contact refers to eating in a manner (time of day, season, food combinations, and so forth) that is contrary to established Ayurvedic dietary guidelines. It also includes contact with poisons and inappropriate medications and drugs.

5. Nose: sense organ for olfaction. Excessive contact includes contact with overly pungent and irritating smells such as those of chemicals like ammonia and sulfuric acid. Negligible contact includes insufficient contact with pleasing and "nutritionally fortifying" aromas such as those of essential oils that may be therapeutic and helpful in balancing the *doshas*. Olfactory experience considered wrong includes contact with smells such as those of putrefying material and noxious odors such as poisons, fumes, and pollution from trucks, cars, or aircraft.

Close attention to *Asatmyendriyartha Samyoga* and its implications is essential to physical, psychological, and spiritual welfare. In many ways, it encompasses the strategies for optimal living and the cultivation of consciousness that Ayurveda espouses. This model reflects "life wisdom," acts to normalize the negative impact of life stressors, and, in effect, enhances the ease of a life well lived.

AN OVERVIEW OF THE FOUR FUNDAMENTAL MECHANISMS UNDERLYING ALL PATHOGENIC PROCESSES

Disease is a process that occurs over time with multiple contributory factors that have a sequential history. Although all concepts of pathogenesis are complex, the Ayurvedic perspective considers four foundational processes as essential and out of which all disease manifestations occur. They are as follows:

1. *Dosha Utpadaka:* vitiation of the *doshas,*
2. *Agnimandya:* impairment of the digestive fire,
3. *Ama* formation: metabolic impurities formation, and
4. *Samprapti:* pathogenesis proper.

The Ayurvedic concept of disease emphasizes the idea that an individual becomes ill only when the field of the body, *doshas* and *dhatus* (tissues), becomes weakened. This weakened condition is associated with diminished immunity, lowered resistance to illness, and lowered *Ojas,* the physical substance that enhances the immune system and pervades the healthy body. Only when specific areas of the tissues, especially the *srotas* or channels of circulation, are compromised in an appreciable manner can disease actually take hold. Damaged lacunae within the tissues, therefore, become vulnerable to a variety of causative factors, both internal and external, such as microbes, germs, and infectious processes. Psychological factors also have a role of inestimable significance in fostering the development of disease.

CONCEPT OF *DOSHA* VITIATION

The concept of *dosha* vitiation is uniquely Ayurvedic. Vitiation is a condition characterized by impairment, imbalance, abnormal excitation, aggravation, excess proliferation, qualitative disturbance, spoiling, and derangement. Vitiation or perturbation of *doshas,* if not checked, heralds the beginning of the disease process. *Doshas* may be vitiated by innumerable factors, but the most common include diet, season, life-style and behavior, age, and psychological stress.

Dosha vitiation or spoiling refers to *doshas* that are in a state of disturbance. General disturbance is called *utpadaka,* and severe disturbance is called *prakopa. Doshas* may be excessively increased (*vruddhi*), excessively aggravated (*prakopa*), or abnormally low (*dosha kashaya*); the latter is uncommon. *Dosha vitiation* is typically a condition of excessively increased *doshas.* The qualitative impairment of *doshas, dosha* vitiation, is called *dosha dushti.* The central key to maintaining and achieving health in Ayurveda is avoiding *dosha* defilement and *dosha* spoiling. In general, any type of *dosha* impairment is termed *dosha* vitiation.

To reiterate, health correlates with *doshas* that are in equilibrium, that is, having normal quantity, normal quality, and normal balance among *Vata, Pitta,* and *Kapha.* Disease reflects disturbed equilibrium and either excessively high or excessively low levels of one or more *doshas.* Vitiation ordinarily refers to one or more excessively high *doshas* that, in effect, cause imbalance and disequilibrium.

It should be mentioned in passing that the condition of abnormally low *doshas* is an uncommon finding. When present, however, they result from inadequate nutrition, especially selectively diminished ingestion of the Five Great Gross Elements in foods, spices, and herbs. Adequate identification of these deficiencies and dietary remediation is restorative. Some Ayurvedic authorities do not emphasize this approach. They recommend, instead, that addressing the more typical condition of doshic imbalance due to excessive and vitiated *doshas* will, in turn, naturally lead to an overall replenishment of any lowered doshic states. When *doshas* are low, however, they may manifest in the following ways. Low *Pitta* creates a desire for foods with Sour tastes, loss of appetite, feelings of coldness, and skin paleness. Lowered *Vata* may suggest insufficient *Prana Vata* or *Apana Vata* and, in general, may produce symptoms of fatigue or insomnia. Lowered *Kapha* may be related to states of inordinate emaciation and to the wasting diseases. The treatments for lowered *doshas* are usually dietary and may include appropriate herbs.

Lowered *Agni* (*Agnimandya*) (not low *Pitta*) is the beginning of disease onset both in general and in most cases. This, in turn, produces vitiated *doshas*. Only when *dhatus* (tissues), organs, and *srotas* (channels) as a whole (*dushya*) in conjunction with vitiated *doshas* become vitiated does true disease set in. *Srotas* in the *dhatus* must become significantly disordered for illness to occur.

Dosha Vitiation Due to Diet

Dosha vitiation is often caused by dietary factors. This type of vitiation may be the most common and is one significant factor that engenders doshic imbalances. When foods that are not suitable for a specific constitutional type are eaten, they will cause a disturbance in the predominant *dosha* or *doshas* in that *prakruti*. A diet such as this is defined as one having a similar composition, both of the primary Elements and of the specific *doshas,* to that of the individual's *dosha* dominance, the *prakruti*. Examples of this are the following:

1. *Vata*-predominant *prakrutis* are exacerbated by foods that increase *Vata,* such as beans, raw vegetables, mushrooms, soda, dry breakfast cereals, popcorn, and carbonated beverages. Foods and other dietary substances with tastes that are Pungent, Bitter, and Astringent will increase *Vata*. Dietary habits such as fasting and taking more food before the previous meal has been digested increase *Vata*. In the already *Vata*-dominant *prakruti,* these foods are vatagenic; they will further increase *Vata* and cause *Vata* vitiation.

2. *Pitta*-predominant *prakrutis* are exacerbated by foods that increase *Pitta,* such as salt, nuts, hot vegetables (peppers, onions, and tomatoes), alcohol, sour fruits (oranges), vinegar, and very hot spices (red pepper). Foods that have Pungent, Sour, and Salty taste components increase *Pitta*. These are pittagenic.

3. *Kapha*-predominant *prakrutis* are exacerbated by foods that increase *Kapha,* such as yogurt, cheese, ice cream, nuts, red meats, oils, cold drinks, and sweets. Foods with predominantly Sweet, Sour, and Salty tastes increase *Kapha*. These are kaphagenic.

Dosha Vitiation Due to Age

As has been described previously, the season of a person's life brings with it a natural dominance of one of the three *doshas*. *Kapha* predominates from birth through adolescence (*bala*); *Pitta* predominates in adolescence until about age 55 (*madhya*); *Vata* gradually predominates thereafter (*vriddha*). The dominance of a *dosha* according to one's age contributes to an increased susceptibility to that particular *dosha*'s disease tendency. Although this, by itself, is not abnormal, it does predispose to an increased susceptibility to doshic vitiation when other factors such as diet, life-style, behavior, and climate contribute their influence.

Dosha Vitiation Due to Season

The normal seasonal fluctuation of the *doshas* has been discussed. This factor, as that of chronological age, does contribute to doshic vitiation. In general, *Pitta* is most increased in the summer and in any hot climate or environmental condition. *Vata* is increased in dry, cold, windy environments such as are found in the fall season. The fall season tends to exert the most severe stress on all the *doshas* in all *prakruti* types. *Kapha* increases when environmental factors include cold, damp, and dark conditions. As with the doshic increases that accompany age, those that set in with changing climatic conditions exert a real influence, but that influence can be considered only partial in its impact. *Doshas* are most disturbed when an array of multiple influences, especially over a significant period, affect them. Diet and season are the most intense sources of doshic provocation.

Dosha Vitiation Due to Life-Style and Behavior

Life-style encompasses those activities and choices of daily living that include such things as sleep patterns, personal hygiene, eating habits, exercise routines, job and career activity, and recreational preferences, to name just a few. Each of the three *doshas* is sensitive to a particular type of activity. The following is a representative sampling of behaviors that cause specific *doshas* to become vitiated or increased.

1. *Vata.* Any excess physical activity increases *Vata.* Other excess activities include *excessive talking* (*prajalpa*) and excessive traveling, especially because of the jerks and agitation that movement causes. Excessive use of the computer and excessive playing of video games increases *Vata.* The use of illicit drug substances aggravates *Vata.* Insofar as sleep goes, *Vata* is increased when one remains awake at night past about 10 p.m. Another concept unique to Ayurveda is that of the *Vega-dharana* or the 13 natural urges. They consist of eating, drinking, vomiting, belching, inhaling, yawning, sneezing, urinating, defecating, passing flatus, ejaculating, crying, and sleeping. They are all controlled by the various subdoshas of *Vata.* When any of these "natural urges" is suppressed, obstructed, or impaired, its complement of *Vata dosha* then becomes vitiated. This vitiation of *Vata* has many imbalancing consequences. One of the most significant is that of the additional vitiation of the specific channel system (*srota*) involved. This vitiation of a particular *srota* causes impaired functioning that may take the form of a reversal (*pratiloma*) of the proper (*anuloma*) flow, a blockage of flow (*sroto-rhodha*), or a flow outside of the channel and into an inappropriate tissue site (*vimarga gamana*). These abnormal channel impingements create a potential for the disease process to set in.

2. *Pitta dosha* may become vitiated by excessive exposure to heat, whether it is climatic or produced by situations such as radiation, machines, saunas, steam baths, fires, tanning booths, and so forth. Competitive activities, mental or

physical, whether in sports or in the job setting, contribute to *Pitta* exacerbation.

3. *Kapha dosha* is increased by life-styles that are slow, sluggish, sedentary, and inordinately inactive. *Kapha* is also increased by excessive sleep, especially during the morning hours and during the daytime.

Dosha Vitiation Due to Psychological Factors

The psychological sphere has cognitive and emotional dimensions. This domain is complex, and only a brief outline of pertinent factors will be described. Any rajasic (turbulent) or tamasic (dulling) stimuli will elicit *dosha* vitiation. Any stressful life event may contribute to doshic imbalance. A vicious cycle is set up when a stressor increases a particular *dosha* because that vitiated *dosha* then tends to attract or elicit further stimulation by the original event that triggered it. As was alluded to in the Introduction, Ayurveda may be a formidable means of addressing life's everyday stressors and so preventing the chronic stress reactions that have clearly been associated with a range of serious disease states. The following are psychological triggers for specific *dosha* vitiations:

1. *Vata* undergoes disruptive excitation when the following are experienced: anxiety, fear, ambivalence, insecurity, impulsivity, hyperactivity, agitation, mania, mood lability, inattentiveness, loquaciousness, inordinate excitability, fear of self-harm, drug addiction, sexual perversion, sexual excess, and psychosis.

2. *Pitta* is vitiated when the following are experienced: anger, aggression, competition, irritability, and controlling, manipulative, and dominating behaviors; also included are envy, pride, narcissism, lustful desire, hate, violence, destructiveness, lying, and criminality.

3. *Kapha* tends to become vitiated when the following are present: greed, inordinate attachment, jealousy, avaricious lust, rigid materialism, clinging dependency, hedonism, depressions with psychomotor retardation, apathy, inertia, and sloth.

IMPAIRMENT OF *AGNI,* THE ENERGY OF THE DIGESTIVE FIRE

Agni, as it exists in the form of the digestive fire or the *Jatharagni,* is one of the most fundamental concepts in Ayurveda. The health or illness of an individual is almost entirely identified with the state of the *Agni.*

The root cause of all disease within an individual can be correlated to impaired *Agni* on all levels—physical, mental, and spiritual. *Agni* in the physical body must be balanced to permit proper digestion of nutrients. *Agni* in the mind as *Tejas* must be balanced so that desire and envy do not impair *Manas* and perpetuate *Prajna-aparadha* through excessive splitting of experiences and, therefore, result in the forgetting of fundamental unity. A healthy and balanced *Agni* (*sama Agni*) ultimately creates *Ojas,* the proper state of immunity and of resistance to developing disease.

The digestive fire of *Agni* is the essential transformative force that facilitates proper digestion, absorption, and assimilation of nutrients. *Agni* not only refers to the gastrointestinal, tissue, and cellular digestive processes, but also extends to include the digestion, so to speak, of all psychological experience. *Agni* and metabolic transformations, therefore, take place in the gastrointestinal tract, in the liver, and at the tissue and cellular levels throughout the entire body, including the brain. *Agni* powerfully exerts its transformative power in the psychological sphere as well.

According to Ayurveda, *Agni* becomes impaired when the *doshas* become vitiated. Although this includes the *tridosha* (three-*dosha*) group of *Vata, Pitta,* and *Kapha,* the vitiation of *Vata* and of *Kapha* are the conditions that most often impair the digestive fire. *Kapha* excess creates conditions that are cold, damp, and heavy and so contributes to dousing the digestive fire. *Vata* has qualities of cold, exuberant agitation, and mobility that can blow out the flame of the digestive fire. When the digestive fire becomes dulled (*Agnimandya*), all metabolic processes begin to become dysfunctional. Some common dietary and lifestyle causes of *Agnimandya* are the following:

1. Overuse of cold foods and liquids;
2. Overeating or undereating (for example, excessive fasting);
3. Heavy foods;
4. Meat in excess;
5. Eating before the previous meal has been digested;
6. Eating before 7 A.M. or after 8 P.M.;
7. Incorrect food combinations;
8. Dietary factors such as quality of food, food preparation, *prakruti* incompatible foods, chronological and seasonal specifications for proper foods;
9. Suppression of the 13 natural urges;
10. Poor sleep patterns;
11. Motoric overactivity or underactivity; and
12. Psychological stressors.

The above listing is not exhaustive. It reflects, in part, the previously mentioned factors that contribute to the vitiation of the *doshas.* All doshic vitiation tends to create conditions that impair the *Agni.* Lowered, enervated *Agni* (*Agnimandya*) reflects indolent energy. It is the principal condition of *Agni* impairment. Variable, irregular *Agni* (*Vishama Agni*) caused by the influence of vitiated *Vata* is also important. High, sharp *Agni* (*Tikshna Agni*) may also have a destabilizing effect. When the *Agni* is impaired for a significant period, the toxic metabolic product, *Ama,* is produced. The vitiated *doshas,* along with *Ama,* launch the potential disease process. Impaired *Agni* precedes the vitiation of the *doshas.*

AMA

Ama is the Sanskrit word that comes from the root *am* meaning "to harm or to weaken." *Ama* constitutes a diverse group of toxic substances that includes internal metabolic and cellular waste products as well as pollutants and other toxins from the environment that enter the body. The phenomena of free radicals, reactive oxygen species, and free radical damaged cellular and tissue debris are included in this idea. The traditional Ayurvedic concept of *Ama* emphasizes the role of seriously impaired *Agni* and its inability to normally digest and metabolize ingested food. The portion of food that cannot be properly digested and assimilated via *Avasthapaka, Bhutagni, Dhatuagni,* and *Vipaka* processes is considered to be in a "raw" state. This raw, undigested material then stagnates and transforms into a toxic mass of impurities contained both within the gastrointestinal tract and in tissue and cellular sites. The resulting *Ama* is further carried by vitiated *doshas* into the tissue channels of circulation and then pervasively dispersed. Although *Ama* is propelled by *Vata* to travel in the channels of circulation, its erratic movements are accompanied by a sluggish quality primarily due to the sticky and adhering nature of the *Ama* itself.

SAMPRAPTI: PATHOGENESIS PROPER

Samprapti is the heart of the Ayurvedic conceptualization of the development of the disease process. The details of this process of pathogenesis have been formulated over thousands of years, and remain the group of basic propositions that reflect the Ayurvedic concept of pathogenesis. In its view of ill health, Ayurveda places greater emphasis on the dynamic processes that occur over time (*kalakriya*) leading up to the manifestation of the disease rather than on the disease itself, as a discrete entity. The first half of these processes constitute the incipient stages of disease, while the last half reflect its consolidated, clinical manifestations. This view of pathology, therefore, is a more dynamic rather than static one. As has been described previously, the triggers for disease lie in the universal phenomena of *Prajna-aparadha,* which leads to wrong choices in diet, life-style, and behavior. Along with these factors, the influence of seasonal variations and the impact that stressful emotional states and cognitive experience produce together contribute to the vitiation process.

When the *doshas* begin to become increasingly vitiated, the *Agni* becomes impaired and *Ama* is formed. Vitiated *doshas* and *Ama* then spread in the channels of circulation and eventually form significant blockages in weakened channels and tissues. This obstructive process produces the manifestations of disease.

Samprapti, also known as *Shat Kriyakala,* connotes the six physiological states and times during which the disease process develops. The six stages are the following:

1. *Sanchaya:* Accumulation,
2. *Prakopa:* Aggravation,
3. *Prasara:* Spread,
4. *Sthana-Samshraya:* Localization,
5. *Vyakti:* Manifestation, and
6. *Bheda:* Differentiation.

Sanchaya: Preclinical Stage 1

Sanchaya is the gradual accumulation of a *dosha* in the process of vitiation that occurs in that specific *dosha*'s home site within the gastrointestinal tract. This site of origin is called *udbhava sthana.* When vitiated, *Vata* accumulates in the colon, *Pitta* accumulates in the small intestine, and *Kapha* accumulates in the stomach; it may also accumulate in the lungs. Signs and symptoms at this early preclinical stage are vague and subtle. *Vata* vitiation may appear as gas, constipation, and the psychological experience of anxiety or fear. *Vata* may cause an Astringent taste in the mouth. *Pitta* vitiation may appear as the sensation of mild heat or burning with a Bitter taste in the mouth. Bitter taste in the mouth suggests that *ama* is absent (*nirama*). *Kapha* vitiation may appear as nausea and the feeling of heaviness. *Kapha* may cause a Sweet taste in the mouth. As the body attempts to correct these beginning imbalances, the individual instinctively begins to crave foods and conditions that are opposite to the qualities of the accumulating *doshas.* This is the body's initial and instinctive attempt to restore balance.

Prakopa: Preclinical Stage 2

Prakopa is the continued increase of the vitiated *doshas,* in their own site of origin, to the point of maximal intensity. The excited *dosha* now is aggravated and "rageful." Signs and symptoms are still vague, but take on a more intense character. *Vata* aggravation may appear as pain, spasm, and abdominal distension. *Pitta* aggravation may appear as acid regurgitation, thirst, and a Sour taste in the mouth. Sour taste in the mouth suggests that *ama* is present (*sama*). *Kapha* aggravation may appear as the loss of appetite, as excess salivation, and as fatigue and lethargy with a need to sleep during the day. As *Vata, Pitta,* and *Kapha* rise to almost maximal intensity, each of them contributes to further diminish the power of *Agni.* The overall metabolic processes therefore decrease. As this occurs, food cannot be transformed properly and completely into healthy, assimilable nutrients, and, therefore, *Ama* formation begins.

Prasara: Preclinical Stage 3

Prasara is the overflow and spread of the maximally elevated *doshas.* They, along with *Ama,* flow out of their respective sites in the gastrointestinal tract and go into the blood and plasma channels to spread most often into more peripheral body sites. The seriously aggravated *Vata,* in this condition, takes a wild and explosive course (*prakupita*) that is improper and contrary to a normal healthy flow. Signs and symptoms become more intense, although they remain in a preclinical state and are not disease specific. The spreading of *Vata* may appear as joint stiffness, backache, spasm, cough, and the sensation of fullness accompanied by bowel sounds. The spread of *Pitta* may show as diarrhea, bilious vomiting, gingivitis, or pulling and burning sensations. The spreading *Kapha* may be signaled by a low-grade fever, no appetite, and lethargy. These symptoms continue to manifest as vague and ambiguous signs of general malaise.

According to Ayurveda, when the vitiated *doshas* begin to spread, they follow one or more of three distinct pathways (*margas*). Their flow in the channels of circulation is usually away from the center of the body toward the more peripheral, dense, and compact body structures. This outward flow has more disease-producing potential since the vitiated *doshas* are mixed with toxic *Ama* and have a predilection to settle in weakened or damaged tissues. They are both attracted to and tend to want to pool in these vulnerable bodily spaces. The three possible disease paths or tracts are the following:

1. *Antharmarga:* the Inner Pathway of Disease. This consists primarily of the entire gastrointestinal tract (*Maha Srotas*), but also includes plasma tissue (*rasa dhatu*). Imbalances typically start here with impaired digestion of foods. If disease originates here or when, after treatments, vitiated *doshas* and toxins return here, they are relatively easy to eliminate. Many *Kapha*-related diseases take hold in this pathway.

2. *Bayhamarga:* the Outer, Peripheral Pathway of Disease. This is associated with the *shakha* or limbs, skin, and compact tissues. It includes blood, muscle, fat, and some bone tissue. Diseases that settle here are moderately difficult to treat since they have invaded compact bodily tissue sites. *Pitta* diseases, especially associated with blood, follow this path.

3. *Madhyamamarga:* the Central, Deep, or Middle Pathway of Disease. This is composed of the paths to the vital organs and includes the heart and the brain. In addition, the kidneys along with nerve, bone, and reproductive tissues are affected. Diseases in these areas are considered the most serious and are very difficult to treat. Examples include chronic and degenerative diseases such as arthritis and cancer. *Vata*-type diseases typically settle in these sites.

Sthana-Samshraya: Clinical Stage 4

Sthana-samshraya means site of deposition, and this clinical stage of pathogenesis is the stage of the relocation of the spreading vitiated *doshas* and *Ama* into a circumscribed area that has already been weakened or damaged in the past. This localization process is considered one of the most critical events in the course of disease formation. It heralds the birth of what may become the final disease condition. Until this event occurs, the incipient pathogenic process has been preclinical, relatively weaker, and accompanied by vague and less definitive symptomatology, and, as well, is more easily treatable. At this clinical stage, definitive signs and symptoms are set in motion.

In this localization phase, the important role of the tissues and the channels in pathogenesis emerges. In the body over time, various events have produced both physical and psychological traumas in the tissues, the organs, and the channels. Causes of weakened or deformed channels, for example, include any or all of the following factors: genetic, congenital, deformity from past disease, external trauma, accidents, poisons, environmental pollutants, and diet and lifestyle practices contrary to one's *prakruti* requirements. Impairment or damage to the channels is exceedingly critical insofar as this constitutes one of the most significant weakened areas that may act like an attractor and as a potential reservoir for the *Ama*-laden vitiated *doshas*. These susceptible areas of devitalization are referred to as *khavaigunya/ kervaigunya* or weak spots. These weak spots may occur within the *dhatu* (tissue) or the *srota* (channel). These weak spots may result from constitutional endowment or from damage by trauma, infection, improper diet, or life-style over time.

The vitiated tissues, themselves, are called *dusha,* also spelled *doosha* or *dushya*. When the vitiated *Ama*-laden *doshas* find and locate in these *dusha,* this pathogenic merging is called *dosha-dusha sammurchanna.*

Sammurchanna is a pathological amalgamation that produces a new substance that has a qualitatively distinct pathogenic character. This *sammurchanna* causes an overwhelming obstruction within the channels that it attacks and produces the phenomenon of *srotorhodha* or channel obstruction. This event heralds the actual birth of the disease. Impaired flow through any of the innumerable channels of circulation produces an overall impairment of the individual's quality of life. This is felt in symptoms of malaise and dysphoria, and in premonitory signs of impending poor health.

One of the most important therapeutic concepts contained in the understanding of this stage of disease is the overwhelming emphasis on the aberrant or vitiated tissue that is able to attract, receive, and hold the *Ama*-laden vitiated *doshas* in the disease process. Disease is possible only when tissue is devitalized. This takes into serious account the concept of resistance to disease and immunity. Only when resistance and immunity are lowered, that is, when there is sufficient tissue vitiation, will disease take hold. The concept of "germs" that includes invading bacteria, viruses, and other pathogens was known in ancient times and is referred to by the Sanskrit word *krimi* in the *Rig-Veda,* the *Charaka,* and the *Sushruta Samhita* medical texts. While attention was given to these pathogens, the major emphasis in preventing and treating disease was placed on the condition of the tissues. Treatments were aimed at strengthening, restoring, and healing the tissues in order to make them unreceptive and resistant to pathogens. This emphasis on tissue health included not only nourishment and restoration, but went beyond and addressed issues of rejuvenation.

Channel obstruction produces a relatively more specific group of prodromal signs and symptoms called *Purva Rupa.* These premonitory signals appear before the actual distinct manifestations of a disease. They can provide clues to impending disease consolidation, which appears at this stage, especially because the clinical signs and symptoms are now more fixed in location and are not merely in the process of wandering.

An important aspect of this stage in the pathogenic process consists of its organizing capacity. A disease process differentiates and takes on a particular identity specifically because of its channel, organ, or tissue involvement. The same *dosha* or *doshas* may produce different types of diseases. The doshic component, therefore, is nonspecific although necessary. The channel component is the most critical factor in determining the identity of a particular disease. Channels of circulation are an intrinsic part of the matrix of every bodily substance. Any impairment of channel structure or functioning affects not only the channel, itself, but also the tissues, organs, and so forth, that it manages in terms of nutrition and removal of wastes.

Vyakti: Clinical Stage 5

Vyakti is the clinical stage of the actual manifestation of the disease. At this point, the full display of a particular disease makes its appearance; it becomes clearly observable. The actual signs and symptoms of a disease are called *Rupa.* The site of manifestation where a disease displays its signs and symptoms is called the *adhisthana.*

The range of categories of *Rupa* includes the following:

1. *Samanya lakshana:* general characteristics,
2. *Visista:* specific and cardinal characteristics,
3. Invariable signs and symptoms,
4. *Upadrava:* complications, and
5. *Aristha:* prognosis.

Bheda: Clinical Stage 6

The last stage of *Samprapti* is *Bheda,* the stage of differentiation. It is here that the disease process and its manifestation become consolidated and most specific. This differentiation within the disease process usually proceeds along the lines of the predominant *dosha* and its tissue involvement. Disease complications also develop from this stage.

TYPES OF *SAMPRAPTI*

Samprapti may be categorized in two ways. The first is according to the type and number of *doshas* involved. When only one *dosha* is involved, the *samprapti* is called *nanatmaja*. When two different *doshas* are involved, the *samprapti* is termed *samanyaja*. When all three *doshas* participate, the disease process is referred to as *sannipatta*. Ayurveda has also given an estimation of the number of different diseases for each *dosha* predominance. There are 80 *Vata*-predominant diseases, 40 *Pitta*-predominant diseases, and 20 *Kapha*-predominant diseases (see Appendix 2).

The second main classification of *samprapti* is according to the leading features of the predominant *dosha*'s qualities or attributes. This assessment is based on the appearance of the various attributes that are specifically related to the particular *dosha* involved. An example of this would be differentiating the disease of arthritis into either a *Vata* arthritis (with symptoms and signs of pain, coldness, stiffness, and so forth), a *Pitta* arthritis (with signs and symptoms of burning pain, red and hot joints, and so forth), or a *Kapha* arthritis (with signs and symptoms of swelling, edema, and so forth). *Vata* attributes that would be outstanding here are cold, hard, and rough; *Pitta* attributes would be hot and sharp; and *Kapha* attributes would be cold, damp, heavy, and static.

7

HEALTH AND THE DISEASE PROCESS. II

THE AYURVEDIC CONCEPT OF CLASSIFICATION AND DIAGNOSIS OF DISEASE

One of the pillars of the Ayurvedic concept of disease is based on the abnormal functioning of the *doshas,* and its manifestation in the imbalanced state of the *prakruti* (constitutional type) called the *vikruti* (imbalanced constitution). The presence of the *vikruti* connotes an impairment of *Agni* or the digestive fire, an accumulation of *Ama* or toxic impurities, vitiated *doshas,* and a dysfunction of the *dhatus* (tissues), *malas* (wastes), and *Manas* (mental and emotional functioning). The patient feels characteristic symptoms, and the practitioner can ascertain signs of the disease through careful, attentive listening and observation. Subsequently, disease diagnosis can be formulated. At the root of all this, however, is a complicated imbalance (*vyadhi*) of an individual's share in the Elements, the *doshas,* and the *Maha gunas.*

Purva Rupa refers to that group of prodromal signs and symptoms that precede the actual manifestation of the disease. It is at this preclinical juncture, before disease sets in, that Ayurvedic medicine is able to detect an imbalance and intervene to prevent the progression toward disease eruption.

Rupa refers to the cluster of signs and symptoms that accompany the full manifestations of a disease. For disease to actually take hold, not only do the *doshas,* the Elements, and the *Maha gunas* need to be in a state of imbalance, but localized pathology, specifically in deep tissue areas, needs to be present and to be acted upon by the vitiated *doshas.* In effect, disease manifests in a wide variety of discrete disorders as well as in broader syndrome complexes. The complex of physical pain and mental suffering, however, constitutes the ultimate disease condition; and, its incarnations are manifold.

ETIOLOGICAL FACTORS CAUSING DISEASE: *NIDANA*

The term *Nidana* refers to etiology and to diagnosis. It is the broadest umbrella under which the spectrum of disease-causing factors is subsumed. *Nidana* is the term given to an etiological factor, usually when it causes the full development of the disease process; as such, these causes are determined, often retrospectively. As has been discussed previously, three fundamental causes are considered the universal reasons for any disease to occur. They are *Prajna-aparadha* (errors in wisdom), *Asatmyendriyartha Samyoga* (inappropriate contact between the sense organs and their objects), and *Kala-Parinama* (effects of time). These three determinants involve axiomatic propositions and rest heavily on theoretical foundations. While these are at the base of all disease manifestations, additional causes may be regarded as particular variables. Classification of these variables includes aspects of the multiple causative factors of disease considered from varying perspectives such as location, timing, insidiousness, external factors, internal contributory processes, and so forth. A discussion of some of the various classifications will follow.

SPECTRUM OF TERMS DENOTING ETIOLOGY

The commonly used terms describing the more concrete precipitants of disease are *hetu* and *karana*. Other terms with differing connotations are the following. The cause of a disease that specifies its path and spread is called *ayatana*. A cause that shows a close relationship to effect is called *pratyaya*. The root cause of a disease is referred to as *mula,* and the site or origin of a disease is called *yoni*. The term *karta* refers to that which creates a disease; for example, the *doshas* in prominent ways are considered the pragmatic creators of disease. *Utthana* and *samutthana* are causative factors that stimulate dormant *doshas,* activate, and vitiate them.

Vitiation of the *doshas* is the basic platform of disease development. Endogenous causes that vitiate *doshas* are termed *nija;* exogenous causes are termed *agantu*.

As far as strength and time of onset, the causes of diseases fall into four categories:

1. *Sannikrushta* refers to causes that produce disease early on and bypass the accumulation phase of *samprapti*. The *doshas* suddenly become aggravated in intensity and produce symptoms. Examples of this are exposure to cold, producing sudden attacks of sinusitis; allergens producing sudden allergic reactions; or damp spring weather triggering an asthmatic attack.

2. *Viprakrushta* refers to causative factors of longer duration that produce delayed results. Examples include chronic smoking leading to emphysema and chronic alcohol use leading to hepatic impairment.

3. *Vyabhichari* refers to very feeble causes that are not strong enough to produce disease unless other intensifying factors such as chronic duration accompany them.

4. *Pradhanik* refers to causes that are fulminating and produce immediate and serious, life-threatening disease. Examples include accidents, trauma, strong toxins, poisons, and some microbial causes.

Another classification system groups variations of causative factors in the following three ways.

1. *Utpadaka* refers to causes that directly vitiate the *doshas.* This refers most specifically to dietary provocations.

2. *Vyadhi pratyanika* refers to specific causes for specific diseases. Examples are infectious sexual contact possibly causing HIV and hepatitis, pica causing anemia and allied conditions, and close contact with already infected patients transferring bacteria to cause conjunctivitis.

3. *Ubhaya hetu* refers to causes that include both of the above, for example, vitiation of *doshas* and disease-causing specificity. An example illustrating this is the chronic use of alcohol that leads to *Pitta dosha* vitiation and subsequently to hepatic impairment and to cirrhosis.

An ancient classification system, based on three primary locations of the etiological events that produce the disease, is as follows:

1. *Adhyatmika* refers to causation that originates within the body. It is subdivided into three groups:

   a. *Adhibala:* genetic causes,

   b. *Janmaja:* congenital causes, and

   c. *Dosaja:* vitiated *doshas* as primary causative factors.

2. *Adhibhautika* refers to causation coming from external causes such as germs, trauma, and accidents.

3. *Adhidaivika* refers to causes that are considered providential, due to Fate, Karma, and other more esoteric sources.

Some disease categorizations reflect a more general yet dynamic perspective. Accordingly, disease etiology, as *hetu* or *karana,* consists of the following three components:

1. *Nimmitta* refers to the necessary precipitating or hastening causes of disease such as diet, life-style, season (*kalabala*), age (*swabhavabala*), and psychological factors.

2. *Samavayi* are the components that are the matrix that makes up the disease and within which the disease manifests. They would be the *doshas, dhatus, srotas,* and so forth.

3. *Asamavayi* refers to the interaction of the entire spectrum of *samavayi* components, for example, *doshas, dhatus, srotas,* and so forth, which combine and interact to yield the final disease product.

CLASSIFICATION OF DISEASE ACCORDING TO PROGNOSIS

Ayurveda divides diseases into two broad prognostic categories: (1) curable and (2) incurable. Curable diseases are either easily treated or resolve with difficulty. Incurable diseases need either long-term maintenance or they may lead to death.

Curable diseases are termed *sukha sadhya*. Their characteristics include minimal severity, *dosha* and affected tissue being not similar in Elemental composition, the vitiated *dosha* not being part of the patient's *prakruti,* and the vitiated *dosha* not being similar to the current season and climate. The ancient Ayurvedic texts also included the need for the "four essential factors for good treatment" to be present. They are (1) a knowledgeable physician, (2) a caring nurse or attendant, (3) proper medicine, and (4) a compliant patient.

Difficult to cure diseases are more severe, have *dosha* and affected tissue of similar Elemental composition, have *doshas* that are part of the patient's predominant *prakruti,* and occur in a season and climate that exacerbates the already affected *doshas*. *Vata*-dominant diseases are considered the most difficult since *Vata dosha* tends to travel and to penetrate into deeper tissues, for example, bone, nerves, and reproductive tissues and includes aspects of psychological dysfunction. *Kapha* diseases are considered most amenable to treatment, and *Pitta* diseases fall in between as far as severity and prognosis are concerned.

Palliable diseases termed *yappa* require long-term maintenance. They are characterized by the involvement of two or more *doshas* simultaneously, by involvement of the central vital organ tract where deeper tissues are involved, and may require treatments that involve surgical procedures.

Intractable diseases termed *asadhya* have very poor or morbid prognoses. They are characterized by the involvement of multiple *doshas,* tissues, organs, and the deeper, vital structures of the body.

CLASSIFICATION OF DISEASE ACCORDING TO STAGES OF THE DISEASE PROCESS

The major staging classification of the disease process has been described as the sequence of *dosha* vitiation and pathological interaction with the tissue elements, that is, *samprapti*. In *samprapti* proper, at the fourth stage of localization of vitiated *doshas* and *Ama* merging with vitiated tissues, this contaminated and polluted condition of the *doshas* and tissues is termed *sama dosha* and *sama dhatu,* respectively. When the *doshas* are therapeutically cleansed of toxins, they are called *nirama doshas*. There is, therefore, a *sama* stage of disease and a *nirama* stage of disease.

There are additional descriptive stages. When a disease is relatively new, it is referred to as *nava;* when chronic, it is termed *jeerna*. When the disease is more superficial, it is called *uttana;* when deep, it is termed *gambhira*. Superficial diseases usually affect the plasma and the blood; deep disease affects the muscle, fat, bone, nerve, and reproductive tissues. Two phases of the explicitness of a disease are described: (1) *vega,* when the disease is urged to manifest; and (2) *avega,* when the disease is hidden in the *dhatus* (tissues) by the masking power of *Vata.*

SIGNS AND SYMPTOMS OF THE DISEASE PROCESS

The disease process is a gradual development that begins with vitiated *doshas* and eventually affects all the other body's constituents and functioning. Pain, malaise, and discomfort attend all disease. *Vata dosha*'s involvement is usually essential. Pain due to vitiated *Vata* is characterized as sharp, radiating, shifting, shooting, pulsating, and irregular. Pain due to vitiated *Pitta* obstructing *Vata* is felt as burning, cutting, penetrating, intense, and producing heat and redness. Pain due to vitiated *Kapha* obstructing *Vata* is felt as heavy, dull, aching, and throbbing. Pain due to *Ama* obstructing *Vata* usually is felt as dull and very heavy, almost leaden in quality. Signs and symptoms of this evolving imbalanced state, therefore, span a continuum from subclinical to clinical manifestations.

Fever (*jvara*), a reaction to disease, is a nonspecific sign that especially indicates the excessive presence of *Ama. Jvara* also means pain. Fever is a complex physiologic response to disease that, according to Western allopathic medicine, is mediated by pyrogenic cytokines and characterized by a rise in core body temperature, the generation of acute phase reactants, and the activation of complex immune systems. A general orientation describing *dosha* vitiation and some specific and clinically decipherable disease syndromes according to channel vitiation will be reviewed.

Indicators of *Vata* Vitiation

The chief clinical manifestation of *Vata* vitiation in the body is pain. Most of the signs and symptoms that *Vata* produces derive from an intensification of its attributes or *gunas. Vata* vitiation tends to create tissue loss (*dhatu kashaya*) with tissue porosity and dilatation and atrophy, excess movement, and hypersensitivity. In addition, one may find the following: spasm; tremors (*kampa*); horripilation; numbness; contraction; tingling (paresthesias); obstruction associated with atrophy and vasospasm; ptosis; stiffness; constipation; cracking sounds from joints; trembling; dehydration; thirst; rough, dry skin; agitation; Astringent taste in the mouth; and red, black, or brown discolorations (*arunasayava*) of the skin or other tissues. The principal manifestations of *Vata* vitiation in the psychological sphere include anxiety, fear, manic depression or bipolar disorder, agitation, hyperactivity, insomnia, and chronic low energy. The strong *rajasic* (turbulent) components within *Vata* directly contribute to its agitating and disorganizing power in the mental sphere. The intensely driven quality of some psychiatric disorders, for example, hyperactivity, agitated depression, and bipolar mania, are manifestations of this.

Indicators of *Pitta* Vitiation

The chief clinical manifestation of *Pitta* vitiation in the body is inflammation. Aggravated *Pitta* manifests as burning sensations; redness; increased temperature; sweating; hot, sensitive, and oily skin; boils; pus formation; hemorrhagic disorders; hypertension; migraines; necrosis; gangrene; dry mouth and thirst; hyperacidity; Pungent, Bitter, or Sour taste in the mouth; and skin and tissue discolorations of any color other than white or brownish black. Different forms of syncope or fainting may be a sign of *Pitta* aggravation. In the psychological sphere, *Pitta* vitiation may produce moderate insomnia, irritability, anger, envy, inordinate competitiveness, obsessive-compulsive behavior, and states of disorientation as, for example, the intoxicated and inebriated condition. Chronic states of exhaustion may have a strong vitiated *Pitta* component since chronic *Pitta* excesses may tend to "burnout" or begin to damage aspects of the central nervous system, including neurotransmitter functioning.

Indicators of *Kapha* Vitiation

The chief clinical manifestations of vitiated *Kapha* in the body include heaviness, edema, swelling, and obstruction. Vitiated *Kapha* also appears as increased mucous production or phlegm, increased salivation, respiratory congestion, cold sensations, torpor, lethargy, inertia, somnolence, impaired and sluggish digestion, itching of the skin, cold and oily skin, hardening of the tissues (for example, lithiasis, tumor, atheroma, and atherosclerosis), obstruction in the channels due to excesses of blocking substances, white or pale skin color and pallor, and Sweet or Salty taste in the mouth. In the psychological domain, vitiated *Kapha* is reflected in states of severe dependency, greed, jealousy, and in inordinate attachment behaviors. Severe depressions with psychomotor retardation are reflective of the strong tamasic (dulling) component within *Kapha* when it is exacerbated and displayed in the emotional realm.

Disease Manifestations Due to Channel Vitiation

The *srotas* or channels of a system's circulation constitute an integral network throughout the body coordinating the integrity of its functioning. For any disease to exert some significant systemic impairment, not only the *doshas* but also the *dhatus* or tissues and the *srotas* or tissue channels need to be affected and involved in a pathological interaction. An outline of the channels with some common vitiating factors and some characteristic clinical manifestations of impairment follow:

> *Pranavaha Srotas* constitutes the respiratory and *Prana*-carrying channels. They have an intimate connection to the heart, the lungs, the brain, and the colon. Causes of vitiation include malnutrition, wasting diseases, excessive physical

exercise, smoking cigarettes, environmental pollutants, and the suppression of the natural urges (*vega-dharana*). *Vata* vitiation, in particular, adversely affects this channel. Signs and symptoms include any respiratory difficulty such as cough, dyspnea, and asthma; as well as disorders related to energy level and psychological status.

Annavaha Srotas constitutes the entire gastrointestinal tract. Causes of vitiation include impairments of the digestive fire, and improper dietary behavior such as overeating, eating at the wrong times, and eating foods contrary to one's needs. Disturbances include all digestive disorders, appetite dysregulation, vomiting, diarrhea, and constipation.

Ambuvaha Srotas is the water regulatory system. Vitiating factors include exposure to excess heat, alcohol, and salt; dehydration; *Ama* buildup; and the experience of inordinate fear. Signs of disorder include inordinate thirst, edema, blood glucose dysregulation, and diabetes.

Rasavaha Srotas is the lymphatic or plasma channel. Factors that damage these channels include impaired digestive fire with *Ama* buildup, improper absorption of nutrients, excess food and beverage intake, and inordinate stress responses over a long period of time. Signs of vitiation include anorexia, premature wrinkling of skin, premature graying of hair, impotence, lymphatic disorders, and fungal infections.

Raktavaha Srotas is the blood circulatory system. Damaging factors include diets with foods and herbs that are too stimulating (*vidahi*) and hot and by overexposure to intensive environmental heat. Signs of vitiation include all the hematological disorders, skin disorders such as acne and rashes, hypertension, hypotension, arrhythmias, liver and spleen disorders, and hemorrhagic disorders.

Mamsavaha Srotas includes the muscular and integumentary systems. Vitiations are believed to result from overconsumption of foods that are heavy and oily, and incompatible. Frequent sleeping after meals causes excess *Kapha* production and negatively impacts muscular tissue. Impairments of the liver, especially with its *Agnis,* and emotional and physical trauma can also cause muscle problems. Signs of disorder include muscle dysfunction such as excess activity (tremor and spasm), hypoactivity, atony, tissue tears, and tumors.

Medavaha Srotas includes the channels of adipose tissue especially around the kidneys and within the abdominal omental sheaths. Vitiating factors, mainly dietary, include excess intake of foods, especially with a high fat content, excess intake of alcohol, and sleep during the daytime. Signs of disorder include obesity, edema, fatty tumors, hypertension, heart disease, cholesterol and blood lipid disorders, diabetes, and arthritis.

Asthivaha Srotas refers to the skeletal system. Damaging factors include trauma and any food, herb, or physical activity that increases *Vata*. Excessive physical activity to the point of sweating and shortness of breath, for example, aerobic exercise, running, jogging, and strenuous manual labor normally increase *Vata*. This becomes damaging only over a long period of time if *Vata* is not periodically reduced in order to prevent inordinate cumulative effects. This point emphasizes the Ayurvedic ideal of continually attempting to restore balance to imbalanced states since it is natural to engage in activities that may tend toward excess and subsequent dysfunction. Acute stress management, especially by Ayurvedic techniques, is very beneficial. Signs and symptoms, especially those exacerbated by chronic stress, include any bone disorders such as osteoporosis, hypertrophy, arthritis, as well as some disorders of hair and nails.

Majjavaha Srotas refers to the nervous system and aspects of the long bones and joints. Damaging factors include trauma, especially the fracture of the long bones, and the ingestion of what Ayurveda considers "incompatible food combinations" (to be discussed later). Psychological trauma is also considered a vitiating factor. Any high *Vata* or high *Pitta* stimuli is particularly stressful and traumatic. Manifestations of disturbance include pain in the joints, lack of coordination, paresis or paralysis of muscle, convulsion, coma, multiple sclerosis, central nervous system and peripheral nervous system dysfunction, as well as distinctive abnormalities in sensory perception, especially that of touch and temperature.

Shukravaha Srotas refers to the reproductive system, and this usually indicates the male system. In addition to physical trauma, Ayurveda considers chronic stress and other behavioral factors to be vitiating to this system. The range includes excessive and aberrant sexual practices, inordinate suppression of the sexual urge, and trauma from accidents, surgery, or chemotherapy. Close attention is paid to sexual activity because excessive activity is believed to deplete *Ojas* (vigor and immune functioning) that, in turn, increases *Vata* and diminishes longevity. In addition to disorders of impotence and sexual dysfunction, other diseases affecting the immune system such as tuberculosis and AIDS may result.

Svedavaha Srotas is the perspiratory and sebaceous system. Damaging factors include excess physical activity; excess exposure to heat, cold, and wind; ingestion of excessively hot and pungent foods; alcohol intake; as well as psychological factors such as fear and anger. Signs include disorders of perspiration and some skin disorders.

Mutravaha Srotas refers to the urinary system. Vitiating factors include excessive or insufficient intake of fluids, exposure to inordinately hot and dry climates, excess sexual activity, suppression of the urge to micturate, renal diseases, and trauma. Disease is reflected in any urinary disorder, including infection, stones, and tumors.

Purishavaha Srotas refers to the excretory system. Vitiating factors include impaired digestive fire, digestive disturbances, and dietary irregularities. Signs of disorder include constipation, diarrhea, colitis, tumors, hemorrhoids, and any other bowel dysfunction.

Artavavaha Srotas refers to the female reproductive system. Vitiating factors are similar to those that vitiate the *Shukravaha Srotas* and include excessive or suppressed sexual activity, improper dietary practices, and stressful emotional factors such as anxiety, fear, and anger. Signs of disorder include premenstrual tension (PMS), dysmenorrhea, amenorrhea, and menorrhagia.

Stanyavaha Srotas is the female lactation system. The breasts and nipples are the main sites. Vitiating factors are considered to include suppression of breast milk by not breast-feeding and, on the other hand, by excessive breast-feeding. Disorders are thought to include conditions of deficient or excessive lactation, and breast dysfunction such as pain, cysts, and tumors.

Manovaha Srotas refers to the channels that are associated with mental and emotional functioning. Vitiating factors include chronic stress, emotional trauma, illicit substance use, excessive sensory input, and other factors that reflect *vatagenic (Vata*-provoking) stimuli. Manifestations of disorder include the spectrum of psychological disorders. *Vata* disorders manifest as anxiety, fear, and bipolar conditions. *Pitta* disorders manifest as intense anger, irritability, hostility, envy, and aggressive symptoms. *Kapha* disorders manifest as inordinate dependency, greed, pathological jealousy, and attachment problems, and also as retarded depressions.

DIAGNOSTIC EXAMINATION OF THE DISEASE: *ROGA PARIKSHA*

A comprehensive diagnostic assessment requires that the disease itself as it exists within the patient be examined using a variety of parameters. There are five standard approaches that classical Ayurveda uses to ascertain the major components associated with disease. They include an examination of the following:

1. *Nidana:* causative factors;
2. *Purva Rupa:* prodromal symptoms;
3. *Rupa:* actual signs and symptoms;
4. *Upashaya:* suitability of the means of alleviation. This method consists of the use of exploratory interventions used when the more exact nature of a disease is unclear. *Upashaya* procedures involve therapeutic trials of a variety of treatments to assess whether alleviation of the problem or an exacerbation of it results.
5. *Samprapti:* pathogenesis.

DIAGNOSTIC EVALUATION OF THE PATIENT

Diagnosis, in Ayurvedic medicine, is evaluation of the patient's baseline *prakruti* and current *vikruti* as a prelude to employing strategies to balance and restore optimal functioning to the *doshas.* Disease is viewed as any disorder disrupting the proper balance of the *doshas.* The diagnostic assessment delineates the basic *prakruti* and what should be the proper functioning of each *dosha,* alone and in interaction with the body's other *doshas.* In addition, this assessment evaluates the quality of the tissues, channels, organs, wastes, and *Manas.*

Diagnostic evaluation is a comprehensive assessment of the patient using a variety of different techniques. The physician arrives at a diagnostic and prognostic assessment by relying on three facets contributing to an understanding of the clinical examination. They are the following:

1. *Aptopadesha/Shabda,* authoritative knowledge. This information derives from two sources. One is the body of theoretical and clinical information found in the literature of Ayurveda and in the teachings of recognized Ayurvedic physicians. The other involves the historical data gathered by the clinical interview. This includes reports from the patient (*prashna pariksha*), the family, and any other past medical and psychosocial history.

2. *Pratyaksha,* use of the physician's five senses. This is the clinical examination using the physician's direct perception. The functioning of the five senses or *jnanendriyas* is highly regarded in the Ayurvedic system. As such, they have a critically important role to play in diagnostic assessments. The physician becomes, as it were, an instrument, and his five sensory faculties are used as precision tools to explore the patient's presentation.

   Examination using the ear or sense of hearing listens not only to the patient's voice but also to sounds coming from joints, intestines, lungs, and so forth. The physician also uses supplemental devices such as the stethoscope to hear cardiac and respiratory sounds. Examination with the eye or inspection is a visual survey of appearance, demeanor, and functioning. Examination using the nose or sense of smell can detect an irregularity in body odor and give an indication of personal hygiene. Examination by touch or palpation supplies data about skin temperature, turgor, abdominal and thoracic organs, and tenderness or sensitivity to pain. Pulse diagnosis is included here (Lad, 1996). Examination by using the sense of taste usually is not done in the United States.

3. *Anumana,* reasoning based on inference. This involves the analytic and synthetic interpretation of all the data gathered from the physician's theoretical knowledge and the patient's clinical presentation. This process produces a diagnosis and a prognosis and suggests a treatment plan.

All of the above are predicated on the physician spending adequate time with the patient. The patient is central and shown respect by the physician's attentiveness, sensitivity, and taking serious whatever the patient reports. Ultimately, the physician must sort out what is primary from what may be secondary in importance. The astute physician thus carefully assesses the presentation and prioritizes the patient's needs and the interventions that may be appropriate.

DIAGNOSTIC PROCEDURES IN THE CLINICAL EXAMINATION

Ayurveda has formalized the clinical examination and suggested a systematic strategy for surveying important aspects of the patient's strengths and weaknesses. There are two major groups of methodology. They are the following.

Dashavidha Pariksha, The Tenfold Examination

Charaka has advocated a method that encompasses a comprehensive clinical review incorporating the major areas that are of significance to the Ayurvedic system. They are as follows:

1. *Prakruti:* baseline body constitution.

2. *Vikruti:* doshic imbalances.

3. *Sara:* tissue quality. This is a survey and estimation of the excellence or optimal quality of each of the seven body tissue systems. The quantitative and qualitative distribution of an individual's Elemental composition is assessed.

4. *Samhanana:* body conformation. This refers to an assessment of the body build or compactness of the body as a whole. It includes an estimation of symmetry, proportion, nutritional status, general functioning, and movement.

5. *Anguli pramana:* body proportion measurement. This refers to an ancient Ayurvedic concept using mathematical formulas with Ayurvedic measurements called "finger units" to assess the proportions of the body and limbs.

6. *Satmya:* wholesomeness. This represents the patient's adaptability to healthy and optimal diet, herbs, climate, and life-style. *Satmya* assesses the patient's natural inclination to gravitate toward and to incorporate *prakruti* compatible, sattvic food choices and behaviors.

7. *Manas prakruti:* psychological constitution. This is an evaluation of the proportions of the *Maha gunas, Sattva, Rajas,* and *Tamas,* which are constitutionally inherent, motivate the patient, and guide lifestyle choices.

8. *Agni* or *Ahara shakti:* digestive fire. This refers to estimating the power of digestive functioning as a result of the quality of the patient's *Agni.*

9. *Vyayama shakti:* capacity for exercise and energy level. This involves an assessment of the general state of energy and endurance, especially concerning physical activity.

10. *Vaya:* age. The actual chronological age of the patient is compared to his current functional level of health and vitality. In addition, the doshic stage of life, for example, early life (*bala*) *Kapha* predominance, midlife (*madhya*) *Pitta* predominance, and older age (*vriddha*) *Vata* predominance, is taken into account. Age and functional capacity are critical to assess.

Ashtavidha Pariksha, The Eightfold Examination

This is a more current and succinct method that particularly takes into account pulse diagnosis. Since a working knowledge of these procedures requires formal training and actual clinical experience, only a brief but representative description of each follows:

1. *Nadi Pariksha:* pulse diagnosis. Ayurvedic pulse diagnosis is different from Western pulse assessments. *Nadi* here refers to the arterial pulse; usually the radial aspect of the arterial pulse is measured. The physician uses three fingers simultaneously. The index finger is placed over the radial artery closest to the wrist; this area reflects the *Vata* aspect of the pulse. Its sensory impression suggests a characteristic movement (*gati*) resembling that of a snake (*Sarpagati*). When *Vata* is vitiated, the *Vata* pulse is irregular, unsteady, and difficult to detect. It has an insubstantial quality to it. The *Vata*

pulse has a low volume and tension, is subtle, and has the weakest or "emptiest" force behind it. Its snakelike character gives it a feel that is thready, narrow, and thin. It tends to be the fastest pulse of the three.

The middle finger is positioned proximal to the index finger and is over the *Pitta* aspect of the pulse. Its sensory impression suggests the leaping movements of a frog (*Mandukagati*). When aspects of *Pitta* are vitiated, the pulse has qualities that are warm, rapid, and thin. It is the strongest pulse and has the highest amplitude, which noticeably drops after each beat. Its froglike character gives a feel that is wiry, taut, tight, jumping, and bounding in quality.

The ring finger is placed next to the middle finger in the direction of the elbow. This is the *Kapha* aspect of the pulse, and it has the characteristic movement of a swan (*Hamsagati*). When vitiated, this pulse is steady, cold, thick, full, and substantial. Its volume and rhythm are balanced and full. The swanlike character gives the *Kapha* pulse qualities that are slow, wide, broad, large, deep, rolling, graceful, and slippery.

When the pulse is basically healthy, it is said to have the feel of the movement of an elephant, that is, slow, steady, and regular.

Pulse rate (*spandana sankhya*) is approximately 80 to 100 beats per minute for *Vata,* 65 to 80 for *Pitta,* and around 70 and lower for *Kapha.* The most accurate pulse reading occurs first in the early morning before food and exertion. The physician uses the right hand and takes the pulse on the right hand of a male and on the left hand of a female. Pulse diagnosis requires a high level of diagnostic sophistication and requires years of training to obtain proficiency. Nuances of the *prakruti* that include information about the subdoshas are discernible in proficient pulse diagnosis.

2. *Jihva Pariksha:* tongue diagnosis. The size, color, coating, and moisture of the tongue are inspected. Small size, pale color, brown or black coating, and dryness indicate *Vata.* Average size, reddish color, yellow coating, and a tendency to dryness indicate *Pitta.* A large tongue that is pale with a moist and whitish coating indicates *Kapha.*

3. *Drika Pariksha:* eye diagnosis. *Vata* signs are dryness and possible tics or twitches. *Pitta* signs are redness and irritation. *Kapha* signs show as watery eyes.

4. *Sparsha Pariksha:* touch diagnosis. This includes detecting the temperature of the skin and abdominal palpation.

5. *Shabda Pariksha:* voice diagnosis. The *Vata* voice is variable in tone and tends to be breathy and relatively indistinct. The *Pitta* voice is sharp, clear, and precise. The *Kapha* voice has a deep tone and is soft and melodious.

6. *Akriti Pariksha:* general appearance diagnosis. This is an important part of the examination and gives both specific and general information concerning the patient's physical body and psychological demeanor. As applies to the other elements of the clinical examination, a further elaboration of technique is beyond the scope of the present work.

7. *Mutra Pariksha:* urine diagnosis. Ayurvedic medicine uses a unique method in assessing the condition of the patient by examining the urine using the addition of drops of oil to the surface. The behavior of the oil droplets is

associated with the *doshic* quality, the severity, and the prognosis of the disease.

8. *Purisha Pariksha:* feces diagnosis. Stool samples are examined for appearance, color, odor, and behavior when placed in a small amount of water. These data reflect the state of the *Agni,* the *doshas,* and the presence of *Ama.*

COMPLEXITY OF THE DISEASE PROCESS AND OF DIAGNOSIS

Ayurveda acknowledges the complexity of the disease process and the difficulty in arriving at an accurate diagnosis. The *BioPsychoSpiritual* perspective takes into consideration the whole individual as an integral person in an interpersonal field.

Charaka recognized the intricacies and variations of morphology and the dynamic nature of physiological and metabolic processes from the cellular through the tissue, organ, and system levels over 2,000 years ago. Concerning this he says,

When classified according to cause, pain, color, site, form, and nomenclature, the number of diseases becomes really countless. A physician need not be ashamed if he is not able to name all diseases, as there can be no definite standardization for all diseases. The same provoked *dosha* may produce a variety of diseases according to diversity of causes and to location. Therefore, treatment should be initiated after diagnosing the nature of the disease (with the vitiated *dosha* and *dushya*), and any special causative factors.

(*Charaka Samhita,* Sutra Sthana 18.42–44).

8

NUTRITION AND DIET IN AYURVEDA

THE CONCEPT OF NUTRITION IN AYURVEDA: THEORETICAL CONSIDERATIONS

The concept of nutrition (*annapanavidhi*) in Ayurveda, like other fundamental Ayurvedic propositions, is thousands of years old (Mukerjee, 1974). It is based on empirical evidence derived from health maintenance practices and disease interventions using dietary and adjunctive herbal and mineral preparations. Nutrition as dietetics and food intake (*ahara*), the ingestion and digestion of protein, fats, and carbohydrates, is considered one of the three main pillars upon which the life of the body is supported. The other two pillars are sleep and proper regulation of sexual functioning.

Nutrition and diet in Ayurveda have several goals. The general aim of diet is to supply the entire individual with nourishing substances to sustain life. More specifically, nutrition subsumes the following: (1) to supply and to replenish the Five Great Gross Elements to the body, (2) keeping the *doshas* in proper balance to maintain quality of life; foods continuously act to rebalance one's *dosha* portfolio, and (3) using tastes or the *rasa* of foods and substances (botanicals, plant substances, herbs, and minerals) to correct imbalances in the *doshas,* that is, to treat disorders and disease. In addition to its primary aim of nourishing the body, food is also used as medicine. Prescribing an individualized selection of foods (*anna*), specifically with a consideration of their *rasas* (taste qualities), is a chief therapeutic modality. A thorough understanding of the integral nature of Ayurvedic nutritional theory, the theory of the digestive process, and the empirical selection of compatible food choices is essential.

Dravyaguna Shastra (Sharma, 1976), the science of the attributes, actions, and effects of substances on the body when taken internally, is the term for the ancient system formalized to explain the nutritive and pharmacological effects both of food and of medicine. In Ayurveda, these two categories have fluid boundaries and are not mutually exclusive. *Dravyaguna Shastra* constituted a rational attempt at standardization and grew out of the empirical work of practitioners throughout the centuries. Any substance that can be ingested, therefore, such as food, liquids, herbs, minerals, and so forth, is governed by the principles established by this system of physiological and pharmacological action. In Ayurveda, this concept is broadened to include the range of sensory experience (perceptual information) as well as motor activity (action imprints), which is believed to be ingested and taken into the mental faculties as mental nourishment having a cascade of effects.

Dravyaguna Shastra, Ayurveda's Materia Medica, is a rational system that outlines the cellular and physiological mechanisms concerned with the pharmacokinetic and pharmacodynamic processes of the body (absorption, circulation, and tissue and cell effects) after substances are ingested. The Sanskrit term *dravya* refers to a fundamental concept in Ayurveda derived from the *Vaisheshika darshana. Dravya* connotes a substance in the specific sense of describing one fundamental category that is a unit of creation. In terms of describing foods, herbs, and medicines, substance means a distinct particle of matter, a fundamental unit used as a building block. It may denote a mutually exclusive category with relatively indivisible status, as, for example, an atom or a molecule. The Five Great Gross Elements, for instance, are considered fundamental material substances that are virtually indivisible and mutually exclusive. *Drayva,*therefore, denotes a container that houses the unique attributes and actions of a substance. An essential part of the inseparable nature of a substance is the indissoluble marriage of its qualities or attributes (*gunas*) and its actions (*karma*).

Shastra refers to a methodical instruction system (a textbook). Other essential concepts in this system include the idea of *karma,* the action and consequences of a substance; *samanya,* the therapeutic principle of "like increasing like"; and *vishesha,* the therapeutic principle of "opposites curing or balancing each other." The last major proposition in this pharmacological perspective is contained in the Sanskrit term *samavaya,* which refers to the overriding principle of interactive unification, one which carries the substance toward its aim. This means that one substance (*dravya*) contains within itself an inseparable linkage to its inherent qualities (*gunas*) and their necessary actions and effects (*karma*).

The boundaries of meaning and usage in Ayurveda among such diverse categories as those that encompass foods, herbs, drugs, as well as the sensory and motor experience of life-style and behavior are thin and exceedingly porous. Dietary substances or *foods* refer to those ingested materials that give energy to bodily processes, replenish utilized bodily components, and provide overall nutrition and nourishment. Foods are characterized by an emphasis on *rasa* (taste), greater quantitative intake, and the gradual replenishment of the inorganic Elements (Ether, Air, Fire, Water, and Earth), which become transformed into "humanized" or biologically assimilable Elements in order to maintain biological doshic balance (*Vata, Pitta,* and *Kapha*). Foods and spices are for daily consumption.

Anna is the term for food. It is biologically "raw" until full digestion in the Ayurvedic sense takes place in order to make it "cooked" and biologically available to the human organism for assimilation into body, mind, and consciousness. In general, this refers to the highly complex digestive process that is described in detail in Chapter 4. Understanding that extensive discussion is a necessary prerequisite to understanding the material presented in this chapter.

The Ayurvedic concept of digestion is complex. First, raw food is acted upon in the gastrointestinal tract by the *Agni* of *Pachaka Pitta* (*Avasthapaka,* primary digestion). The onset of this ripening process begins to transform it into *ahara rasa,* an unhomologous pool of nutrients. Second, *ahara rasa* is transported into the liver where *Bhutagnis* and *Ranjaka Pitta* transform *ahara rasa* into the homologous, biologically available *poshaka* (precursor nutrient) called *asthayi* (unstable) *rasa* and finally *sthayi* (stable) *rasa,* which floats all over the body and bathes each tissue. Third, the *sthayi rasa* acting as a transport medium propelled by *Vyana Vata* carries *asthayi* tissue precursors that are in the process of forming to the sites of their specific tissues where each is acted upon by its respective *dhatu Agni* to become the *poshaya* that is *sthayi* (stable mature tissue nutrient) for that specific *dhatu.* This is an important aspect of *Vipaka* digestive assimilation. *Sthayi rasa* as well as the *asthayi* form of each tissue float all over the body. Only when the latter becomes positioned and then stationery in its respective tissue does it become *sthayi* (stabilized) *dhatu* (tissue).

The formative cascade of the seven tissues begins with *rasa* and *rakta.* For example, initially within about five days, the *asthayi ahara rasa* undergoes various *Agni* digestive transformations to form two end products simultaneously: (1) *sthayi rasa dhatu* (stable or mature plasma) and (2) *asthayi rakta dhatu* (immature blood). After about ten days, the stable plasma helps *asthayi rakta dhatu* to become transformed by its *Raktadhara kala* (blood tissue holding digestive membrane) to become *sthayi rakta dhatu* (mature blood), the second *dhatu* in the cascade. The formation of the plasma or *rasa* is the substratum out of which arises the formation of all the other bodily tissues. Subsequently, as *rasa* travels out of the liver to each specific tissue site, it facilitates the formation of and also partly transforms into stable *rakta,* then *mamsa,* then *meda,* then *asthi,* then *majji,* then *shukra,* and ultimately, *Ojas.*

In Western physiology, most blood formation occurs in the bone marrow, although the liver, the spleen, the lymph nodes, and the thymus are also important sites. In Ayurveda, the liver and the spleen assume central significance in the formation of plasma and blood.

Drugs, in the Ayurvedic sense, refer to any ingested medicinal substances (botanicals, herbs, plant substances, and minerals) that perform in an active therapeutic manner *to induce* doshic balance in the presence of significant imbalance, to restore vitiated tissues, and to alleviate disordered conditions. Botanical and mineral drugs act to dynamically rebalance vitiated *doshas.* Unlike foods, drugs are taken into the body in very small quantities. Foods primarily nourish the *dhatus* (tissues), while drugs harmonize and balance the overall structure and functioning of the body.

Foods and drugs have four fundamental bodily effects: *rasa* (taste), *virya* (energy), *vipaka* (postdigestive effect), and *prabhava* (idiosyncratic effect). The *rapid and powerful* therapeutic action of Ayurvedic medicinal substances (herbs, minerals, and drugs) is dominated mostly by the *virya* (potency and energy) of the substance. A drug's efficacy and effectiveness is directly related to the specific and unique *virya* that emerges from its particular composition of Elements. *Virya,* it is to be remembered, refers to the energetic hot-cold spectrum of a substance; it is one of the most fundamental *gurvadi gunas,* that is, an attribute that defines what a substance is and how it performs. *Virya* pulls its potency from the *Jatharagni, the central digestive fire.* The concept of *virya* holds a very special place in Ayurvedic pharmacology because the hot (*ushna*) attribute of a substance targets the activation of *Agni* within the body both generally and at very particular sites (cells, tissues, organs, and channel systems) in a direct and powerful way.

In terms of the actions of a drug, the *vipaka* (postdigestive effect) is also more important in eliciting a therapeutic effect than its *rasa* (taste). The *prabhava,* a substance's special, unusual, and idiosyncratic medicinal action, however, overrides all else. A substance with a special *prabhava* does not work on the *doshas* in general. It targets a specific tissue, organ, symptom, or disease—almost in an isolated fashion. Various examples of substances with special *prabhavas* are the following: emetics, laxatives, cardiac stimulants, vermifuges, narcotics, ghee and milk combinations, and the action of basil, gems, crystals, and mantras.

Consequently, this requires consumption of much smaller quantities of drugs and substances that have peculiar *prabhavas* because of their greater intrinsic therapeutic potency and their ability to destroy *Ama* (toxins) and to pacify vitiated *doshas.* This chapter, then, in covering the principles of Ayurvedic nutrition as it pertains to dietary food intake, also covers the fundamental theoretical principles of *Dravyaguna Shastra* and medicinal substances.

THE MAJOR CONSTITUENTS OF FOODS, HERBS, AND MINERALS

In Ayurveda, the fundamental properties of foods, herbs, and minerals are conceptually analyzed and understood as consisting of four categories of component parts. Although these four classes are virtually inseparable in a substance, for academic purposes, they can be distinguished. They are the following:

1. *Maha gunas.* This consists of the major subtle qualities of *Sattva* (purity), *Rajas* (turbulence), and *Tamas* (inertia) that are contained in a substance. Through experience and the analytic methods of *Dravyaguna Shastra,* each food article and each medicinal substance have been recognized as having a predominance of one of these universal, binding factors. A substance actually evokes a particular *Maha guna* increase in an individual rather than merely containing it apart from human contact. In other words, some foods are more

sattvic and wholesome than others and so in turn act to enhance an individual's consciousness and spirituality.

2. *Gurvadi gunas.* These are the ten pairs of opposite attributes (hot/cold, heavy/ light, oily/dry, stable/mobile, hard/soft, clear/cloudy, rough/smooth, gross/ subtle, dull/sharp, and liquid/dense) that characterize all substances. These impart meaning through perceptual information. Ayurveda considers that virtually every manifestation in the created world can be described using several of these fundamental properties. They expose stylistic form on substantive Elemental content. These attributes have physical and tangible status as well as having internal pharmacological actions. Of all the *gurvadi gunas,* the hot (*ushna*)/cold (*shita*) pair of thermal attributes holds special prominence. The heat of a substance powerfully affects *Agni* on all levels in the body. This *virya,* which is rooted in the *Jatharagni,* is quintessential to the potency of a substance, particularly to a drug. In addition to the primacy of the effects of *virya,* other pairs of food qualities that have important effects on the *doshas* are heavy (*guru*)/light (*laghu*) and oily (*snigdha*)/dry (*ruksha*).

3. Elements. The Five Great Gross Elements or *Mahabhutanis* (Ether, Air, Fire, Water, and Earth) are the elemental building blocks of all material substances. The Elements are the principal *dravyas* in food and are important components in the effects of medicines. The Elements make up all material substances, inorganic and organic, inanimate and animate. These Elements are the chief templates that impart substantive identity to a physical substance. Every substance contains all five Elements, but only one or two Elements predominate. In a given substance, the Elemental composition varies in its proportions. The characteristic Elemental composition of any substance is the material bedrock upon which all other phenomena such as attributes, taste, and actions operate. Each Element contains a subtle half known as its "subtle essence" or *Tanmatra.* This constitutes a significant nutritional component that feeds the individual on an energetic level. *Manas* is fed in this way.

4. *Rasa.* This Sanskrit term has several meanings; some of which are *taste, plasma, essence,* and *sap.* In terms of nutrition and medicinal substances, *rasa* refers to the predigestive taste, specifically to one or more of the six primary tastes: Sweet, Salty, Sour, Bitter, Pungent, and Astringent. Taste is a major constituent of food and also exerts a major effect within the body. Within each different taste or *rasa,* two Elements predominate. Each taste, however, contains all five Elements, and this virtually infinite blending of Elements emerges as the taste of a substance. The concept of taste, in fact, has a corollary meaning, that is, the subjective taste experience evoked within the individual by the ingestion of a food or herb. Dietary and medicinal materials, themselves, however, are considered to have some intrinsic taste qualities, in part, determined by their Elemental composition. Taste or *rasa* in the operational Ayurvedic sense is virtually identified with the nexus between the objective taste nature of ingested materials and the subjective taste experience that they evoke. *Rasa* as taste both directly and indirectly (via *Pitta* and *Agni*) affects and modulates the *doshas. Rasa,* food as nutrition, and maintaining *dosha* balance all act in conjunction with one another.

THE FOUR EFFECTS OF INGESTED FOODS AND DRUG SUBSTANCES

Ayurveda is unique in having formulated a fourfold scheme of the actions of foods and drug substances once they are ingested. Once taken into the mouth and then swallowed, each substance may be analyzed according to its *rasa* (taste), *virya* (potency), *vipaka* (postdigestive effect), and *prabhava* (idiosyncratic effect). Unlike the major constituents of foods, which are a description of their compositional categories, the four effects denote their actions inside the body.

It should be mentioned, however, that these four different terms and concepts reside on differing levels of discourse. *Rasa* as taste and *virya* as potency are more descriptive of the nature and properties of a substance as well as on their effects on the *doshas* and the body. The emphasis in the concept of *Vipaka,* by contrast, is on a highly complicated series of physiological actions and functions within the colon and at cellular and tissue sites. *Vipaka* denotes mechanisms of action and transformative operations. *Prabhava* denotes the unique and, oftentimes unexplainable, effect that a therapeutic substance exerts within the body.

THE NATURE OF TASTE OR *RASA* ACCORDING TO AYURVEDA

As has been described, the phenomenon of taste is a leading descriptor in Ayurvedic nutritional classification. All substances have the additional characteristic of therapeutic potency, and although this potency is contained in dietary foods, it is most important when considering therapeutic herbs and minerals. The taste aspect is more dominated by the influence of a substance's Elemental composition. Taste denotes the predigestive experience (Sweet, Sour, Pungent, Astringent, Bitter, or Salty) of a substance when put on the tongue. Taste is mediated chiefly by the functions of *doshas: bodhaka kapha* in the mouth, *prana vata* in the brain, and *sadhaka pitta* in the brain.

Ayurveda places the subjective and the objective experience of taste in a premier position. The taste experience, in large measure, is the ongoing, daily, and repetitive contact that the individual makes with the outside world. Satisfaction, pleasure, and survival result. Western medicine has delineated an extensive neurophysiologic mapping of the mechanisms underlying taste and has included the interdependent mechanisms of the sense of smell, the olfactory system, in describing these sensory functions. While a thorough review of this complicated area is beyond the scope of this book, a brief outline of some basic principles will be given for the sake of perspective and clarity.

The olfactory function, the sense of smell, is considered relatively more important and overriding in the Western view of gustatory experience. Aromas of ingested substances are produced by their volatile components and picked up by the sense of smell that is experienced as the "flavor" of food. An almost infinite number of distinct flavors are differentiated in the process of ingesting a substance, and these are mainly the result of the substance's aromas stimulating the olfactory cranial nerves. The sense of smell is mediated by the chemosensory system that includes the nasal olfactory neuroepithelium containing olfactory sensory receptors that, in turn, travel through the first cranial nerve, the olfactory nerve. To a smaller extent, the fifth cranial nerve, the trigeminal, is also involved. The smell experience determines the flavor and the palatability of foods.

The gustatory function, the sense of taste, is considered to have important significance, but its functions play a relatively secondary role in overall taste perception since Western medicine views olfactory sensation as more overriding in its interplay with the sense of taste. Gustatory coding is believed to consist of gross and of finer discrimination. There are five major groupings of taste buds with taste receptor cells. Four of these are anatomically located on the tongue; the fifth is more diffuse and has sites on the palate, the epiglottis, the larynx, and the esophagus. The sense of taste is mediated chiefly by the seventh cranial nerve, the facial nerve, which has its distribution on the anterior two-thirds of the tongue. The ninth cranial nerve, the glossopharyngeal, and the tenth, the vagus, also play a part. These nerves terminate in the part of the brain stem called the nucleus tractus solitarius and produce, according to the Western view, the experience of the two leading tastes, Sweet and Salty. The other two tastes that are recognized, Sour and Bitter, result from the combined olfactory and gustatory interplay.

In Western nutrition, a large part of the taste of foods is related to their phytochemical content. These phytonutrients are often polyphenol antioxidants and contain pigments that impart bright colors to fruits and vegetables. Some examples are lutein that makes corn yellow, lycopene that makes tomatoes red, carotene that makes carrots orange, and anthocyanin that is responsible for the blue color of blueberries and the purple color of eggplant. A subgroup of phytochemicals is the group of flavonoids in berries, herbs, and vegetables. Although these phytochemicals are not regarded as essential to normal metabolism, recent studies suggest a beneficial role in promoting improved immunity, reducing inflammation, neutralizing free radicals, and preventing forms of cardiovascular disease and cancer. The top phytonutrient-rich foods are soy, tomato, broccoli, garlic, flax, citrus, blueberries, sweet potatoes, chilies, and legumes such as beans, peas, and lentils.

The tastes are perceived at various areas on the tongue. Locations may vary. The following is a general orientation. Sweet taste is sensed at the tip; Sour taste at the anterior, lateral front sides; Bitter taste at the posterior, middle, and lateral sides; Salty taste at the more posterior, lateral sides; Pungent taste at the anterior, middle third; and Astringent taste at the posterior area.

Ayurveda regards the predigestive *rasa* (taste) of a substance as the culmination of its integrated blend of *Maha gunas, gurvadi gunas,* and Elements. While each individual taste contains all five Elements, usually only two predominate. Sweet taste has Earth and Water, Sour taste has Earth and Fire,

Salty taste has Water and Fire, Pungent taste has Air and Fire, Bitter taste has Air and Ether, and Astringent taste has Air and Earth.

In Ayurvedic nutrition, the essence of food is contained in the innate qualities that are experienced as its taste. The meaning of the essence of food is understood as having a dual nature. The apparent material nature of food is considered to contain its gross food essence. This is composed of some combination of the Five Great Gross Elements (*Pancha Mahabhutanis*), which is gustatorily perceived as food's taste or *rasa*. The ingestion of this aspect of food primarily nourishes the physical body.

The other aspect of food's nature is understood to be its subtle food essence. This is composed of the subtle halves of the Great Gross Elements, the *Tanmatras*. These subtle essences, not directly perceived by taste, are taken in along with the gross food essences. They are also taken in psychologically through each of the five senses (hearing, touch, vision, taste, and smell). These *Tanmatras* are ingested by *Manas* (mind) and contribute to mental nutrition as well as to overall bodily nutrition, especially to that of the *doshas*.

In Ayurveda, therefore, proper nutrition rests solely on the adequate intake of the Five Great Elements (*Pancha Mahabhutanis*) and their five subtle, energetic essences (*Pancha Tanmatras*). The *Maha gunas* (*Sattva, Rajas,* and *Tamas*) reside within the container of the Elements and the *Tanmatras*. The gross or combustible portions that can be reduced to ash are important but of secondary order. The reference point in Ayurvedic nutrition is the experience of taste. Nutrition, therefore, is based on a complex delineation of the taste properties of foods. The almost infinite permutations and combinations of differing quantities and qualities of the Elements produce a spectrum of degrees of specific tastes, and these, in turn, combine to produce distinctive subjectively perceived flavors.

Ayurveda considers that it is the *rasa,* the taste of a food or herb when put on the tongue, that exerts an immediate and localized effect. The launching of this process occurs before digestion proper begins. Since the Ayurvedic term *rasa* signifies both taste as well as the plasma of the body, the intimate association between the two pervades a discussion of each and of their interdependent functioning. In Ayurveda, the mechanisms of taste begin to operate first through the medium of water (saliva, *Bodhaka Kapha*), then circulate through channels to reach the brain and mind in order to initiate the complicated process of digestion. Taste is the key point of contact and entry of the unhomologous external world into the internal world. The aim of optimal digestion is to facilitate *Agni*'s adequate transformation of unhomologous Elements into homologous Elements that are capable of being assimilated and then providing nutrition to support the *dhatus* (bodily tissues).

Ayurveda recognizes six basic and mutually exclusive tastes. Every ingested substance has a predominance of one or more of these tastes. While every substance contains a portion of each of the five Elements, yet only a few predominate just as only a few essential tastes predominate in any one substance. It may seem quite simplistic, if not reductionistic, to use such a seemingly narrow taste range as the foundation for a broad nutritional concept. The Ayurvedic literature recognizes this, and in a conspicuous fashion, distinctly acknowledges the immense complexity involved in the taste phenomena as well as in the taxonomy and mechanisms of *Dravyaguna Shastra*. The descriptions presented here, therefore, represent a basic introductory approach to a very complicated pharmacognosy and pharmacological body of knowledge, which applies to all ingested substances including foods, herbs, and medicines.

Foods and medicines are primarily classified according to their taste composition. The six tastes are Sweet (*Madhura*), Sour (*Amla*), Salty (*Lavana*), Pungent (*Katu*), Bitter (*Tikta*), and Astringent (*Kashaya*). Each taste has an Element, *Maha guna,* and *gurvadi guna* (ten pairs of opposite qualities) makeup. The Elements in the substance are the chief source of nutrition to the tissues of the body. They restore the body's used-up Elements that are dissipated into energy through the metabolic processes. *Rasa* (taste) is the instrument used to ascertain the Elemental composition of a food or herb. *Rasa,* therefore, is understood to be the taste perception of the specific manner in which the Elements combine in a given food or substance.

The *gurvadi guna* attributes, especially their thermal *virya* dimension, of a substance contribute to balancing the *doshas* of the body especially when these *doshas* are vitiated or aggravated. The influence of these *gurvadi gunas* is so powerful that their action supersedes or overrides the general effects of the overall taste action of a substance. The *guna* attributes, in fact, have significantly greater efficacy and potency both on the physiological and on the pharmacological level.

The *Maha guna* effect of a substance affects the individual's quality of consciousness. Sattvic substances refine and enhance consciousness, rajasic substances tend to agitate, and tamasic substances tend to constrict. None of these trends acts unilaterally; they act in concert with one another and only one *Maha guna* predominates.

TASTE AND ITS EFFECT ON THE *DOSHAS*

In Ayurveda, one of the primary methods of affecting doshic balance is through the medium of taste. The Elements or Primary Pentads in foods act to gradually feed the tissues and more slowly, to increase or to decrease the *doshas*. By virtue of the taste (*rasa*) properties of drugs, especially their hot-cold *guna* and *virya* spectrum, the *doshas* are more rapidly affected. The taste profile of a substance directly affects the *doshas* (*Vata, Pitta,* and *Kapha*) by contributing either to their increase or to their decrease. The Elemental dominance of a particular taste also contributes to the rise or fall of a *dosha*.

Each *dosha* has a predominance of two Elements, one of which may be considered primary and the other secondary. *Vata* (propulsion) has Air as its primary Element and Ether as its secondary. *Pitta* (transformation) has Fire as its primary Element and Water as its secondary. *Kapha* (consolidation) is generally considered to have Water as its primary Element and Earth as its secondary.

Vata in the body is increased by foods that have any of the following tastes: Bitter, Astringent, or Pungent. This is due to the predominance of the Air Element in these three tastes. The secondary Elements in these tastes are Ether in Bitter taste, Earth in Astringent taste, and Fire in Pungent taste.

Pitta is increased by foods that have any of the following tastes: Sour, Pungent, and Salty. Each of these tastes has Fire as its primary Element. The secondary Elements for these tastes are Earth for Sour, Air for Pungent, and Water for Salty.

Kapha has substantial amounts of Water as well as the Earth Element. The three tastes that increase *Kapha* with their associated Elements, respectively, are Sweet with Earth and Water, Salty with Water and Fire, and Sour with Earth and Fire.

The tastes that decrease the levels of the *doshas* in the body are the following: Salty, Sour, and Sweet tastes decrease *Vata;* Bitter, Astringent, and Sweet tastes decrease *Pitta;* Pungent, Bitter, and Astringent tastes decrease *Kapha.*

Taste, therefore, contributes to the modulation and functioning of each *dosha;* taste, in effect, has a general therapeutic action. Proper and healthful diet and nutrition can be achieved only by the correct matching of one's individual *prakruti* (constitution, body/mind type) needs with the corresponding foods and herbs. These needs include a range of components such as optimal doshic levels, Elements, *gurvadi gunas,* and *Maha gunas.* The essential idea for optimal health is the ongoing maintenance of equilibrium proper to the optimal functioning of the individual's *prakruti.* Daily attention to this is emphasized since daily needs regularly change. This is, in part, due to the natural utilization and dissipation of the aforementioned components in the course of growth, maturation, and development. In addition, a therapeutic need for restoration results from the processes of depletion (for example, the Elements) or vitiation (for example, the *doshas*).

An adequate nutritional level of the range of the five Elements is the single most significant and necessary factor needed to maintain overall equilibrium. These five Elements are the building blocks of the *doshas, dhatus* (tissues), and *malas* (wastes). Foods provide ongoing nutrition. Herbs act as healing drugs and medications. Proper nutrition and diet customized to one's *prakruti* and doshic needs keep the *doshas* balanced and optimally functioning. This, in turn, promotes healthy tissues, organs, and psychological well-being. Diet, therefore, is directly related to the quality of health and to the disease process. The Ayurvedic concept of nutrition strongly emphasizes these considerations. The nutritional perspective of Western medicine that deals with foods and their protein, carbohydrate, fat, and vitamin components is recognized as important, but is not a major focus in the Ayurvedic view.

THE CONCEPT OF *VIRYA:* POTENCY OR ENERGY

The *virya* aspect relates to the energy of a substance and to its capacity to produce a significantly strong and substantial effect. The concept of *virya* may be likened to the dual pharmacological concepts of drug efficacy and drug potency. *Virya* is that aspect of a nutritional or medicinal herbal substance that exerts its primary effect during digestion proper. *Virya,* the dimension reflecting a substance's energetic temperature, is subsumed within the ten pairs of opposite attributes or *gurvadi gunas* but retains a special position in nutrition and herbology. *Virya* is rooted in the *Jatharagni.* It derives its efficacy from this primary transformative energy. The therapeutic potency of many herbs, for instance, relates to their *virya* status.

Although the concept of *virya* includes a range of diverse characteristics, the leading attributes identified with it are on a spectrum with designations ranging from hot to cold. The hot end denotes increased potency toward activation, and the cold end denotes increased potency toward reduction. This reflects the specific action of *virya* on the *Agni,* the transformative energy of the body as a whole. A direct effect on the biological *Pitta dosha* is closely tied into this. For example, when the *virya* of a food choice appropriately matches an individual's constitutional needs, it produces a positive enhancement of the entire digestive process. In terms of a hot *virya,* the Salty taste is warm, the Sour taste is warmer, and the Pungent taste is hottest. In terms of a cold *virya,* the Sweet taste is cool, the Astringent taste is cooler, and the simple Bitter taste is coldest. The Bitter taste most powerfully lowers *Pitta dosha* and *Kapha dosha.* The Sweet taste most powerfully increases *Kapha dosha* and decreases *Vata dosha.* Finally, many factors contribute to the *virya* of a substance. These include its growing location, season of growth, harvesting time and technique, handling, age, and processing.

THE CONCEPT OF *VIPAKA:* THE FINAL METABOLIC, POSTDIGESTIVE TASTE EFFECT IN TISSUES (THE SECOND PART OF PRIMARY DIGESTION)

The concept of *Vipaka* (postdigestive effect) or *Isthapaka* in the process of digestion as understood in Ayurveda has the sense of digestive cooking and occurs after the primary macrodigestive process (*Avasthapaka*) is completed within the gastrointestinal tract.

Vipaka represents the delayed, systemic whole body digestive effect, the end phase and result of digestion. This metabolic conceptualization, part of an entire spectrum of the metabolic-digestive process, is unique to Ayurveda. The *vipaka* effect of a food occurs after all the digestive processes have occurred when the properly prepared nutrients (*ahara rasa*) are ready to be assimilated into cells and to become part of the tissue substance. *Vipaka* occurs both in the colon and at the cellular and tissue levels.

Vipaka may be understood as the final assimilative process of microdigestion that represents the culmination of the entire digestive process and yields a bottom line cellular effect within the tissues and the organism as a whole. *Vipaka* represents the dynamic action that uses the essence of foods and herbs in a nutritive manner to support and maintain the body. The *vipaka* of a substance is also more powerful in exerting a therapeutic effect on the tissues than is that substance's primary *rasa* or taste.

In summary, as Charaka (c. 700 B.C.) has explained in his medical treatises, *vipaka* is understood to refer to one of three end results of digestion. These are described in terms of postdigestive tastes. (1) Foods with either Sweet or Salty tastes remain sweet at the culmination of all digestion. This has a cooling effect, increases *Kapha,* significantly contributes to the nutritive buildup of all seven bodily tissues, and aids in healthy elimination. Many tonic substances have this Sweet *vipaka.* (2) Foods with a predominantly Sour taste produce a Sour postdigestive effect that is somewhat heating, increase *Pitta,* contribute to the buildup of all bodily tissues except the reproductive tissues, and produce a small eliminative enhancement. (3) Foods with tastes that include Bitter, Pungent, and Astringent aspects have a Pungent postdigestive effect that is catabolic, increases *Vata,* and does not contribute to the buildup of bodily tissues or to enhanced eliminative processes. Substances whose *vipaka* is Pungent are beneficial in that they act as digestive stimulants and help to reduce *Ama.*

Sushruta speaks of only two *Vipaka* results: (1) Sweet *vipaka, Brimhana* or building up the tissues and (2) Sour and Pungent *vipaka, Langhana* or lightening the tissues.

THE CONCEPT OF *PRABHAVA:* THE IDIOSYNCRATIC PHARMACOLOGICAL EFFECT BEYOND *RASA, VIRYA,* AND *VIPAKA*

Although Ayurvedic nutrition and herbology are essentially covered in the concepts of *rasa* (taste), *virya* (potency), and *vipaka* (postdigestive effect), the effects of certain foods and herbs transcend comprehension using these categories. When such a substance with a recognizable set of tastes, energies, and postdigestive characteristics does not behave accordingly, it is said to contain a unique *Prabhava.* This special action is usually very pointed in its targeted effect. *Prabhava* aims itself at a specific tissue, organ, or disease. The *prabhava* quality of a substance frequently is related to a unique energy, potency, and hot/cold quality, although this is not invariably uniform. The Bitter predigestive *rasa* is the taste most associated with *Prabhava.*

An illustration of *Prabhava* is the uniqueness of ghee (*Ghritam* in Sanskrit meaning to shine). For example, both milk and ghee share a Sweet *rasa,* a cold *virya,* and a Sweet *vipaka.* Only ghee, however, beneficially optimizes *Agni* while reducing excess *Pitta.* Another example of *Prabhava* is the herb

Tulsi or basil. It is heating in *virya* but acts to reduce fever. Black pepper has a Pungent *rasa* and a heating *virya* but reduces *Vata* along with reducing *Kapha*. Black pepper burns *Ama,* but this pepper must be used judiciously since it is very *rajasic.* Meat is Sweet in *rasa* but has a heating *vipaka. Amalaki* has a Sour *rasa* but a cooling *virya.* The pomegranate (*dadima*) used by the ancient Zoroastrians of Persia and also used in Ayurveda has a Sweet and Sour taste in its fruit and an Astringent and Bitter taste in its unripe fruit and in its root bark; its *virya* is hot. Yet, its *Prabhava* is to decrease *Pitta.*

Prabhava as an unexplainable special healing effect has also been attributed to gemstones, crystals, and mantras.

THE SIX BASIC TASTES: THEIR COMPONENTS, EXPRESSION IN FOODS, AND ACTIONS IN THE BODY

Madura: The Sweet Taste

The subjective sense of the Sweet taste includes characteristics of being pleasant, mild, full, and flowing. Sweet is composed of Earth and Water Elements, and its main attributes include cool, heavy, and unctuous (a soft, flowing, liquidy feel just short of being oily). *Unctuous* is the English rendition of a traditional Ayurvedic term that has no direct English equivalent. An approximate meaning would suggest the term *moist.* The temperature appellation *cool* refers to *virya,* the immediate energetic effect of taste on digestion. Substances with a Sweet taste increase *Kapha* and decrease both *Vata* and *Pitta.* These substances, therefore, have an anabolic and nourishing overall effect on the body and are associated with satiation of hunger and thirst. This tissue-building effect is termed *brimhana* and is, perhaps, the most essential nutritional component of a healthy diet. Most foods, for example, carbohydrates, proteins, and fats, have this *madura rasa* as their primary taste. Herbs with a Sweet taste and Sweet *vipaka* are considered tonic and restorative. In Ayurveda, there are significant correspondences between specific tastes and body organs and emotional states. The Sweet taste is associated with the pancreas, the stomach, and the lungs. In addition, there is a correspondence with feelings of satisfaction, well-being, love, and attachment. In excess, dullness, inertia, greed, and greedy desire may be produced. The food groups that primarily contain a predominance of the Sweet taste are carbohydrates, sugars, fats, and proteins. This includes dairy products, grains, fats, oils, nuts, seeds, meat, and fruits.

Amla: The Sour Taste

The Sour taste produces a feeling of some stinging and puckering in the mouth and tends to increase salivation. There is an aperient or appetizing, refreshing, and cleansing effect produced. The Sour taste is composed of the Earth and Fire Elements with attributes that include slightly heavy, hot, and unctuous or moist. Sour increases *Kapha* and *Pitta* and decreases *Vata.*

Foods with an acid content tend to be Sour and supply minerals to the body. Some examples of the Sour taste found in foods include acid, citrus fruits, acid and nightshade group of vegetables (such as tomatoes, potatoes, egg-plant, and peppers), spinach, alcoholic beverages such as wine, yogurt, vin-egar, pickles, and fermented items. The Sour taste strengthens *Pitta* and enhances digestion. The Sour *vipaka* also promotes good elimination of wastes in urine and feces. The pacification of *Vata* tends to promote a reduc-tion in spasm and tremor and may be related to the high mineral content of many sour foods. The Sour taste is associated with the small intestine, the stomach, and the liver. The emotional states associated with the Sour taste are described as a feeling of being refreshed and of increased alertness and attention. In excess, envy, jealousy, and irritability are said to be stimulated.

Lavana: The Salty Taste

The Salty taste is composed of the Fire and the Water Elements and has attributes of being heavy, hot, moist, and sharp. Salt also contains a signifi-cant portion of the Earth Element. The hygroscopic nature of salt causes it to attract water and facilitate solubility. The Salty taste tends to stimulate, soften, and loosen. Digestion and movement are enhanced and elimination is increased. An overall cleansing action is produced. The Salty taste is asso-ciated with the kidneys (*vrukkau*). The significance of salt holds a special place in all concepts of nutrition. At times under conditions where *prakruti, vikruti,* and the season require, salt's Water Element has a nutritional or therapeutic effect that is cooling and hydrating. Conversely, when conditions require, the Fire Element may exert its predominant effect and heat the body thus increasing *Pitta dosha*. Both these aspects of salt have medicinal and therapeutic implications. It should be added that, although the current Ayur-vedic literature does not emphasize the Earth Element in salt, this important and real property has significant therapeutic implications since it may act to decrease *Vata* and increase *Kapha* acutely in the short term and so produce a downward or sinking action within the bodily tissues. In proper amounts, the Salty taste is considered to have a grounding emotional effect. In excess, especially chronically used over the long term, it can aggravate *Pitta* and blood, increase *Vata,* dry out circulatory *rasa dhatu,* cause premature aging, and cause laxity of the bodily tissues. Psychologically, excesses enhance tendencies toward avarice, greed, and hedonistic pursuits. Foods with a Salty taste supply a variety of minerals to the body and include the range of natural salts from the earth and the sea, as well as foods like the variety of seaweed.

Katu: The Pungent Taste

The Pungent taste is composed of the Air and Fire Elements and has the characteristic attributes of being hot, dry, light, and oily. The Pungent taste is often referred to by the terms *spicy* and *aromatic*. Pungent tastes can be caustic or burning. When ingested, pungent substances produce a tingling sensation on the tongue, increase the flow of saliva and other fluids both in the gastrointestinal and in the respiratory tract, and may cause some lacrimation. The Pungent taste decreases *Kapha* and increases *Vata* and *Pitta*.

Pungent substances are carminative (reducing flatulence), expectorant (liquefying bronchial secretions), anticoagulant, antiseptic, and enhance digestion by increasing *Pitta* and enhancing *Agni*. Their strongly transformative actions tend to increase catabolism and the reduction of bodily substances (*langhana*). They strongly increase *Pitta* and consequently tend to be very drying. Included in this large group are the spices, aromatic herbs, and some essential oils. The Pungent taste is associated with the liver. The emotional aspects produced by and associated with the Pungent taste are those related to stimulation and increased awareness. In excess, irritation, anger, envy, and aggression may be provoked.

Tikta: The Bitter Taste

The Bitter taste is composed of the Air and Ether Elements. Its basic attributes are light, cold, dry, subtle, and penetrating. Bitter tastes are often acrid. Bitter tastes, which are either simple or tannin, reduce *Kapha* and *Pitta* and increase *Vata*. Bitters tend to diminish the flow of saliva and dry the mouth. The chemical vehicles of Bitter are the alkaloids and the glycosides. The effects of the Bitter taste are pronounced in the body. They include a drying, reducing (*langhana*), catabolic, and purifying effect. The Bitter taste is linked with the gallbladder, hence its action on bile and on cooling the liver.

The Bitter taste is strongly detoxifying. The Ether and Air Elements in the Bitter taste act to separate *Ama* from the tissues. This is partly due to the action of Bitter *rasa* to increase *Samana Vata*. It aids in the process of *Ama Pachana*, the reduction and palliation of *ama* toxicity. This helps to transform *sama* (with *Ama*) *doshas* and *dhatus* (tissues) to *nirama* (freed from *Ama*) *doshas* and *dhatus*.

Pungent or aromatic Bitters such as turmeric, fenugreek, and calamus have a mostly hot *virya,* increase *Agni,* increase *Samana Vata,* and reduce *ama*. This taste component strongly stimulates digestion through an enhancement of *Vata,* which has a cleansing action on the digestive process. This is related to the action termed *Ama Pachana* (*ama* digestion) and *ama* reduction.

Simple Bitters such as gentian, neem, chicory, dandelion, coptis, chrysanthemum, jasmine, vetiver, and red clover have a mostly cold *virya,* decrease *Pitta,* and are both anti-inflammatory and antibacterial. Tannin and astringentlike Bitters such as aloe, bhringaraj, yellow dock, devil's claw, henna, barberry, and golden seal have a mostly cold *virya* and are antibacterial. Simple and tannin Bitters cool the toxically hot liver conditions (hepatitis, hypertension, and migraines, for example) and reduce body heat.

Some Ayurvedic authorities say that the Bitter *rasa* is the best one of the six tastes. This is based on the idea that it helps to balance and to return to normal all of the other five tastes if they are out of balance.

The Bitter taste is associated with a strong trend toward mental clarity, the opening of consciousness, and a sense of sobriety. In excess, it may produce a sense of coldness felt both physically and emotionally and experienced as grief, sorrow, or depression. The Bitter taste is a component of some botanical, plant, and vegetable substances including some herbs. For example, vegetables that are considered predominantly Bitter are dandelion, chicory, endive, Chinese (*ku gua*) and Indian (*karela*) bitter melon (*Momordia charantia*), romaine lettuce and artichoke; most beers are primarily Bitter in taste. Some olives have a slightly Bitter taste component. Some herbs with significant Bitter taste aspects include turmeric, fenugreek, and aloe vera. Burdock root (*gobo*) is Bitter and Pungent with a cool *virya*. The grain rye has Bitter properties. Bitter herbs are noted for their potent *Prabhava* effect. This has medicinal utility. Bitter tastes cool the heat in the liver, regulate metabolic processes in the pancreas, and are recommended for conditions such as diabetes, headache, and hypertension. Some Bitter tastes have powerful *Prabhava* medicinal effects.

Kashaya: The Astringent Taste

The Astringent taste is composed of the Air and the Earth Elements. Its chief attributes are slightly heavy, cool, and dry. The Astringent taste produces a sense of stiffening, contracting, and puckering in the mouth and throat, dryness, and reduced saliva flow. The chemical vehicle for astringency is usually found in the tannins. This taste is relatively uncommon and is usually consumed in very small quantities. Western medicine, at this time, differentiates only four taste groups: Sweet, Salty, Sour, and Bitter; the Astringent taste in not considered a distinct taste class. Ayurveda describes the actions of the Astringent taste to include those of drying excess secretions, some anti-inflammatory effects, a general healing tendency, and acting to provide some needed minerals. This taste is linked to the kidneys. Psychologically, when in proper balance, it has been associated with asceticism and a general reduction of emotionality, fear, and fright. In large excess, astringent foods may cause increased bodily dryness, constipation, possible impotence, and decreased physiological functions. Some common foods and other edible substances that have astringent qualities are cabbages, potatoes, teas, lettuce, sprouts, raw vegetables, some grasses, pomegranates, cranberries, quince, some apples, and unripe bananas.

PRACTICAL NUTRITION: GENERAL DIETARY GUIDELINES

Practical nutrition comprises guidelines (*upayoga samstha*) for the proper preparation and consumption of foods as well as the proper choice of foods based on one's *prakruti,* age, the season, and current needs. The following delineates some fundamental guidelines for an optimal and healthy diet:

1. A balanced diet includes all six tastes to be ingested as appropriate to one's constitution and also in moderation each day.

2. Dietary choices should be compatible with one's individual *prakruti*.

3. One's diet should generally include foods with qualities that are opposite to one's predominant *dosha* or *doshas*.

4. All foods should be of high quality and should be wholesome (*satmya*).

5. Foods should be fresh, freshly prepared for each meal, and should be cooked and eaten warm or hot. Occasional salads, of course, are eaten raw. The cooking process tends to maximize digestibility and to minimize adverse effects.

6. The largest meal of the day should be eaten around noontime.

7. No food should be eaten until the previous meal has been adequately digested.

8. Close attention to the qualities of each food and to the size of each portion is very important. In general, everything in moderation, as well as moderation itself, is a solid guideline to follow. Intermittent excursions from the norm are beneficial.

9. The quantity and types of foods consumed should match the state of one's digestive fire, the *Agni*.

10. The quantity of food consumed at a meal should be about three-quarters of the stomach's capacity.

11. Incompatible food combinations and improper food mixing should be avoided. The chief examples of this include the following: Milk should not be consumed with any other food except grains. The most undesirable combinations are with bananas, fish, or sour fruits. Eggs should never be eaten with cheese or with potatoes. Melon should always be eaten alone. Yogurt as well as eggs should also be eaten by themselves. Honey should never be cooked. One should never eat honey and ghee in equal proportion. One should never eat a mix of hot with cold foods together.

12. One should generally avoid eating foods that are excessively heavy and cold or excessively dry.

13. Very cold beverages and iced water are not recommended.

14. One's eating demeanor and setting should be pleasant, congenial, and quiet. One should not eat when emotionally upset or rushed. There should be minimal talking and maximal focus and concentration on the food and the eating process. One should try to appreciate the eating experience using all five senses. After eating, one should walk for about 20 minutes. In fact, contemporary Western medicine has clearly demonstrated that such exercise after a meal significantly lowers blood glucose, a very beneficial action. One should avoid heavy *Kapha*-like foods such as yogurt, ice cream, and sesame products after sunset. No food should be eaten within two hours of going to sleep.

15. Large quantities of yogurt, ice cream, cheese, and meat are not recommended. If consumed, they require the addition of spices to act as "antidotes" to prevent excessive adverse reactions. Some examples of these

include the following: Yogurt should be consumed with small amounts of ginger or cumin. Ice cream should be eaten with small amounts of cardamom or cloves. Black pepper or cayenne pepper should accompany cheese; they act to balance excess *Kapha.* If meat is eaten, some added cayenne pepper and some turmeric will make it more digestible. If alcohol or coffee is consumed, cardamom or cumin will counter some of its adverse effects.

16. *Chyavanaprash.* This is, perhaps, one of the most famous general tonics in Ayurveda. It is a medicated paste or jam (*avalehas*) chiefly composed of the *amla* (Hindi) fruit, which is *Phyllanthus Emblica,* also termed *Emblica officinalis. Amla* has a sourlike taste, but *Chyavanaprash* is sweet since it is made with a multitude of other herbs, minerals, raw sugar, honey, and ghee. There are standard compositions of *Chyavanaprash* as well as customized formulas suitable for specific *prakrutis* and particular conditions. Although daily consumption of small amounts is ordinarily beneficial, certain precautions are advised. Those with *Kapha* dominance, excess *Ama,* diabetes, or lipid dysfunctions should seek professional advice before using. Excessive use of very large amounts is not recommended. Use of *amla,* itself, such as in powder or capsule form, however, is very beneficial.

The *amla* fruit is also called Indian gooseberry (English) and *amalaki* (Sanskrit). The *amla* tree is held in legend to have been the first tree created in the universe. Its *rasa* is composed of Sour, Sweet, Pungent, Bitter, and Astringent; there is no Salty taste. Its *virya* is cool, and its *vipaka* is Sweet. The vitamin C concentration in *amalaki* is extraordinarily high and stable, especially to heat. *Amalaki* or *Amla* is called *Dhatri,* the Sanskrit word for nurse or mother who nurtures, protects, and restores. It is a strong rejuvenative, especially for *Pitta dosha.*

Special mention must be made in regard to *Nigella sativa,* black seed oil. This substance is referred to by a variety of names: kalonji (Hindi), Habbatus Sauda and Kamun Aswad (Arabic), shoneez (Persian dialect), kezah (Hebrew), and charnushka (Russian). In *Unani Tibb* medicine, it is regarded as a holy and blessed oil with universal application as an antimicrobial, a digestive stimulant, an immune system booster, and a general restorative. The recommended dosage is about 2.5 ml or ½ teaspoon twice daily.

Special attention needs to be given to the concept of *satmya* (wholesomeness) concerning foods and herbs. *Satmya,* which embodies a high degree of *Sattva* (essential goodness), refers to the degree of optimal quality and purity that a substance, activity, or process contains. Dietary choices need to be carefully considered since only substances that are *satmya* are beneficial to consume. Foods, spices, and herbs need to be fresh, unadulterated, and not or only very minimally processed. The concepts of "organic," "natural," "free from pesticides and herbicides," "hormone-free" and "not genetically engineered" are representative of trends toward *satmya* substances and their production.

AYURVEDIC FOOD GROUPS

Ayurveda recognizes about a dozen different food groups. This differentiation is based on empirical experience and is not necessarily restricted to the carbohydrate, protein, and fat model of modern organic chemistry. The following constitute the Ayurvedic food groups:

1. Cereals and grains (*sukadhanya*);
2. Legumes, beans, and lentils/pulses (*samidhanya*);
3. Meat (*mamsa*);
4. Vegetables (*saka,* and *harita varga* for raw);
5. Fruit (*phala*);
6. Nuts;
7. Milk and dairy (*gorasa*);
8. Water (*ambu*);
9. Wine and spirits (*madya*);
10. Sugars (*iksuvikara*);
11. Spices, minerals, fats, oils, and condiments (*aharayogin*); and
12. Cooked food preparations (*kritanna varga*). This category is made up of various preparations that include soups, fruit juices, and cooked milk products.

AYURVEDIC AND WESTERN NUTRITIONAL ASPECTS OF COMMON FOOD GROUPS

Food, in general, supplies basic nutrition to the tissues and to the whole body. As a whole, food is considered to have a primarily Sweet taste, a neutral energy, and a Sweet postdigestive effect. A commonly accepted modern classification of food groups is the following: fruits, vegetables, grains, beans, nuts, dairy products, meat, sugars, oils, and spices or condiments. While it is beyond the scope of this book to address all aspects of foods in general and in great detail in terms of their nutritional and medicinal qualities, the following brief outline presents a basic overview. Practical cookbooks and food guides using Ayurvedic principles are relatively few in number but are available (Fallon, 1999; Douillard, 2000; Morningstar & Desai, 1990; Yarema, Rhoda, & Brannigan, 2006). Sally Fallon's book is highly recommended. In the last year, several new ones have been published.

In this section, both Ayurvedic and Western perspectives on nutrition are presented. It is to be remembered that the Ayurvedic concepts were formulated in the climate of India, which tends to be warmer, hotter, and more humid in general. There, nutrition is much closer to nature, that is, fresher and less processed. Western nutritional understanding is both European and U.S. based and so reflects cooler, colder, and drier climate requirements in general. Western nutrition is more removed from nature; there is much more emphasis on processing, long shelf lives, and "instant" or microwavable foods. In general, 1,500 kcal/day (kilocalories per day) (especially for those about 100 to 125 pounds) and 2,500 kcal/day for those up to 200 pounds are best in terms of total caloric intake. Certainly, all the suggestions in this chapter require individualized considerations and customized tailoring.

Most fruits are considered to have a Sweet taste, a cool energy, and a Sweet postdigestive effect. *Vata* and *Pitta dosha* are slightly decreased, and *Kapha* is increased. This produces a balanced condition if fruit is taken in moderation. In excess, the digestive fire is diminished and *Kapha* may increase to produce excess fluid and, possibly, *Ama*. Fruit is considered to be highly sattvic and pure. Sweet fruits are highly recommended for those with *Vata* or *Pitta* predominance. Fruit in moderation is acceptable for *Kapha* persons. Apples may be the best choice for *Kapha* predominance. Fruits, such as blueberries, are cool in nature and are best eaten in moderation during the spring, summer, and early fall seasons.

Vegetables are more of a heterogeneous group of foods than fruit. Their taste may range from Sweet (root vegetables, for example) to Astringent (leafy greens, cruciferous, and beans, for example) to Pungent (onions, eggplant, and chilies) to Bitter (dandelion and chicory, for example), to Salty (seaweeds), and to Sour (some nightshade vegetables). Their energy tends to be neutral, and their postdigestive effect is usually Sweet. Including large amounts of the vegetable and plant food group is beneficial for almost all constitutional types. For example, lettuces tend to have a neutral *virya* but are believed to invigorate the subtle life force, *Prana* or *Qi*. For *Pitta* and *Kapha prakrutis,* salads are beneficial; for *Vata prakrutis* or to reduce excess *Vata* in any constitutional type, steamed lettuce, perhaps with a little oil, is soothing and valuable. An example of a vegetable that has been shown to have strong free radical fighting properties is eggplant. Although originating in India, the American variety has a deep purple skin that contains *nasunan,* an anthrocyanin phytonutrient with antioxidant effects. In addition, the phenolic compound *chlorogenic acid* with strong free radical scavenging action is found in eggplant. In general, eggplant has Bitter and Pungent tastes. The American variety is cooler in *virya,* and the Indian small green variety is hotter. Eggplant contains about 10 percent fiber and 8 percent potassium. Its glycemic index (the lower the better on a scale of 100 for pure sugar) is about 15, similar to most nonroot vegetables, and hence, is blood glucose–friendly. Okra, another valuable vegetable, has a low glycemic index and is rich in mucilage and minerals. It is called *bhindi* in India and *bamyah* in the Middle East. Vegetables should constitute a very large portion of total dietary intake.

Grains are considered to be Sweet in taste, neutral in energy, and Sweet in postdigestive effect. Basmati rice is considered a balanced grain and beneficial to all *dosha* types. It should be consumed in moderation. Wheat is heavier and so tends to be more *Kapha* increasing. It is recommended for *Vata* and *Pitta* types. Barley, especially pearl barley, is a useful grain, especially suitable for *Pitta* and *Kapha* constitutions. *Kapha* constitutional types also tend to do well with rye and millet. All grains are best used as whole grains. These are referred to as "complex carbohydrates." These tend to stabilize blood glucose levels and to manage the problem of insulin resistance, which in full measure equates with diabetes. Whole grains along with beans and legumes and vegetables supply fiber to the diet. Most Western authorities suggest a fiber intake of between 20 and 40 grams per day. Two main fiber categories are (1) soluble fiber (beta-glucans, gums, mucilage, and pectin) found mostly in fruits, vegetables, oats, and beans and (2) insoluble fiber (cellulose and lignins) found mostly in grains.

Beans and legumes (peas and pealike seeds) tend to increase *Vata* and so are not recommended, in general, for *Vata* types. Those with strong *Kapha* body types do well with moderate amounts of beans and legumes. Split yellow mung/moong beans are unusual because they are tridoshic (beneficial to all *doshas*) and so are recommended for all, even *Vata*. In general, *Vata* types should not eat legumes except mung beans. *Pitta* types may eat all legumes, especially brown lentils; kidney beans are also best only for *Pitta* types. Common American lentils are also referred to as Continental or European brown lentils; they are cool in *virya* and best only for *Pitta*. Lentils are considered a pulse legume and are one of the oldest cultivated legumes in history dating back about 6,000 years. *Kapha* types may consume all legumes. Chickpeas are legumes, pods with pealike seeds. In moderation, they are very good for *Kapha* and *Pitta* types. Hummus/hommus, which is a combination of chickpeas and sesame seed tahini, is a good source of complex carbohydrates. Aduki/adzuki beans are good for *Pitta* and *Kapha* constitutions.

Beans and legumes are complex carbohydrates that stabilize blood glucose and are beneficial in managing proper insulin levels. Consuming up to 4 ounces (½ cup or about 100 grams) per day is reasonable.

Although there are no officially recommended dietary allowances (RDAs) for carbohydrates and fats, complex carbohydrates such as beans, grains, and vegetables should constitute about 50 percent of one's total caloric intake. This very roughly typically hovers around 200 to 300 grams per day, usually more. If one chooses to consume only between 20 and about 60 grams per day, metabolism is shifted to a weight loss mode similar to that used in contemporary very low carbohydrate diets. It must be emphasized, however, that Ayurveda maintains that balance in all aspects of one's life is essential. A balanced, wholesome (*pathya*) dietary life-style that changes according to one's age, the seasons, and other expected and unexpected life events is best.

Nuts and seeds are considered Sweet in taste, warm in energy, and Sweet in postdigestive effect. They are sattvic in nature and are especially recommended for those with *Vata* predominance. *Pitta* and *Kapha* may eat nuts and seeds in small quantities.

Dairy products are considered to be Sweet in taste, cool in energy, and Sweet in postdigestive effect. In general, all dairy products tend to be sattvic in nature and very nutritive. Before the modern era, milk was not homogenized, pasteurized, or produced from cows treated with hormone and

antibiotic drugs. Animal feed was more organically produced in that synthetic herbicides and pesticides were unavailable. In order to eradicate the
transmission of milk-borne diseases, pasteurization at high temperatures
became a public health necessity. Pasteurization may be necessary nowadays
to provide disease-free dairy products on a wide scale. Ayurveda believes
that dairy products currently produced on farms that do not use more natural,
organic methods and use homogenization are safe but substantially less beneficial to health since they contribute heavily to the production of *Ama*. Recommendations are for limited milk use, in general, especially in adulthood.
When milk is used, it is suggested that it be warmed to a gentle boil with a
pinch of ginger or turmeric in order to reduce its *Ama*-provoking qualities.
Charaka has compared the nature of *pure* milk to that of *Ojas,* the essence
of life, and considered it a major *rasayana* (rejuvenative tonic). Milk is best
taken alone, or with some grains (cereals), or with ghee. Milk should never
be consumed with fruits, especially bananas. Ghee, which is clarified butter
from cow's milk, is one of the most sattvic foods and is recommended almost
unreservedly by all Ayurvedic authorities when used in moderation and in a
context of monitoring of blood triglyceride and cholesterol levels and any
other obviating metabolic or cardiac concerns.

Meat, chicken, and fish are considered to have a Sweet taste, a warm
energy, and a Sweet postdigestive effect. The ancient Vedics used meat.
Ayurveda uses meat and meat products judiciously. Systems of Yoga tend
to encourage vegetarian practices since meat is considered rajasic (agitating)
and highly tamasic (dulling) in nature as well as contrary to the principle of
ahimsa or nonviolence. Since meat is a highly nutrient packed food, it will
increase *Kapha* if used excessively. It will also increase *Pitta*. Meat decreases
Vata and may be a part of *Vata*-predominant diets when necessary. Depending on an individual's overall life-style and personal preferences, the inclusion of some meat in the diet may be beneficial in order to balance *Vata*
excess and to restore a sense of overall grounding. Meat in the form of soups
and stews that are cooked with vegetables, oils, and spices into a homo-
geneous blend are considered best. Since meat (like nuts) is a highly concentrated food that resists easy digestion throughout the gastrointestinal tract,
large quantities at any meal are not recommended. Viewing the use of meat
more as a condiment may be a good choice. The nature of eggs is a special
case of a concentrated food derived from the animal world. Eggs have strong
nutritive, restorative, and reputedly aphrodisiac properties; they may
decrease *Vata* and increase *Kapha* as well as stimulate *Rajas*. The consumption of eggs, therefore, is considered acceptable but needs to be judicious and
not excessive.

According to Western medicine, the recommended dietary requirements
for protein are weight adjusted and correlate with growth rate; this protein
need decreases from infancy until adulthood. Good kidney function is
required to properly use protein. The following amounts per day are suggested: 2.2 g/kg (grams of protein for each kilogram of body weight) in

3-month-old infants, 1.2 g/kg in 5-year-old children, and 0.8 g/kg in adults. These protein requirements correspond to essential amino acid requirements. In general, protein should constitute about 15 to 20 percent of total caloric intake, in the range of about 50 to 100 grams per day.

Oils and fats are chiefly contained within foods, as a natural part of their composition. Oils and fats may also be added to foods in cooking or in a complementary manner such as their use in salads or vegetable dressings or in dips. Oils and fats, also in the form of supplements, which are considered required, that is, unable to be made or to be made in sufficient quantity in the body, are termed "essential." Fats are considered to be Sweet in taste, warm in energy, and Sweet in postdigestive effect. The best oils and fats for consumption according to *dosha* are the following: *Vata:* all oils, especially sesame and ghee; *Pitta:* olive, sunflower, and ghee; *Kapha:* a minimum of all oils; sunflower, mustard, flaxseed, and ghee in moderation are acceptable; modest amounts of olive oil may be beneficial. Ayurveda advises that every individual consider judiciously incorporating an appropriate amount of oil and ghee into the daily diet. Substantial elimination of all dietary fats, in other words, very low fat diets, is thought to be unwholesome. All dietary vegetable oils, including ghee, are best consumed uncooked, that is, added in the raw state to foods; light cooking is acceptable. Since heating to high temperatures diminishes the nutritional quality of oils and ghee, they should be consumed in their natural and uncooked state or in as minimally cooked a condition as possible. Animal fats (saturated fats) in meat and chicken soups and stews need to be cooked.

From a Western perspective, vegetable fats and oils are usually polyunsaturated in the form of omega 6 fatty acids (linoleic acid or LA); these omega 6 fatty acids are essential and should be consumed in a balanced fashion by using about twice (or more) as much of the other category of essential fatty acid, omega 3 fatty acids (alpha-linolenic acid or LNA), which are primarily those contained in fish body oils; flaxseed oil is also an omega 3 oil, but it is not as readily assimilated as fish oils. Early on in the history of Western nutrition (1923), these essential fatty acids, omega 3 and omega 6, were referred to as Vitamin F. Omega 3 fatty acids are also found in eggs, walnuts, soy, pumpkin, algae, and some green plants with fish such as salmon, mackerel, sardines, and anchovies being the most readily available sources that are also biologically assimilable. Omega 3 oils, especially from marine sources, produce two of the most important essential fatty acids that the body requires. They are eicosapentaenoic acid (EPA) and docosahexaenoic acid (DHA). Perilla leaves (*Perilla frutescens*), also called green *shiso* and the beefsteak plant, commonly found in Japanese sushi dishes, contains up to 60 percent of alpha-linolenic acid, omega 3 fatty acids similar to flaxseed oil. The form of omega 6 called gamma-linolenic acid (GLA) is found in seeds such as borage (24 percent GLA content), black currant (17 percent), evening primrose (9 percent), and hemp (2 percent). It is used in capsule form as a nutritional supplement. Both omega 3 and omega 6 fatty acids are often taken as gelatin capsules in supplemental form since typical dietary intake is usually small. Omega 9 fatty acids are needed but are not regarded as essential. These monounsaturated fats are found in olive oil, cashews, macadamia nuts, all tree nuts, pecans, sesame oil, peanuts, and avocados.

Healthy fat and oil intake should constitute about 25 to 30 percent of total caloric intake. Omega 3 fatty acids foster the production of prostaglandin 3, which is beneficial to health. Omega 3 fats decrease triglyceride levels, have antiplatelet actions, lower fibrinogen, and act as mood stabilizers by increasing serotonin and, perhaps, by decreasing excessive testosterone. Omega 6 fatty acids foster the production of prostaglandin 1, which is anti-inflammatory; they also decrease prostaglandin 2, which in excess is associated with blood clotting, vasoconstriction, and sodium retention. Healthy levels of omega 6 fatty acids, especially GLAs, decrease cholesterol, are anti-arthritis in their anti-inflammatory role, and may act to regulate the irritability, anxiety, mood swings, and fluid retention associated with premenstrual tension. It is important to remember that both types of fatty acids are essential, but that their appropriate proportional intake and proper balance in the body makes for good health.

Requirements for essential fatty acids (EFAs)—omega 3 and omega 6—vary by age. Current Western nutritional authorities state that adults require amounts of linoleic acid equal to at least 2 percent of total caloric needs, and linolenic acid (marine fish oil and flaxseed oil) equal to at least 0.5 percent. Total healthy fat intake can be up to about 60 grams per day, with about 45 grams being unsaturated. The author can only recommend that, in general, added fats and oils as culinary accompaniments to foods should ideally be in the form of extra virgin olive oil and small amounts of ghee. Chapter 10 discusses the benefits of ghee. Ghee, for example, increases *ojas,* immunity, and intelligence and helps all substances penetrate deeply into the tissues. Adding flaxseed oil to foods is beneficial but the flax oil must be raw, expeller pressed, and very fresh since it has a tendency to become rancid quickly after several weeks or months, especially if kept outside of refrigeration. This suggestion is aimed primarily at those in the United States, especially because of climatic conditions. Olive oil is primarily Sweet in taste but has an important Bitter (detoxifying) component. It is warm in energy and Sweet in postdigestive effect. Its qualities include softness and lightness.

Sweeteners are usually recommended for different doshic types. Those with *Vata* predominance may use all types of sweeteners in moderation. *Pitta* constitutions do well with the use of maple syrup since it is cooling. *Kapha* body types may use honey since it is warming and has diuretic properties.

The choice of condiments and food spices depends on constitutional type. *Vata* types may use all spices that are moderate in intensity. Examples of this include ginger, cinnamon, cardamom, cumin, basil, and fennel to name just a few. Salt and vinegar in moderation are also acceptable. *Pitta* body types require only mild spices such as coriander, cumin, cinnamon, cardamom, fennel, and turmeric, to name just a few. Salt and vinegar are not recommended.

Those with a *Kapha*-constitutional predominance may take all spices in large quantity. Hot and intensely Pungent spices reduce excess *Kapha*. Salt and vinegar are not recommended. Coffee and regular teas have some Bitter qualities and may be used by all *dosha* types in small amounts without harmful effects. Alcoholic beverages are not forbidden. Excessive use, however, evokes rajasic turbulence and usually increases *Pitta dosha* to an inordinate degree. Some medicinal herbal and wine preparations taken in moderation are beneficial. Adequate consumption of water throughout the day is recommended.

DIETARY CHOICES ACCORDING TO *PRAKRUTI*

One's innate constitutional type reflects the predominance of one or more *doshas* and the characteristic qualities that they impart to the structure and physiology of the body. Digestive capacity or *Agni* is one of the major functions of *prakruti*. Dietary food choices, therefore, should be closely aligned with *dosha* predominance. Traditionally, a range of choices has been found to best suit each *prakruti*. While these suggestions have been proven over time, they are not rigidly mandated. They act as guidelines that need to be adapted to the nuances and variations of each individual body type.

Vata-Predominant *Prakruti*

Vata-dominant *prakruti* constitutions require dietary regimens that are opposite to the chief attributes that characterize *Vata*. The attributes of *Vata* include cold, dry, light, airy, rough, subtle, clear, mobile, and agitating. Diets should be regular, grounding, and moderately substantial, warm, and moist. The temperature of foods should not be too hot or too cold. Raw foods should be kept at a minimum, especially apples. It is also best to avoid beans, lentils, raw vegetables, cabbages, broccoli, Brussels sprouts, lettuce, mushrooms, and dry foods such as popcorn, potato chips, and pretzels. Freshly prepared soups, stews, warm beverages, and moist, moderately oily foods and food combinations are best. The tastes that are best to emphasize in the diet are Sweet, Sour, and Salty.

Foods that balance *Vata* include sweet, moist fruits, lemons, mangoes, some cooked vegetables, grains such as basmati rice, oats and wheat, mung beans, all nuts and seeds, and all oils and fats. All dairy products and all sweeteners, except honey, are good. All spices that are moderate in intensity are recommended, as is a moderate amount of salt and of vinegar. Animal products such as meat, fish, and eggs are good in moderation. Nuts and seeds, however, should be restricted in cases of diverticular disease of the colon.

Pitta-Predominant *Prakruti*

Pitta-predominant *prakruti* constitutions require nutritional regimens that are opposite to the inherent qualities of *Pitta*. *Pitta* has hot, dry, light, penetrating, and oily qualities. The digestive capacity of *Pitta* types is usually very good, but overheating and overacidity may be a problem. Dietary choices should avoid hot and pungent foods. The following foods should be kept to a minimum: sour and citrus fruits, bananas, nightshade vegetables (tomatoes, potatoes, peppers, and eggplant), onions, garlic, hot spices, salt, vinegar, nuts, honey, meat, and black, red, and tur lentils; fried foods, peanut butter, and alcohol should be avoided. Foods should be eaten warm or cool.

Pitta constitutions do well on fresh, sweet fruits, most vegetables especially artichoke, celery, asparagus, dandelion, chicory, and escarole, basmati rice, barley, some beans such as mung and chickpeas, oils such as olive and sunflower, ghee, most dairy products, all sweeteners except honey, mild spices such as coriander, cumin, fennel, turmeric, mint, and a small amount of cardamom, and mild light fish and meats (chicken). Chickpeas (*Cicer arietinum*), also called garbanzos, *chana,* gram, and ceci are believed to have been first domesticated in Jericho and ancient Turkey almost 10,000 years ago. They have a Sweet and Astringent taste and a cooling *virya.* They are slightly drying and reduce internal dampness. From a Western perspective, their glycemic index value is low (similar to nonroot vegetables) and thus are very desirable for all diets, especially diabetic regimens. Azuki red beans are neutral in energy yet have a mildly cooling effect. They are believed to augment adrenal, kidney, and spleen energy and are very beneficial in diabetic diets. Limes, coriander leaves, and neem leaves are beneficial. Raw vegetables and salads are recommended in moderation. Foods that are cooling, light, and calming are best. Chinese winter melon (*tong gua*), also called white, ash, and wax gourd, is known in India as *petha.* It is a cooling vegetable that clears heat, detoxifies, and is said to relieve irritability. It can be made into a soup in any season. Sweet, Bitter, and Astringent tastes, in general, should be emphasized in the *Pitta* diet.

Kapha-Predominant *Prakruti*

Kapha-predominant *prakruti* constitutions are strong, grounded, and robust by nature. The optimal *Kapha* diet should be opposite to the chief qualities of *Kapha;* these are cold, heavy, oily, soft, and dense. Because of the heavy nature of *Kapha,* diets should be light and stimulating. In general, the following foods tend to be heavy and should be minimized: dairy products, meat, wheat, oats, nuts, fats, oils, as well as sweets, salt, and vinegar. The consumption of heavy, starchy vegetables like sweet potatoes, the nightshade family of vegetables (tomatoes, potatoes, and eggplant), and okra should be minimized in general. Eggplant, however, when prepared with warm spices, reduces excess *Kapha.* All cold or iced foods should be avoided.

The best diet for this constitutional type is light, warm, dry, and stimulating. The best fruits are apples, cranberries, and pears; some lemon and some dried fruits are good. Most vegetables, for example, celery, garlic, onions, cabbage, and green leafy ones, other than the heavier ones such as potatoes, are excellent choices and a *Kapha* dietary mainstay. Grains such as barley, buckwheat, and rye are good. All beans including red and tur lentils are recommended. Very small amounts of oils and fats are recommended. Ghee, sunflower, mustard, and flaxseed oils are good choices. The best sweetener is honey. Small amounts of meat as well as eggs are acceptable. *Kapha* types do very well with large amounts of all spices, particularly the hotter ones like black pepper, ginger, and red pepper. Pungent, Bitter, and Astringent tastes should predominate in the diet.

GENERAL DIETARY CHOICES ACCORDING TO THE SEASONS

Although one's diet should be shaped to fit one's basic *prakruti,* seasonal variations play an exceptionally important part in affecting individual *doshas* and the interplay of the *doshas* in the constitution. Each season has its characteristic attributes and qualities, and one's dietary choices should tend to be opposite to the characteristics of the current season. This is an important dietary guideline and, in general, partially overrides or should take greater precedence, to a judicious degree, over dietary choices than choices based on one's constitution alone. An optimal diet tailors one's individual *prakruti* needs with the features of the environment at any given moment.

Ayurveda has divided the year into two broad seasonal periods: (1) *Adana Kala,* a period of relative weakness and (2) *Visarga Kala,* a period of relative strength for all biological life.

In India where there are six seasons, *Adana Kala* occurs roughly from mid-January through mid-July. It is a time of relative dryness and exerts a dehydrating quality to nature and to man. During this period, all biological organisms are relatively weakened, less energetic, have less available strength, and diminished digestive power (*Agni*). This generally hot, dry period is broadly associated with a predominance of solar forces and is called *Agneya.* In the United States where there are four seasons, the window for this period begins at the vernal equinox, around March 21, when the number of hours of day equals that of night; its decline occurs near the end of September well after the summer solstice, around June 22. *Adana Kala,* thus, occurs from spring through summer.

Visarga Kala follows this and goes from the end of September through the end of March. It is a period of increased moisture, less heat, growing strength for both man and other biological organisms, and stronger *Agni.* During this period, for instance, vegetables become richer and more nutrient packed. This span of time has been called *Saumya,* the cooling, moist time of the year dominated by lunar forces. In the United States, it begins at the autumnal equinox, about September 22, and begins to decline at the winter solstice, about December 22, when the sun is farthest from the equator. It ends at the vernal equinox in late March. *Visarga Kala,* thus, occurs from autumn through winter.

Dietary Choices in the Fall

Fall is a *Vata*-dominant season characterized by cool, dry, windy weather that tends to be irregular and changeable. The autumnal equinox, occurring around September 22, is an especially significant junctional transition and is considered an important stressor for man in the Ayurvedic system. The irregular weather changes between hot and humid and then cool and damp is confusing to one's doshic balance and can become severely aggravating and disruptive. All constitutional types, therefore, should tend to employ diets that are cooked, warm, moist, grounding, and slightly heavier during this fall season. Foods that are pacifying to *Vata* should be emphasized. Spices that are exceptionally good at this time of year include cardamom, cinnamon, fresh ginger, basil, fennel, rosemary, and asafetida. Asafetida is an uncommon spice in the West but is a common Indian spice. It is very strong in aroma and is used in small amounts.

Dietary Choices in the Winter and Early Spring

Winter is a *Kapha*-dominant season characterized by cold, dark, heavy, and damp conditions. There is a pointedly still, constricted, frozen, almost inert quality that pervades these months. All constitutional types benefit from diets that are warm to hot, substantial, and stimulating. Cold weather strengthens the digestive processes, and the *Agni* is enhanced and able to handle heavier foods. Foods that are consistent with balancing *Kapha* should be emphasized. Spices that are best include black pepper, red pepper or cayenne, dry ginger, and sage, to name just a few.

Early spring is the season in which the cold, dense qualities of *Kapha* are beginning to be assuaged by the burgeoning heat of the approaching *Pitta* summer season. Accumulated body *Kapha,* at this time, naturally tends to soften and liquefy. The looming warmth of this season requires foods that are cooler, lighter, less oily, and less Sweet and Sour in taste. Bitter vegetables such as dandelion, chicory, and artichoke are of great benefit.

Dietary Choices in the Summer

Summer is the time of *Pitta* predominance. Heat and dryness prevail. The digestive powers represented by the condition of *Agni* are diminished at this time. Foods, therefore, should have characteristic lightness, coolness, and calming rather than stimulating qualities. Cooling fruits and some dairy products are best if one is able to digestively handle dairy products. This is the time of year when aloe vera is most beneficial taken both internally and applied externally. Beneficial cooling spices include coriander, some cumin, turmeric, and peppermint.

Dietary Choices at Times of Heavy Rain

Whenever heavy rains occur (spring, late summer, and early fall in the United States; July and August in India), their coolness tends to chill and aggravate both *Vata* and *Kapha*. The dampness, humidity, and possible acidity present in the rain, as well as intermittent heat, tends to aggravate *Pitta*. The heavy rains that usually occur around the autumnal equinox (September 22) are especially distressing because this juncture between summer and autumn exerts the most direct and stressful impact on the individual as a whole. This is related to the weakened condition that normally results from the previous hotter and drier period of the year, and the usual *Ama* buildup from inside the body. At these times of tridosha irritation, the use of honey is ideal. Warm teas to which honey is added are beneficial to reduce dampness and add warmth. Fresh ginger root used in teas and in foods is cleansing and pacifying. Grains such as barley and rice, along with freshly prepared light to medium vegetable soups, are recommended.

DOSHA COMPATIBLE DIETARY CHOICES

Dietary food choices that induce and maintain *dosha* balance are termed pacifying.

Vata-Pacifying Diet

General: Warm foods and beverages that tend to be moist and moderately oily; Sweet, Salty, and Sour tastes should predominate.

Fruits: Sweet fruits, apricots, avocado, bananas, berries, cherries, coconut, dates, fresh figs, grapefruit, grapes, lemons, mangoes, sweet melons, oranges, papaya, peaches, pineapples, and plums.

Vegetables: Cooked vegetables, asparagus, beets, carrots, cucumber, garlic, green beans, okra, onions, parsley, sweet potatoes, radishes, watercress, zucchini, and salads with oil.

Grains: Basmati rice, cooked oats, and wheat.

Legumes: No legumes except mung beans, warm tofu, and black and red lentils.

Meats: Chicken, turkey, and seafood.

Nuts and seeds: All nuts and seeds.

Dairy: All dairy products in moderation.

Oils: All oils especially sesame.

Sweeteners: All sweeteners except white sugar.

Condiments and spices: Cinnamon, cardamom, fennel, cumin, basil, fresh and some dry ginger, cloves, small amounts of black pepper, salt, and mustard seeds are preferred.

Avoid or reduce excessive amounts of the following: light, dry, and cold foods; foods with Pungent, Bitter, and Astringent tastes; barley, corn, millet, rye, and buckwheat; dried fruits; raw vegetables, cabbages, broccoli, celery, eggplant, mushrooms, peas, white potatoes, and tomatoes; apples, pears, cranberries, pears, and watermelon; and all beans.

Pitta-Pacifying Diet

General: Warm foods that have a predominantly Sweet, Bitter, or Astringent taste.

Fruits: Sweet fruits; apples, avocado, coconut, figs, grapes, limes, mangoes, pears, pineapples, plums, pomegranate, prunes, and raisins.

Vegetables: Asparagus, broccoli, Brussels sprouts, cabbage, chicory, cucumber, cauliflower, celery, cilantro leaves, dandelion, escarole, green beans, leafy greens, artichokes, mushrooms, okra, peas, green peppers, potatoes, sprouts, small amounts of yucca root, zucchini, and Daikon radish.

Grains: Barley, cooked oats, basmati rice, and wheat.

Legumes: All legumes and beans except black, red, and tur lentils.

Nuts and seeds: No nuts except coconut; no seeds except sunflower and pumpkin.

Meat: Chicken and turkey.

Dairy: Ghee, cottage cheese, and milk.

Oils: Olive and sunflower.

Sweeteners: All sweeteners except honey and molasses.

Condiments and Spices: Coriander, cinnamon, cardamom, fennel seeds, turmeric, peppermint, small amounts of cumin, black pepper, and fresh ginger.

Avoid or reduce highly spiced foods, hot spices; foods with predominantly Pungent, Sour, and Salty tastes; yogurt, sour cream, cheese, and buttermilk; honey and molasses; sesame, almond, and corn oils; corn, millet, rye, and brown rice; black, red, and tur lentils; sour fruits; hot peppers, radishes, tomatoes, eggplant, garlic, onions, spinach, and beets; nuts; beef, seafood, and eggs; salt; vinegar; and alcohol. Peanut butter is exceptionally *Pitta* provoking.

Kapha-Pacifying Diet

General: Light foods and diet that is dry and warm with tastes that are predominantly Pungent, Bitter, and Astringent.

Fruits: Apples are best; apricots, berries, cherries, cranberries, dry figs, mangoes, peaches, pears, persimmons, pomegranates, prunes, and raisins.

Vegetables: Most vegetables are very desirable, especially asparagus, beets, broccoli, Brussels sprouts, cabbage, cauliflower, celery, eggplant, garlic, leafy greens, lettuce, mushrooms, okra, onions, parsley, peas, peppers, radishes, spinach, sprouts, and watercress.

Grains: Barley is best; basmati rice, corn, millet, dry oats, buckwheat, and rye.

Legumes: All legumes and beans except cold tofu.

Nuts and Seeds: No nuts; no seeds except some sunflower and pumpkin.

Meat: Chicken and turkey.

Dairy: Minimal dairy except ghee, goatmilk, and skim milk.

Oils: No oils except sunflower, flaxseed, and small amounts of virgin olive oil.

Sweeteners: No sweeteners except honey.

Condiments and Spices: All spices except salt; dry and some fresh ginger is very beneficial.

Avoid or reduce overeating; avoid foods that are cold and oily, and those with predominantly Sweet, Sour, and Salty tastes; avoid all dairy products and oils other than very small amounts; avoid all nuts and pork; avoid large amounts of beef and seafood.

BENEFICIAL HERBS, SPICES, AND FOODS RELATED TO THE ORGANS AND TISSUES

The following are general guidelines for the use of herbs, spices, and some foods that target specific organs and tissues. These are generally supportive and nutritive but also have some therapeutic effect in the sense of maintaining doshic balance and preventing the buildup of *Ama*.

Brain: Basil, calamus (*Acorus calamus*), and gotu kola; ghee.

Thyroid: *Trikatu,* kelp, and Irish moss (*Chondrus chrispus*).

Lungs: Ginger, pippali, bamboo, figs, and persimmon.

Breast: dandelion, fennel, fenugreek, and shatavari.

Heart: Hawthorn, saffron, lotus seed, arjuna, and mulberry.

Liver: Aloe vera, turmeric, barberry, gentian, sillymarin/milk thistle, chicory, dandelion, artichoke, Daikon radish, bitter melon (Chinese *ku gua*), cilantro leaves, lime, banana, asparagus, pears, and chrysanthemum tea.

Spleen: Neem, turmeric, and azuki red beans.

Pancreas: Turmeric, dandelion, pomegranate; azuki red beans; bitter melon (Chinese *ku gua*) and bitter gourd (Indian *karela*); *shilajit.*

Stomach: Coriander, cumin, fennel, dill, peppermint, bay leaves, orange peel, ajwan, black pepper, and ginger.

Small intestine: Cumin, ghee, and aloe vera.

Large intestine/colon: Triphala, rhubarb, psyllium, asafetida, and banana.

Kidneys and Adrenal: Gokshura (*Tribulus terrestris*), Chinese red dates (*jujube*), walnut, chrysanthemum tea; black (turtle) beans; azuki red beans. *Shilajit* is a black mineral pitch derived from the Himalayan tundras. It is Pungent and Bitter in taste with a warm *virya*. In addition, it has some Sour and Astringent properties. It is said to alleviate all three *doshas, Vata, Pitta,* and *Kapha.* It has special rejuvenating properties related to the kidneys. Its chief use is in diabetes, sexual impotency, and obesity. It is considered a restorative tonic that slows down the aging process while having antistress, analgesic, and anti-inflammatory properties.

Female reproductive: Shatavari, aloe vera, myrrh, and raspberry.

Male reproductive: Saw palmetto, gokshura, ashwagandha, bala, garlic, and walnut.

Fat: Honey, guggul, and boswellia.

Bone: Boswellia (*shallaki*), guggul (Commiphora mukul) (*shuddha*), castor oil, turmeric, ghee, and organic dairy products.

Finally, the color of food is generally associated with targeting various bodily organs. The associations are the following:

White foods nourish the lungs and colon.

Black, dark blue foods nourish the kidneys.

Green foods nourish the liver and the gallbladder.

Yellow and orange foods nourish the stomach, the spleen, and the pancreas.

Red foods nourish the heart and the small intestine.

9

LIFESTYLE AND BEHAVIORAL REGIMENS IN AYURVEDA AND IN YOGA

AYURVEDIC REGIMENS FOR OPTIMAL HEALTH: LIFESTYLE *RASAYANAS*

Health maintenance is essential for promoting balance and integration throughout the bodily, mental, emotional, and spiritual dimensions of each individual. This presumes maintaining a rigorous reality sense, which constitutes the ability to differentiate in a skillful fashion both the grosser and the finer distinctions within nature, to rank their relative positions in the scheme of reality, and to reasonably discern their differing levels of meaning and significance. This discriminative understanding then guides one in selecting and implementing suitable choices within the fabric of everyday living.

Ayurveda addresses these needs in its guidelines for food and nutrition (*anna*), lifestyle and behavioral practices (*vihara*), and herbal supplementation (*aushadha*). The Sanskrit word *swastha* means healthy, and the state of optimal health is called *swasthavritta*. This is understood to constitute a "harmonious abiding in one's own nature," living in harmony with one's constitution during the changing course of the life cycle as well as that of the seasons. A fundamental sense of satisfaction and confidence both psychologically and felt in the body results from increasingly balanced and optimal functioning.

Life-style includes the manner in which one's life is viewed and conducted. It is a style or mode of living that reflects values, attitudes, choices, and standards as well as habits of consumption. Ayurvedic regimens for optimal health may be thought of as "Lifestyle *Rasayanas*," which connote the vehicle or path that one travels in order to regenerate, renew, restore, and enhance the vital essence of *rasa*. It is rejuvenating one's overall quality of life. *Rasayanas* are Ayurvedic formulas, usually herbal preparations, which are considered to have special antiaging and rejuvenative properties. The suitable conduct of one's life may also be restorative. The concept of a healthy life-style includes particular consideration in regard to three aspects of one's overall values, conduct, and behavior: (1) *dinacharya,* the daily regimen; (2) *ritucharya,* the seasonal regimen; and (3) *sadvritta,* one's ethical outlook and behavior.

Dinacharya or daily regimens are closely allied to personal hygiene routines. *Din* means day and *acharya* means to follow or to be close to. These guidelines take account of times to arise and to go to sleep, breathing routines, elimination, washing and bathing, oil massage, physical exercise (*vyayama*), meditation, diet, study, work, travel, and leisure pursuits, all during the course of a day. They include optimal times to awake (before sunrise when the environment is most *Sattvic* and pure), care of the mouth with special attention to the teeth and tongue, and care of the eyes, nose, ears, and skin. Care of the tongue is especially important and involves routine morning mild scraping with a special tongue utensil that produces both a cleansing effect and a stimulating action. Morning routines include attention to cleansing procedures as well as regular bowel habits, breathing exercises, stretching and Yoga exercise routines, some massage, and bathing.

In relation to dietary choices, careful attention to one's constitutional needs is vital. Yet, for example, all *prakrutis* may benefit from a light breakfast that includes a cooked apple (second best: a small amount of natural, unsweetened applesauce) with a very light sprinkling of black pepper, turmeric, and cinnamon. If sweetness is desired, some pure maple syrup may be added. Alternatively, *Kapha prakrutis* may prefer two hardboiled eggs with black pepper. Soy-based foods are also a good option. Protein, rather than carbohydrate, is best for breakfast. A warm to hot beverage such as tea or, in moderation, one cup of coffee is not unreasonable since the Bitter *rasa* of coffee affords the system this underutilized taste, which is so beneficial to internal cleansing and detoxification. A small amount of a hot, nourishing soup may also be a breakfast option. Lunch is *Pitta* time, and it is recommended that it be the most important meal of the day. Specific dietary options have been discussed in Chapter 8. After each meal, a short walk of up to 20 minutes is suggested.

Physical exercise is very important in maintaining the body's energy flow, circulation, flexibility, and overall tone. Exercising at one-fourth to one-half of one's capacity is recommended. Some Ayurvedic authorities have suggested that exercise should stop when one begins to perspire. This point has been called *ardhashakti* and includes significantly increased heart rate, respiration, and temperature. Sweating in this sense refers to the excessive perspiration that results in large amounts of sweat coming from the head. Normal perspiration such as occurs in sweating under the armpits and a little on the back is expected. Each constitutional type (*prakruti*) responds to a different mode of physical exercise as will be discussed later. It should be noted that, in general, *Vata* is increased by motion, especially produced by cardiovascular training such as treadmill work and running, and by the use of other exercise machines. In addition to individual motions, health club members are also exposed to the bobbing up and down and sometimes frenetic movement of those around. This visual input can exacerbate an already overly stimulated *Vata*.

Excessive, not moderate, exercise predisposes to high *Vata,* which, in turn, causes mental agitation (anxiety, poor attention and concentration, and moodiness). Those who are *Vata* dominant, therefore, should constrain excessive activity and chose milder pursuits such as Yoga, Tai Chi, walking, and swimming. *Pitta*-dominant metabolic types are naturally competitive and so should balance this tendency by exercises that are either team oriented or more solo such as hiking and backpacking. *Kapha*-dominant constitutions do best with vigorous exercise; cardiovascular and weight training are good choices. The popularity of health clubs and gyms makes careful attention to one's choice of physical activity an important lifestyle consideration. Martial arts training is beneficial for promoting self-discipline, impulse control, and respect for one's partner. It is a good choice for children and adolescents, especially when adults emphasize the negative impact of violence and the proper regulation of aggression both from an interpersonal and a social perspective.

Ritucharya or seasonal routines include dietary choices and activity recommendations proper to the season. In general, the best time to engage in active exercise is the *Visarga* period in fall and winter. One's strength is optimal at this time. In addition, one's diet should be relatively greater in quantity since all foods at this time are believed to be imbued with greater energetic and nutritional components. The *Adana* period in spring and summer is a time for less exercise and less food intake. This period is considered to be one of diminished overall energy and strength and should be used for greater rest and activities that require less physical exertion.

Sadvritta or ethical regimens include recommendations for the examination and the refinement of one's values and behavior, especially interpersonal and social aspects. Emphasis on this reflects the importance that Ayurveda gives to areas of one's life extending beyond those pertaining only to the single individual and to the care of the material body. The Ayurvedic literature stresses that these guidelines are not merely considered to be moral dictums nor believed to be solely culturally based. They are understood as universally applicable principles of proper conduct for all people in all circumstances. Ayurveda, by its internal nature, neither discriminates against, rejects, nor summarily excludes differing worldviews, either Western or Eastern. Ayurveda is inclusive. It does put exceedingly heavy weight on meditative techniques and consciousness-enhancing viewpoints that have a proven record of accomplishment and efficacy. The ancient sages laid unreserved emphasis on this. While the conceptual framework and styles surrounding these do have a distinctly Eastern flavor, Ayurvedic health regimens, nonetheless, are expressly applicable to all religious, nonreligious, spiritual, philosophical, and humanistic orientations.

Sattvic (pure, balanced, and good) qualities in thought, feeling, and action are directions considered valuable to strive toward, embrace, and attempt to achieve. These include self-discipline, proper management of the five sensory faculties, impulse control, regulation of desire, avoidance of harm to self and others, honesty, truthfulness, and working to achieve health in body, mind, and consciousness. All endeavors, therefore, that aim at enhancing refined consciousness, harmony, balance, intelligence, compassion, and mental equanimity are considered to be valuable, meritorious, and in the service of producing excellence.

These proposed healthy lifestyle regimens must arise from an individual sense of personal responsibility for work on the self. Membership in groups or organized bodies that help to facilitate this self-work is always important, although self-work on an individual basis must continue to remain primary. Parents and all caregivers, however, are in vital positions of influence and nurturing. Direction and guidance, especially by modeling, example, and quality, mutually interactive dialogue, provide indispensable and organic sustenance for the welfare of the next generation. Child-rearing techniques, accordingly, may find Ayurveda to be a valuable resource. Ayurvedic lifestyle regimens are a well-suited accompaniment to all child-care practices.

Attention to sexuality, for example, is important both in childhood and in adult life. In raising children, parents or loving caregivers should consider the chronological and developmental age of the child and the adolescent and offer ongoing developmentally appropriate and sensitive dialogues. These should include discussions about male and female anatomy, the sexual organs, respect for the sexual organs, and sexuality in its widest implications —intimacy, love, procreation, and the family. All of this applies, accordingly, to a loving and respectful attitude toward self, others, and the larger social context.

In due course, a new person, man or woman, one with enlightened wisdom, can be generated thereby. Individuals of this higher spiritual caliber then contribute to the establishment, in a true sense, of a new nation of integral human beings whose real wealth is firmly and rightly established on enduring spiritual insights. Power, influence, and authority then manifest not in relation to others but as the empowerment of the self. Life wisdom thus engendered is predicated on a deep sense of gratitude with heartfelt compassion and is not constricted by historical or theoretical legalisms and narrow dogma. This enrichment (*vibhuti*), brought about by the deepening of consciousness, can act to raise, in a significant way, the quality of life for all people in every walk of life.

Faithfulness to the individual pursuit of self-discipline, therefore, is primary. Out of this base, moreover, compassion and concern for others may naturally emerge. A balanced relationship between individual ethical conduct and its further expression in the shared care and helping of others constitutes the optimal moral position. Faith and good works, together, are essential.

LIFESTYLE REGIMENS BASED ON *DOSHA* PREDOMINANCE

Lifestyle regimens generally address what are considered to be the "three pillars of life": (1) food, (2) sleep, and (3) the management of sexual activity. These represent fundamental and biologically based needs. In addition, we may add guidelines that address occupation, exercise, and aspects of the psychological life of man, that is, mental health. All recommendations derive from an understanding of *prakruti,* one's constitutional body/mind type, as it operates within a particular environmental context. Guidelines for each of the three primary doshic types are outlined to serve as broad directions to be further customized and appropriately combined in order to suit mixed constitutional types. Since there are, in fact, as many different *prakruti* types as there are people in the world, these recommendations are to be considered as rough blueprints that require ongoing individualized adaptation to changing conditions: stage of the life cycle, season, particular stressors at a given time, and so forth.

Vata Predominance

The *Vata dosha* (principle of propulsion), considered the strongest *dosha* (bioenergetic principle regulating the body), is also the most sensitive and may easily become disturbed or vitiated. This is true for all *Vata*-dominant *prakrutis,* and for the *Vata* component within all individuals. To maintain balance, *Vata*-dominant individuals require regular meals preferably with the main meal taken around noontime. Smaller regular feedings may be required. This is acceptable since *Vata* innately tends toward variability, which may be addressed therapeutically by habits aimed at regulating the tendency toward irregular, inconsistent behaviors. Extremes should be recognized and avoided. Foods should be taken warm, moist, moderately oily, and consist of moderately heavy items. Stews or cooked mixtures of a variety of different food items prepared together are beneficial and more easily digested. Fasting, in general, should be avoided.

Sleep (about eight hours) should strive for regularity. One should awake by sunrise and go to sleep relatively early. Sleeping or naps during the daytime are permitted when necessary. *Vata* becomes aggravated when an individual stays up very late into the night. This is an Ayurvedic fact of exceeding importance. It affects the *Vata* component in everyone and results in a multitude of physical and mental difficulties, which are potentially preventable.

Exercise should be regular and moderate. As is true for all doshic predominances, one should exercise only to half of one's capacity. In addition, when one begins to perspire, exercise should be stopped. Those with *Vata* dominance tend to be driven, hyperkinetic, and prone toward frenetic, maniclike activities. Exercises such as aerobics, running, jumping, and jogging are highly aggravating to *Vata* and are not recommended. Mild, regular activities such as walking, stretching, golf, horseback riding, and sailing are preferable. Tai Chi is especially soothing for *Vata*. Yoga exercises will be described later.

To maintain mental health and prevent the natural tendencies toward anxiety, fear, mood swings, mania, and feelings of insecurity, *Vata* types should strive for regular, balanced hobbies, study, and meditation. In addition, the *Vata* component, naturally present to some extent in every individual, also may be benefited by implementing these trends at times during which inordinate stress exacerbates *Vata dosha*. *Vata*-dominant persons tend to generate original and creative ideas, although they require pacing and discipline to remain focused and follow tasks to completion. These people do well in professions that are compatible with this trend. Regular oil massage reduces excess *Vata* in both body and mind and is highly recommended as a routine practice. The best climate is one that is both hot and humid.

Since specific stresses and activities tend to aggravate *Vata* in very serious ways, the following is a partial list of some main culprits. These include exposure to wind and cold, traveling, especially on airplanes, and excess exposure to highly stimulating sensory inputs such as television, radio, loud music, cinema, and computers; excessive exercise increases *Vata*. *Vata* is specifically aggravated by loud and harsh sounds. Excessive talking both aggravates and also reflects vitiated *Vata*. Less talking, periods of silence, and more extended periods of attentive silence are health promoting and are restorative to *Vata*.

Regarding sexual activity, it is believed that *Vata* persons require less frequency and degree of intensity than do those of other *dosha* predominance. While the central importance and nuances of human sexuality are an intimate part of life, a detailed survey here is beyond the scope of this book. It, nonetheless, must be said that this area, innately prone to excesses, is often perceived and dealt with in too casual a manner. Improper management seriously impairs aspects of the *Vata dosha* in all persons regardless of specific constitutional dominance. That disturbance in *Vata,* in turn, causes further turbulent cascades of derangement in *Pitta* and *Kapha*. Judicious attention to this heavily counted area is an important consideration for the wholesome conduct of any life-style. All of these recommendations control aggravated *Vata* (*Vatshamak*).

Pitta Predominance

Pitta dosha (principle of thermogenesis) is associated with the strength of transformation and the penetrating intensity of intelligence. Preferences should be for foods that are cool, calming, and minimally stimulating. *Pitta*-predominant constitutions do well when eating salads and a moderate amount of raw vegetables. Alcohol and very hot spices should be avoided. The largest meal should ideally be taken around noontime when *Pitta* is naturally strongest and digestive capacity is optimal.

Sleep is usually sound and regular. A moderate requirement of about six to eight hours is usual. If *Pitta* becomes aggravated, sleep may become disturbed with typical awakening at around 1 to 2 A.M.

Exercise preferences usually tend toward competitive sports. This should be avoided since it will aggravate *Pitta*. Sports that are more team oriented or performed alone are preferred. Recommended exercises and sports include swimming, canoeing, sailing, hiking, archery, and skiing; hobbies such as gardening are soothing and beneficial. Tai Chi and Yoga are conducive to a balanced activity regimen.

Pitta is the *dosha* of heat, and all things associated with excess exposure to heat are not recommended. Outdoor exposure to the sun, sunbathing, steam baths, and hot climates, in general, should be avoided.

In order to maintain psychological health and to reduce irritability, anger, hostility, envy, unduly critical attitudes, jealousy, inordinate competitiveness, and controlling tendencies, *Pitta prakrutis* should try to avoid heat-engendering situations (foods, spices, competition, and so forth). The *Pitta*-predominant person tends toward deep, penetrating intellect and sustained attention directed toward task completion. Careers and occupations that require this degree of mental organization, fastidiousness, and precision are *Pitta dosha* compatible, for example, engineers, detail managers, physicians, attorneys, professors, and so forth. The best climates in which to live are those that are both cool and temperate.

Kapha Predominance

Kapha dosha prakruti, in balance, is strong, stable, grounded, and steady. Food choices should tend to be light, warm, dry, and stimulating. All cold, frozen, and iced items should be avoided. The main meal should be around noontime, and all food intake should cease by early evening.

Those with *Kapha* predominance require the least amount of daily sleep. Six hours may be sufficient for the adult. Infancy, childhood, and a large part of adolescence constitute the developmental period of *Kapha* dominance. Infants and children naturally require substantially more sleep, and adolescents require no more than eight to nine hours. The adolescent predilection for staying up late into the night and then sleeping into the late morning hours is particularly deleterious and should be carefully monitored and avoided. Parental guidance is advised, if not critically important, in safeguarding the welfare of children and adolescents whose healthy upbringing is predicated on such responsible and vigilant parenting. Awakening by or shortly after the time of sunrise (at least by 8 to 9 A.M.) is recommended since it may ensure or, at least, create conditions for optimal functioning. This admonition is one of the *single most important safeguards* that responsible parents can and should implement in caring for the young, especially adolescents. Another is extra careful monitoring between the hours of 4 P.M. and 8 P.M. when the propensity for at-risk behaviors is highest.

Sleeping during the daytime hours is considered very unhealthy, especially for those of a *Kapha* constitution, since it strongly increases *Kapha dosha*. Staying awake relatively later into the night but going to sleep before or by midnight is acceptable. Since sleep has an intimate connection with the quality and quantity of *Kapha dosha,* those with this constitutional type are especially prone to oversleeping. The negative consequences of this are numerous and result in pervasive lethargy, indolence, and passivity both physically and psychologically.

Staying awake late into the night, therefore, is exceedingly deleterious. It not only disturbs *Kapha,* but the added disturbance in *Vata,* that is, restlessness, impulsivity, and evoking a penchant for thrill-seeking activities, compounds the magnitude of the vitiation. When anyone, for that matter, stays awake late into the night, a vicious cycle is set up that predisposes to oversleep in the morning. Sleeping later into the morning hours tends to increase *Kapha* to abnormal amounts, and this has a ripple effect that tends to disrupt both *Vata* and *Pitta. Prana Vata* has an intimate connection with clarity of consciousness, fundamental balance, and sound health. Disturbances of *Vata,* therefore, are most important to avoid or to minimize.

Kapha dominance is the only *dosha* type that benefits from very intense, rigorous exercise. Strong aerobic exercises, weight lifting, running, jogging, bicycling, as well as all strenuous physical activity is beneficial and recommended. In addition, moderate exposure to the sun and judicious sunbathing are acceptable.

In order to prevent excess *Kapha* from accumulating, *Kapha*-dominant types should avoid exposure to excess cold in foods and environments, too much sleep, procrastination, and inordinate bouts of physical and mental inertia. Psychological health maintenance also will curb *Kapha*'s natural and default tendency toward lethargy, complacency, greedy and possessive attachments, and depression. Pursuits that are more intrinsically active, such as those requiring stimulating study, travel, and healthy action-oriented pastimes are most beneficial. This *dosha* dominance performs well in caring, nurturing, counseling, and administrative endeavors. The best climate is one that tends to be hot and arid.

YOGA AND MEDITATION

Yoga and Ayurveda: Their Differing Emphases

The practice of Yoga and meditation may be considered part of the system of Ayurveda insofar as both may complement and enhance Ayurvedic practices. Classical Yoga is an orthodox *darshana* that highlights consciousness-enhancing virtues and daily performance practices. It is much more than merely physical exercises aimed at physical fitness.

Although they share some similar, yet not identical, origins with some historical parallels, there are important differences between the two. Ayurveda as a whole is more ancient and is derived from the ancient Vedic foundational texts, particularly the *Rig-Veda* and the *Atharva-Veda*. It also draws from the older orthodox and nonorthodox *darshanas*. Traditional or Classical Yoga theory and practice, codified by Patanjali, is at least 2,000 years old and thus relatively younger than the *Vedas* (Condron, 1991; Dasgupta, 1989). Patanjali, author of the *Yoga-Sutra,* the source text of Classical Yoga, may have lived in the second century A.D., although Hindu tradition identifies him with the famous grammarian of the same name who lived 400 years earlier.

While sharing many similarities, Ayurveda and Classical Yoga contain some significant and qualitatively differing emphases. Whereas the Yoga system has stronger dualistic themes underlying its ideology and practice, Ayurveda tends to be relatively more monistic in that a *BioPsychoSpiritual* integration is advanced. Yoga systems tend to suggest trends toward ascetic renunciation (*tapas*) of the flesh and of the material world (Condron, 1991; Dumont, 1980; Kaelber, 1989; Olivelle, 1992). Ayurveda, on the other hand, puts more positive emphasis on the physical body and the material aspects of the environment as they contribute to health and well-being. In many ways, Ayurveda can be regarded as having a more "full bodied" rather than "disembodied" espousal of all aspects of life and living. This robust emphasis on the positive value of the body within nature is a primary focus in Ayurveda.

Among the goals of Ayurveda, a central theme is the attainment of a healthy and progressively purified body since it is the physical aspect and expression of its mental and consciousness dimensions. When the body is maintained in optimal balance, psychological and spiritual experience is enhanced. A delicate balance between being in the world versus being identified exclusively with the world, that is, materialism and hedonism, restructures in a positive sense the meaning that attachment (*upadana*) to material reality plays in the Ayurvedic worldview. Although man's spirituality is considered primary and significant, Ayurveda's first attention begins with the spirit's material counterpart, the physical body. The Vedic goals of life, personal and social duty (*dharma*), necessary material wealth (*artha*), sexual and material pleasure (*kama*), and enlightenment (*Moksha*) are intrinsic to Ayurvedic values. While Ayurveda is the basis for the practice of a healing profession, the application of its principles and values by individuals in a personal way can optimize general health and overall well-being in all aspects of daily living.

Yoga, on the other hand, is a self-enhancement system primarily practiced by the individual, mostly in a private manner, as the decisive method for self-development and spiritual advancement through purification of body and mind (Eliade, 1973; Mishra, 1959, 1963; Sarkar, 1993; Vishnudevananda, 1960). Unlike Ayurveda with its distinctly medical orientation, Yoga disciplines are usually not a primary means for health maintenance and addressing specific medical problems and illnesses. In Yoga systems, more emphasis is given to mental and spiritual hygiene, disciplining the mind and enhancing consciousness, per se. In the initial stages of Yoga studies, that is, *Hatha*

Yoga, a familiar and commonly pursued activity virtually synonymous with contemporary Yoga in the West, physical postures (*asanas*), breathing exercises (*pranayama*), and, oftentimes, an attempt at meditative practices (*sadhana*) constitute the entire Yoga practice. Advanced Yoga techniques (*Samyama*), while incorporating the aforementioned preliminary procedures, lay much greater emphasis on mental training, deepening constraint, and the refinement of consciousness. While Yoga practices allot ample attention to the needs and care of the physical body, the meditative experience, taming of the inherently unstable mind, and rigorous disciplining of the senses constitute the highest values and become the primary focus of work. The literature both of Ayurveda and of Yoga, however, shares common terms and has a similar conceptual and theoretical framework although the emphases, methodologies, and procedures of each differ.

Yoga: Its History in the Ancient *Vedas* and Later Development by Patanjali

In a manner similar to that of Ayurveda, the historical roots both of Yoga and of meditation originated from Vedic sources (Feuerstein, 1998). Precise historical dating relating to the development both of Ayurveda and of preclassical Yoga, including its meditative practices, is ambiguous at best. Preclassical Yoga postures have been identified in the meditative poses documented before the time of Patanjali. Ayurveda, therefore, has a relatively more explicit written textual rather than oral foundation. The ancient Vedic origins of the oldest forms of Yoga can be traced using later Vedic texts. The *Upanishads* (c. 600 B.C.–300 B.C.) appear to contain explicit and clear references. The earliest *Upanishad,* the *Brhadaranyaka,* may contain the earliest historical reference to meditation in its description of admonitions for the stilling of the mind in order to concentrate its focus inwardly for the purpose of perceiving the true self or spirit (*atman*). Although there are many early references, historians consider the first use of the term *yoga* to have occurred in the *Katha Upanishad.* This early work also relates a classic metaphor that embodies the sense and aim of the yogic pursuit.

In a famous dialogue between a man named Nakiketas and the personification of death, Yama, man is likened to a chariot driven by horses and steered by the individual person. The chariot represents the body, the horses represent the senses, and the charioteer represents the self or spirit. In this analogy, the life of man is seen as a journey powered by potentially wild and unbridled instincts that require discipline and guidance in order to ensure a direct path to a destination. The destination is reached by the journey to the core of the self that transcends the ordinary state of merely existing in the world in an unquestioning and nonintrospective manner. The highest value is considered to reside in the deepest understanding of the true nature of the self, and this, in turn, becomes identified with an understanding of the ultimate nature of all existence.

The famous epic literature of India, the *Mahabharata* (c. 400 B.C.–A.D. 300) as well as the *Bhagavad Gita,* contains descriptions of Yoga practices and of schools with differing emphases such as the pursuit of knowledge (*jnana*), of action and service (*karma*), and of love and devotion (*bhakti*). The most famous of the Yoga *Upanishads* (c. 100 B.C.–A.D. 300), the *Yogatattva,* describes four kinds of Yoga: (1) *mantra yoga,* the repetition of sacred sounds; (2) *laya yoga,* the activation of the *Kundalini* energy that enhances consciousness; (3) *hatha yoga,* the practice of body postures and breath control; and (4) *raja yoga* (the best or royal yoga), which became the comprehensive system *later* elucidated by Patanjali and his school (c. 100 B.C.–A.D. 500). The preclassical Yoga schools before Patanjali emphasized the goal of individual union and identity with the universal, immanent spiritual ground of existence.

The modern-day system of Classical Yoga practice with its eight branches is essentially derived from Patanjali's *Yoga Sutras* (Condron, 1991; Feuerstein, 1989). These writings codified the Classical Yoga system as we know it today and outlined what were considered its eight limbs (*asthanga*). It is said that the *Hatha Yoga* that gives particular prominence to the *asanas* or yogic postures as a primary means of cleansing the body was formally organized only about a thousand years ago by its most popular teacher, Goraksha (c. tenth century A.D.) born in Punjab. Up to this time, most Yoga practices were aimed at mental and spiritual cultivation through meditation and less focused on the physicality that is correlated with Hatha practices. Only in more recent times has the Hatha dimension been rekindled into prominence. Krishnamacharya (1880–1989), born in South India and working for much of his life in Mysore, is considered a modern grand master. His deep study of the older Yoga traditions resulted in a reorganization that brought them into the modern mainstream both in India and in the West. Swami Vivekananda (1863–1902) was the first to bring Hinduism and Yoga to the West in the very early 1900s. B.K.S. Iyengar (b. 1923) is also a modern Yoga master whose influence both in India and in the United States is well recognized. Indra Devi (1899–2002), who came to the United States in the 1930s, and Paramahansa Yogananda (1893–1952), author of *Autobiography of a Yogi* (1946) who began the Self-Realization Fellowship in California, were influential figures in bringing Yoga to America.

Yoga's mental and physical practices aim at clarifying consciousness by disciplining the naturally wandering mind and training it to become more focused and singular (*ekagrata*). This activity over time would then lead to a union or *yug* between individual consciousness (*atman*) and the universal consciousness (*Purusha, Brahman*). The result of this is the state termed self-realization (*samadhi*). In turn, liberation and enlightenment (*Moksha*), in fact, complete transcendence (*Kaivalya*), a total separation from the material world, would be achieved. Classical Yoga, therefore, seeks extrication from the material world in contrast to Ayurveda's emphasis on embracing, purifying, and refining the material dimensions of experience.

The Eightfold Path of Union, the *Asthanga Yoga* (eight limbs or steps of Yoga), was comprised of the following in ascending order of refinement or purity of consciousness. These steps have been referred to as "Raja Yoga" or the royal path. This connotes the universal path that is to be traversed in some way in order to attain ultimate freedom of choice, in essence, *Moksha.*

The *Asthanga Yoga* has an intimate identity with the Eightfold Path (*Asthanga Marga*) aimed toward refining consciousness and toward ultimate liberation (*Nirvana*) at the heart of all Buddhist teachings. The Eightfold Path constitutes the last pillar of the four foundational propositions in Buddhism, the Four Noble Truths (*Arya Satya*). The *Asthanga Marga* of Buddhism outlines the methods to be used to manage, attenuate, and extinguish (*nirodha*) human suffering (*duhkha*), whose principal cause resides in desire (*trishna*).

In *Asthanga Yoga,* Yama or the regulation of the self in relationship to itself and to others initiates this process. The last three phases, *Dharana, Dhyana,* and *Samadhi,* are referred to as the *Samyama.* This achievement heralds the ultimate release of attachment and of bondage to an unconsidered, passive, and mechanical existence. It connotes a state of silence or being within unfettered consciousness.

1. *Yama:* mental restraint, self-control virtues, and ethical interpersonal behavior. The five fundamental guidelines included *ahimsa* or nonviolence, *satya* or truthfulness, *asteya* or not stealing, *aparigraha* or nonoverindulgence and detachment from material and worldly things and activities; this covers desire, craving (*trishna*), hankering, lust, envy, greed, and jealousy; and *brahmacharya* or regulation of sexual experience. *Yamas* are abstentions and "do not" guidelines. Within the Buddhist Eightfold Path are the *shila,* guidelines for ethical conduct akin to the Yogic *Yama.*

2. *Niyama:* personal observances, practices, religious rituals, and disciplines. These attitudes of devotedness included cleanliness and purity of body, senses, and heart; serenity and contentment; austerity and ascetic practices (*tapas*); study of sacred texts (*svadhyaya*); and devotional surrender to the highest good (*bhakti* and *prapatti*). *Niyamas* are suggestions for positive action; they are "do" guidelines.

3. *Asana:* physical yoga postures.

4. *Pranayama:* the intentional and regulated management and expansion of breathing in order to normalize it and thus, in turn, quiet and still the mind.

5. *Pratyahara:* the withdrawal of attention experienced in the sensory faculties from their outward sensory objects; an introspective refocusing.

6. *Dharana:* narrowing the mind by focusing and concentrating.

7. *Dhyana:* the process of meditation.

8. *Samadhi* or *Satya Buddhi:* the ultimate union of the microcosmic self with its origins, macrocosmic consciousness. *Kaivalya,* total extrication from matter, is *samadhi*'s superlative achievement.

The system of Yoga in all its variations and differing modalities is a time-honored endeavor to help regulate, enhance, and develop body, mind, and consciousness. It was devised to highlight and to address the natural unruliness and untamed quality of the mind, its passions, inclinations, and oftentimes unhealthy life choices. It continues to be a necessary and beneficial path for those to whom it provides a suitable vehicle for serious self-examination and work. Although Ayurveda and Yoga constitute different disciplinary fields, they are compatible and can be mutually enhancing. As was alluded to previously, there are both some obvious and some more subtle differences. In order to further explicate the differences that are significant yet more subtle, some nuances of each are highlighted. This may help to distinguish each in terms of its respective general perspective, emphases, metaphysical values, and material practices.

Classical Yoga as a discipline stresses a contemplative and meditative mode of experience and action. In its metaphysical worldview, Yoga begins with a strongly dualistic frame of reference. This view sees man as a potentially realized self who needs to overcome his inherently unstable and disorganizing tendencies. The worldly environment, in effect, is viewed as potentially hostile. Aspirants on the Yogic path, therefore, may see themselves as strivers or even warriors struggling to fight and to oppose bondage (*bandha*) to the sense objects of the material world. Yoga practices aim at controlling, disciplining, and virtually eradicating the range of desires and the power of the bodily instincts that fuel desire and thus perpetuate worldly attachments. Renunciation is given a high value. It is achieved by *tapas,* that is, rigorous discipline, mortification, asceticism, and *dhuta,* which is the gradual shaking off all aspects of bondage to the world. *Tapas* denotes fierce willpower and superefforts. The idea of the continual striving for detachment to worldly experience pervades traditional Yoga systems. There is a subtle sense of this constituting an underlying negative world bias or socially negating attitude. The strict self-discipline (*Samyama*) that concentration, meditation, and striving for *samadhi* requires connotes a progressively introspective journey. The ultimate achievement is called *Kaivalya,* that is, the absolute liberation from connectedness to anything.

Purity, in the Yoga sense, is equated with the withdrawal of the spirit from the flesh. The Classical Yoga of Patanjali was profoundly associated with the formalization of ascetic and renunciate cultural movements. This, in part, may be interpreted as having been a "reaction formation" taken to extremes as a result of the innate difficulty of managing oneself with equanimity in a diverse world in which pleasure, wealth, envy, greed, desire, and human frailty was (and is) part of daily living. Classical Yoga systems offered a means of addressing this problem. This classical separatist paradigm, however, had exceptions, notable of which was the Integral Yoga school (Aurobindo, 1976) advanced by Sri Aurobindo (1872–1950).

This characterization of such a subtle propensity in Yoga, it is hoped, is not meant to oversimplify or to reduce the profundity and value of the enduring contributions that Yoga has made to man's striving for meaning and for self-development. The main thesis of the highlighted contrasts between Ayurveda and Yoga, however, does have a firm basis in the substantiated history and texts of the Yoga tradition. Along with the significant contributions to personal development and to well-being that Yoga philosophy and procedures have made and continue to provide, one is impressed with an indisputably fervent spiritual and, at times, almost antimaterial or other worldly leaning pervading the Classical Yoga corpus. In contrast, one cannot overlook the fact that Yoga may be more accessible and attractive to the general population at large, especially in the West. The seat (*asana*) of Yoga begins with *Hatha* Yoga postures. This has great appeal as a user-friendly means to physical exercise, stretching, and flexibility. Yoga, as ordinarily perceived in the West, presents itself as these forms or postures. Yet, Yoga is more. It offers a path to self-reflection, quietude, physical and mental poise, and then a union or *yug* that extends beyond these preliminary beginnings.

Recognizing this, accordingly, in the context of the immense contributions that Yoga and its practices have made to man's search for meaning and self-development, its judicious integration, in a balanced and complementary fashion, into Ayurvedic health practices can only enhance, if not strengthen, the value of both approaches. The renowned Ayurvedic physician Charaka, in his foundational medical text *Charaka Samhita,* has extolled the merits of Yoga practices as being conducive to the attainment of *Moksha* (enlightenment and freedom).

YOGA PROCEDURES ACCORDING TO *DOSHA* PREDOMINANCE

Yoga procedures include yoga postures (*asanas*), breathing techniques (*pranayama*), and purification practices (*shuddhi kriyas*). There are specific postures and breathing techniques that are suitable for maintaining the health of the body and contributing toward the balancing of doshic irregularities. As in the study and practice of Ayurveda, the guidance of a qualified teacher is essential.

Some of the more important Yoga practices that are specifically applicable to the three broad classes of *prakruti,* the *Vata, Pitta,* and *Kapha* constitutional types, are outlined. A full elaboration of the six yogic purification practices is beyond the scope of this book, but they are mentioned in brief. They have their parallel in the Ayurvedic *Panchakarma* system of intensive bodily purification, which will constitute a complete discussion later in Chapter 10. Since the scope of Yoga practices is broad and includes a vast vocabulary unique to its own point of view and system, only simple English terms will accompany their Sanskrit equivalents in the text. These, along with other terms specific to Yoga theory, will not be included in the glossary but can be found in other texts devoted to Yoga practices (Condron, 1991; Mishra, 1959, 1963; Vishnudevananda, 1960). The *Shuddhi Kriyas* comprise the following six procedures:

1. *Neti:* nasal cleansing;
2. *Dhauti:* stomach cleansing;
3. *Nauli:* abdominal contractions;
4. *Trataka:* cleansing the eyes;
5. *Basti:* enema cleansing (not therapy) of the colon; and
6. *Kapalabhati:* forceful exhalation, abdominal contraction, and inhalation.

Vata-Dominant Constitution

The *Vata*-dominant *prakruti* requires procedures that are mild to moderate in intensity and have regular, relaxing, and stabilizing features. Some beneficial Yoga postures include the *sukhasana* (easy pose), the *siddhasana* (perfect pose), and the *padmasana* (lotus pose). These three *asanas* help regulate the *Vata* subdoshas of *Prana* and *Udana.* The *shavasana* (corpse pose) balances all the *Vata* subdoshas, and the *vajrasana* (kneeling pose) helps regulate the *Apana Vata* subdosha. The best breathing technique is the *nadi shodhana pranayama* (alternate nostril breathing). The *nauli* (mild abdominal contractions) help *Samana Vata* subdosha. *Apana Vata* subdosha is responsive to Yogic *basti.*

Pitta-Dominant Constitution

The *Pitta*-dominant *prakruti* requires procedures that are moderate in intensity and tend to be cooling and calming. Some beneficial Yoga postures include the *bhujangasana* (cobra pose), the *sarvangasana* (shoulder stand) that helps regulate *Pachaka Pitta,* the *halasana* (plough pose) that helps *Ranjaka Pitta,* and the *shirsasana* (headstand) that helps *Sadhaka Pitta.* The *shitali kumbhaka* (cooling breath) is a very gentle and beneficial breathing exercise. Another breathing technique, done in great moderation to avoid overly cooling the body, is called *chandrabheda* (lunar *pranayama*) and consists of left nostril breathing techniques. The *Alochaka Pitta* subdosha is benefited by the cleansing techniques of *trataka* and *kapalabhati.*

Kapha-Dominant Constitution

Kapha-predominant *prakrutis* require strong, intense, and forceful procedures. The *suryasana* (sun salutation exercise) and series of postures, the *paschimotasana* (sitting with forward stretching posture), and the *yogamudra asana* (symbol of yoga posture) are all helpful for *Kapha dosha.* The best breathing exercise is *suryabheda pranayama* (solar breathing). This is especially useful for regulating the *Avalambaka Kapha* subdosha. Other useful breathing techniques include *ujjayi* (loudly victorious breathing) and *bhastrika* (bellows breathing) technique. *Dhouti* stomach cleansing benefits the *Kledaka Kapha* subdosha. *Neti* (nasal cleansing) helps the *Bodhaka Kapha* subdosha.

10

AYURVEDIC THERAPIES, *PANCHAKARMA*, AND MATERIA MEDICA

AYURVEDIC TREATMENT: THE RANGE OF THERAPEUTIC INTERVENTIONS

The range of treatments in Ayurveda is broad and comprehensive. It includes dietary, herbal, lifestyle, behavioral, psychological, meditative, exercise, Yoga, and *Panchakarma* therapeutic interventions (Joshi, 1996; Lele, Ranade, & Qutab, 1997; Ranade, 1993, 2003). *Panchakarma* is a group of five specialized techniques used to cleanse and detoxify the body of *Ama* (toxins) and vitiated *doshas* (bioenergetic regulatory substances). The entire spectrum of Ayurvedic therapy, however, aims at restoring the normal balance and functioning of the *doshas* and the mind. This entails attention to optimizing the digestive fire or *Agni*. In addition, treatments, as well as daily routines for health maintenance, attempt to reduce accumulated *Ama* and to prevent its initial buildup. The matrix of treatment rests on proper nutrition, and this serves as a base upon which all therapeutic interventions are structured. Restoring balance, therefore, coupled with customized nutritional and lifestyle prescriptions covers the scope of all treatment.

As with the classification of disease and the assessment of diagnosis, the range and nuances of specific therapies can be immense and complex. A brief survey, therefore, with only an orienting discussion is presented here. A brief but representative discussion of commonly encountered clinical presentations and their treatments from the Western and Ayurvedic perspectives is found in Appendix 3.

BRIMHANA AND *LANGHANA*

The famous Ayurvedic physician Vagbhata (c. seventh century A.D.) categorized all medical treatments in two broad categories: (1) *Brimhana* (tonification) and (2) *Langhana* (reduction).

BRIMHANA

Brimhana methods tonify, nourish, strengthen, enrich, fortify, and supplement. The term *tonification* is widely used in most contemporary herbal texts to describe the range of these toning, enriching, supplementing, and nutritive interventions. *Brimhana* therapy is also termed *santarpana* (therapy that is indulgent and that gladdens). The primary Elements of Earth and Water constitute the predominating Elements of the substances used since they contribute to an increase in substance, mass, and the *Kapha dosha* (principle of consolidation). The *Brimhana* category has three subdivisions: (1) *Brimhana* diet and herbs (tonification proper), (2) *Snehana* (oleation), and (3) *Stambhana* (therapy).

Brimhana Diet and Herbs

Therapies that tonify aim at increasing body weight and strength. They are used in conditions that include debilitation, weakness, convalescence, and malnutrition. *Vata* (principle of propulsion) disorders tend to cause weakness and are most responsive to tonifying procedures. *Pitta* (principle of transformation) disorders may sometimes benefit from supplementation, but *Kapha* (principle of consolidation) disorders usually do not require this type of treatment. Tonification or toning therapies are contraindicated in conditions marked by inordinate toxicity, *Ama,* or fever. Diets that tonify are rich and nutritious and include foods such as milk, ghee, raw sugar, almonds, and rice. Some herbs with marked toning properties include ashwaghanda, shatavari, bala, and amalaki. A life-style with little stress, very gentle exercise, and rest is recommended.

Snehana

Snehana therapy uses oils and fats both internally and externally for lubrication. This is termed oleation. Ayurveda stresses the importance of an adequate intake of fat, as, for example, in the form of ghee, olive, and flaxseed oils to maintain proper nutritional balance. The Sanskrit term *sneha,* in fact, has multiple meanings that include both material and psychological references. *Sneha,* for example, denotes (1) material stickiness as in oil and fat and (2) emotional attachment as in affection and love. These varied meanings hold enormous value in Ayurveda. In many ways, they denote the sense of gravity, connectedness, grounding, and soothing balance. Ghee (a special form of highly clarified butter), for example, is considered a primary and essential food and medicine. It calms, soothes, and pacifies both *Vata* and *Pitta,* and, in moderation, is beneficial and supportive to *Kapha.* These actions optimize the digestive fire, *Agni,* and enhance physiological functioning and, in addition, promote tranquility, intelligence, and compassion both to self and to others.

When various cleansing and detoxifying procedures are done, large doses of prescribed, medicated oils are taken along with specific external oil massage routines. *Vata* disorders are particularly responsive to heavy oleation. *Pitta* disorders require mild oleation, and *Pitta* is especially responsive to treatment with *ghee*. Disorders characterized by significant *Kapha* excess are treated sparingly and parsimoniously with oleation since this will intensify *Kapha* and excessive oleation thus will exacerbate the *Kapha* condition.

Stambhana

Stambhana or astringent methods are less commonly used in therapy. *Stambhana* is an action (*karma*) that promotes contraction (*sankochanam*) and constriction of vessels containing bodily fluids such as blood and lymph. Herbs and mechanical methods (cold sheets) may be used. Those with *Pitta* excess are candidates for these interventions. When used, they act to stop or limit excess discharges from the body such as in bleeding disorders, hemorrhage, or diarrhea.

LANGHANA

Langhana Proper

Langhana or reduction therapies include three subtypes. They are (1) *Langhana* (reduction proper: *Shamana* and *Shodhana*), (2) *Rukshana* (drying), and (3) *Swedhana* (sudation). *Langhana* therapies make use of three major Elements: Ether, Air, and Fire. These contribute to processes that reduce, break down, detoxify, and cleanse the body of excess accumulations, toxins, and vitiated *doshas*. Since these reducing procedures are somewhat rigorous, require self-discipline, and may be experienced as difficult, *langhana* treatments have also been referred to as *asantarpana* (therapy that demands abstinence and is discontenting).

Reduction therapy proper (*langhana*) has two major and clinically significant subdivisions first enumerated by Charaka (c. 1000 to 760 B.C.), considered the father and one of the greatest of all Ayurvedic physicians and scholars. They are *Shamana* (palliation, alleviation, and reduction) and *Shodhana* (purification and elimination). *Shodhana* is virtually synonymous with the five procedures of *Panchakarma*.

Shamana

Shamana procedures are commonly used as a part of everyday health maintenance. They are also used in more highly specific ways as individualized treatment interventions and as preparatory procedures (*Purvakarma*) before *Panchakarma* (radical detoxification and elimination therapy). *Shamana* therapy aims at reducing toxic buildups of *Ama,* calming vitiated *doshas* at their respective sites, and at supporting the energy of *Agni*. Palliation may be divided into seven methods:

1. *Agni dipana:* stimulating the digestive fire to burn up and to destroy *Ama*. This is a central and fundamental procedure used therapeutically for *Panchakarma* proper and also for ongoing health maintenance. Fasting, by itself, increases *Agni*. Drinking plain hot water increases *Agni*. A number of herbs are used for optimizing the energy of the *Agni*'s optimal transformative power (*dipana*). Pungent herbs with a hot *virya* are specifically used to increase *Agni* and to burn out and to destroy *Ama*. Herbs that are mild include fennel and calamus; stronger herbs include dry ginger, plumbago, turmeric, cumin, asafetida, and the combination called *Trikatu,* a famous Ayurvedic digestive formula containing black pepper, pippali, and dry ginger.

2. *Ama pachana: Ama* digestion and detoxification, that is, to cleanse *Ama* from the body. This is another central and fundamental procedure used both therapeutically and for maintenance. Bitter or aromatic herbs (often but not always possessing a heating *virya*) are specifically used to reduce and to cleanse *Ama*. These include guduchi, cilantro leaves, coriander, fenugreek, tarragon, turmeric, calamus, Echinacea, burdock, chamomile, calendula, elder flowers, hops, myrrh, St. John's wort, and even coffee in moderation. The Bitter *rasa* is the principal moiety that acts to increase *Samana Vata* and so to fan *Agni*. This Bitter *rasa* acts to separate *Ama* from *doshas* and from tissues so that *Ama* may be digested and reduced, and so that *doshas* and tissues may be cleansed. The hot *virya* of guduchi and of turmeric increase *Pitta* and burn *Ama*. Pungent herbs are used to burn and to destroy *Ama*. There are several herbs used to burn *Ama,* but the main ones are dry ginger, black pepper, and *Trikatu.*

3. *Khust:* fasting from food. Fasting, by itself, increases *Agni*.

4. *Trit:* fasting from water or limiting fluid intake.

5. Exercise and Yoga.

6. *Atapa-sevana:* exposure to sun and heat.

7. *Maruta-sevana:* exposure to wind and fresh air.

Shamana is a moderate regimen for general detoxification. It may be practiced daily as a preventative to disease. It is not a radical intervention like the five procedures of classical *Panchakarma*. *Shamana* primarily *reduces* the buildup of toxic *Ama* at its respective sites in the various peripheral bodily tissues (*shakha*) and organs (*marmas, madhyama*) along with *calming down aggravated doshas*. These aggravated *doshas* are still partly contaminated with *Ama;* that is, their condition is one of being *Sama*. These vitiated *doshas* still remain largely not expunged or eliminated. Reducing *Ama* and calming aggravated *doshas,* however, is beneficial since both the reduction and the calming processes diminish the likelihood of excessive *Ama* buildup and the initiation of the disease process. Appropriate and regular use of *Triphala* according to one's *prakruti* is very beneficial in fortifying *Apana Vata* and enhancing proper bowel elimination. This also helps to keep toxins from accumulating.

The cleansing action of *Shamana* is in sharp contrast to *Shodhana Panchakarma,* which is primarily the *radical elimination* of vitiated, *aggravated doshas* that, after careful preparation (*purvakarma*) have traveled from their sites in the *dhatus* back to the central location *in the gastrointestinal tract* (*koshta*) from which they can be eliminated. The condition of these cleansed yet still vitiated *doshas* in the gastrointestinal tract is termed *Nirama,* which denotes that they have been freed from and contain no *Ama,* although they remain aggravated or vitiated. It is contraindicated to use formal *Panchakarma* to expunge *doshas* that are still significantly contaminated with *Ama,* just as it is contraindicated to do *Panchakarma* when *Ama* is within the gastrointestinal (GI) tract. *Ama* in the GI tract is reflected in conditions of acute fever.

Shamana is palliation, that is, a moderate, less intensive, attempt at (1) reduction and calming of vitiated or aggravated *doshas,* (2) reduction of toxic *Ama* accumulation, and (3) a *partial* yet significant clearing within the *srotas* of these blocking *Sama dosha* substances. *Shamana* is periodic and prophylactic detoxification that must be done at the junctures of the seasons, especially, the end of summer and the beginning of autumn, and the transition from spring to summer. In addition, whenever one feels a subjective malaise that has elements of bodily, psychological, or spiritual uneasiness, *Shamana* procedures may be used.

The essential components must include moderate fasting or reduction of food and liquid intake, drinking hot water every few hours, along with the ingestion of ghee, *Agni*-optimizing herbs (such as *Trikatu*), and herbs (such as turmeric) that aim at the reduction and destruction of toxic *Ama* buildup. The duration spans from three to seven days.

Shamana as a "mini-detox" that is more than mere palliation but less than radical elimination may be completed by the ingestion of castor oil (one to three tablespoons) and ginger on the last night. This partial purgation helps rid the gastrointestinal tract of whatever *Nirama* vitiated *doshas* have been transported there. This addition to *Shamana,* therefore, produces a partial rather than radical elimination.

Shodhana

Shodhana, intensive purification, specifically refers to *Panchakarma* therapy. It is the premier set of techniques that Ayurveda employs to radically eliminate excess vitiated *doshas.* This is usually done under supervision in a therapeutic setting. It is a series of specific treatments with a circumscribed course ranging in time from about ten days to one month for completion. *Panchakarma* proper is discussed at length later in this chapter.

Rukshana

Rukshana (drying) consists of ingesting foods and herbs that may have diuretic properties in addition to the use of dry massage with herbal powders.

Kapha diseases such as obesity and diabetes are partially responsive to *ruk-shana* interventions.

Swedhana

Swedhana (sudation, fomentation, and sweating) refers to therapies that induce an increase in body heat, vasodilation, and cause subsequent sweating. This may involve external applications of dry heat or steam, or the ingestion of herbs such as ginger, cinnamon, and the compound *Trikatu. Vata* conditions marked by cold and dryness are responsive to steam applications. *Kapha* conditions that are cold and damp respond to the ingestion of herbs that have hot and dry qualities.

To reiterate, two major therapeutic categories each having three subdivisions are the following: (1) *Brimhana* (tonification, supplementation, and enrichment): (a) *Brimhana* diet and herbs, (b) *Snehana,* and (c) *Stambhana;* and (2) *Langhana* (reduction): (a) *Langhana Shamana* and *Shodhana,* (b) *Rukshana,* and (c) *Swedhana.* These six subdivisions have been called *Shad Upakramas* or sixfold treatment. The internal and contrasting symmetry of the group reflects the fundamental Ayurvedic principles of treatment: "like increases like" (*samanya*) and "opposites balance and so cure each other" (*vishesha*): *Brimhana* (enrichment) versus *Langhana* (reduction), *snehana* (lubrication) versus *ruksjana* (drying), and *stambhana* (constriction) versus *swedhana* (dilation). These therapeutic actions cover the entire field of Ayurvedic treatments.

PANCHAKARMA AND AYURVEDIC MATERIA MEDICA

Ayurveda historically has been and currently remains an empirical science. As "life wisdom," it is first and foremost pragmatic in outlook. Its theoretical propositions guide its clinical application. The direct implementation of theory, in a concrete fashion, applied to man living in the world, is the premiere goal-directed action of Ayurveda. As previously outlined, there are a variety of treatment modalities and preventative methods commonly used to maintain health and correct imbalanced states. *Panchakarma,* however, is considered the ultimate purification treatment, unique to Ayurveda. Unlike *shamana* (palliative therapy), which may and should be a part of one's daily health maintenance home routine, *Panchakarma* is considered *shodhana* (radical purification and elimination therapy) and, in fact, requires the close supervision of a qualified Ayurvedic physician. Many procedures need to be performed in the monitored confines of an Ayurvedic clinic. This therapeutic environment becomes an interpersonal space that is protective, caring, empathetic, sensitive, and nurturing. These psychologically sensitive conditions foster efficacious treatment since all aspects of the person are given due and appropriate attention.

Contraindications for *Panchakarma*

As with all recommendations presented in this book, they are guidelines whose actual implementation is best undertaken under the direct guidance of a qualified health professional. Since *Panchakarma* is a radical group of procedures, it is not suitable for everyone. In general, the following conditions are contraindications for *Panchakarma:* active infection, internal bleeding, acute fever, alcoholism, cancers, congestive heart failure, HIV/AIDS, infectious diseases, premenstrual period and active menstrual period, morbid obesity, pregnancy, and uncontrolled hypertension. Those under 12 years and over 80 years of age are generally not candidates.

Persons who are obese and have strong *Kapha* constitutions should avoid oleation. Those with strong *Vata* or *Pitta* constitution and bleeding problems should avoid sweating procedures. *Vamana* (therapeutic emesis) should not be done by those with strong *Vata* constitutions, upper GI bleeding, or heart disease. *Virechana* (therapeutic purgation) should be avoided by those with chronic diarrhea, lower GI bleeding, and prolapsed internal organs. *Basti* (therapeutic enemas) should be avoided by those with diarrhea or asthma. *Nasya* (nasal treatment) should be avoided by those with bleeding disorders.

Oleation should not be done after *Panchakarma*. *Virechana* should not be done until three days after *Vamana*. *Nasya* should not be done immediately after oleation, *Vamana*, *Virechana*, and *Basti*.

CLASSICAL *PANCHAKARMA*

Classical *Panchakarma* treatment consists of three phases: (1) *Purvakarma*, preparatory actions; this is, in fact, *Shamana* with the addition of intensive oleation (*snehana*) and intensive sweating (*swedhana*); (2) *Pradhanakarma*, the five principal actions of *Panchakarma* proper; and (3) *Paschatakarma*, also termed *Uttarakarma*, post-*Panchakarma* actions.

I. *Purvakarma: Shamana* to Increase *Agni,* to Reduce Excess *Doshas,* and to Cleanse *Ama*

Purvakarma, the first phase of the *Panchakarma* process, is essentially a series of *shamana* (reduction) procedures. These preparatory activities have several objectives. These include reducing and destroying as much *Ama* as possible, increasing the gastric fire (*Agni*), calming and reducing vitiated and excess *doshas,* and then allowing these processed *doshas* that are now free from *Ama* to flow back from the compact body tissues (*shakha*) to the more central areas of the body, namely, the gastrointestinal tract and the lungs (*koshta*). These preliminary procedures thus permit the vitiated *doshas,* which have been freed of *Ama* (*Nirama*), access to centrally located anatomical areas from which *Panchakarma* proper procedures can be used to eliminate them.

Dietary and Herbal Preparations and Behavioral Recommendations

Purvakarma consists of three parts: (1) dietary and herbal preparation and behavioral recommendations to increase *Agni* and burn off *Ama,* (2) oleation (*snehana*), and (3) sudation (*swedhana*). Although precise prescriptions can be given only for a particular and individual patient undergoing treatment, a very general outline suggesting customary treatment trends provides a map showing direction and landmarks.

Preliminary procedures usually begin about two weeks before *Panchakarma* proper. The dietary component requires the patient to consume a light diet that avoids heavier foods such as meats, dietary fats, complex carbohydrates, dairy, as well as alcohol. Light soups of basmati rice and vegetables are best. A monodiet of *kichari,* a mixture of basmati rice, split yellow mung dal (lentils), and mild spices, such as cumin, coriander, turmeric, and fennel seeds, is often suggested. If possible, one should avoid unnecessary drugs, medications (discussion with one's medical doctor is recommended), alcohol, and all nonprescribed dairy products. In addition, one may use a simple three-day light diet of only basmati rice with ghee and either cumin, coriander, and fennel, or cinnamon, allspice, and tomato paste. Hot water should be consumed throughout the duration of this diet. On the last day, one to three tablespoons of castor oil with one teaspoon of ginger is to be taken before bedtime. This modest purge helps eliminate toxins, *Ama,* and the vitiated *doshas* that return to the gastrointestinal tract. This procedure is a partial, not radical, detoxification.

Selected herbs that reduce and destroy toxic *Ama* buildup are consumed. Some representative ones are the following: ginger, black pepper, cumin, chitrak, asafetida, and red pepper. Herbs, such as ginger, fennel, and pippali, which optimize the digestive fire (*Agni*), are also given.

This therapeutic dietary and herbal cleansing is essential to target the *Ama* impurities present in cells and tissues in order to neutralize or "burn" as much *Ama* as possible. Any *Ama* residing in the gastrointestinal tract also needs to be detoxified in this way. At this stage, two important preliminary reducing actions are accomplished: (1) attempts to decrease and to destroy (*Ama pachana*) as much *Ama* as possible and (2) optimizing the energy of the gastric fire (*Agni dipana*) in order to improve metabolism thus preventing further *Ama* production.

Rest, relaxation, and avoidance of exercise and exposure to cold and wind are highly recommended in order to therapeutically curtail any excess actions of *Vata*. One is advised to stay warm, consume warm to hot foods and beverages, and avoid all cold foods and environmental conditions. Drinking plain hot water every two to four hours while awake optimizes the cleansing process. This process of dietary and lifestyle preparation should span up to seven days.

Snehana: Oleation

With the above *shamana-purvakarma* procedures in place for at least one week, the next step entails attempts at reducing, calming, and mobilizing the vitiated *doshas* that reside in and are bound pathologically to the tissues. The two primary methods used to accomplish this are oleation (*snehana*) and sudation (*swedhana*). This step is a critical juncture in the attempt to mobilize lodged vitiated *doshas* that are embedded in the tissues. This pathological amalgamation requires this therapeutic series of interventions to disengage the vitiated *doshas.*

The oleation process consists both of the internal consumption of oily substances and of their external (*abhyanga*) application. [Oil enemas (*basti*) are discussed further on in this chapter as part of formal *Panchakarma.*] This oleation step has been classically referred to as "turning the wheel of dryness into the wheel of life."

The therapeutic ingestion of ghee is used in most cases since it both calms excess *Vata* and increases *Agni.* Other oils such as sesame, flaxseed, sunflower, or mustard, to mention only a few, may be used depending on the specific case to be treated, especially if the clinical condition requires a more heating or drying intervention. Factors such as constitutional type (*prakruti*), the nature of the imbalanced *doshas,* and the season are taken into consideration when making individualized selections concerning the use of specific oils.

Ghee (*Ghritam*) has been used in Ayurveda for thousands of years. Ghee is butter (best from cow's milk) that is cooked in order to remove both its initial water content (18 to 20 percent) and its milk solids (about 2 percent). This renders it relatively stable, lactose-free, and able to keep indefinitely without added preservatives or refrigeration. Its use has been considered therapeutic rather than only dietary, although it has many essential and beneficial nutritional functions. According to Ayurveda, ghee plays many vital roles in the body. Some of its more important functions include (1) stimulating and optimizing the energy of *Agni* (digestive fire and metabolism); (2) reducing all three *doshas,* especially *Pitta* to normal levels; and (3) promoting longevity, intellect, memory, strength, eyesight, and the soundness of the integumentary or skin system. The taste of ghee is considered to be Sweet, its energy is cold, and its *vipaka* (postdigestive effect) is Sweet.

Among the very healthy saturated fats within ghee are butyric acid (3.09 percent), capric acid (2.38 percent), and lauric acid (2.72 percent). These have been shown to have antimicrobial and antifungal properties. Ghee also contains phenolic antioxidants. All of these factors make ghee resistant to free radical damage and rancidity. It does not require refrigeration. Ghee contains about 5 percent polyunsaturated fats, among which linoleic acid constitutes 3.82 percent. Conjugated linoleic acid (CLA) has been shown to increase lean body mass and optimally metabolize body fat. Ghee is a pure, nonhydrogenated fat about one-third monounsaturated and about two-thirds saturated consisting of about 90 percent short chain fatty acids. This profile suggests that it can be beneficial to health since the preponderance of short-chain fatty acids is known to bring about full assimilation and metabolism resulting in energy production. Saturated long-chain fatty acids found in animal fats and red meats, on the other hand, have been shown to be associated with cardiovascular disease, blood clots (thrombosis), and a proneness to carcinomas. Monounsaturated fats, moreover, have been demonstrated to be associated with the prevention of heart disease and cancer. Trans fatty acids are manufactured, processed fats. They are found in hydrogenated fats, margarine, and many commercially prepared baked goods. They have been positively associated with the development of coronary heart disease; ghee contains no trans fatty acids. Elevation of the low density lipoprotein (LDL) fraction of blood cholesterol is believed to be one of many (for example, smoking, hypertension, obesity, and the Metabolic Syndrome) major risk factors for atherosclerotic cardiovascular disease. While beneficial fats in the form of essential fatty acids such as fish, flax, and some plant-derived oils are nutritionally necessary, the total saturated fat intake should not exceed between 7 and 10 percent of all dietary calories or about 10 to 20 grams per day.

For safe and salutary dietary and nutritional maintenance, up to one (5 grams) to two teaspoons of ghee per day is suggested; this may be added to food or taken with herbal preparations and preferably should be uncooked. Each teaspoon contains about 45 calories. For therapeutic oleation *on a short-term basis,* about 1 to 5 ounces per day in the morning on an empty stomach is customary; this requires drinking hot water or hot ginger tea during the entire course of the oleation procedure. These suggestions for ghee ingestion are for those who have no specific cholesterol or triglyceride abnormalities, no cardiovascular disease, and who have obtained clearance from a qualified medical doctor after appropriate physical examination and laboratory investigations.

External oleation is termed *snehana* when it is used as part of a therapeutic procedure such as *purvakarma*. Some examples of other terms for oil massage that are less medically oriented are *abhyanga* (whole body), *shirodhara* (oil drip to forehead), and *shirobasti* (oil retention on top of head). For external oleation a variety of types of oils is used depending on the specific conditions involved. Some representative oils used are sesame, almond, castor, coconut, and ghee. Small amounts of essential oils having specific therapeutic properties may also be added to the aforementioned for an enhanced *dosha*-balancing effect (Miller & Miller, 1995).

The duration of internal oleation ranges from three days to seven days; longer than this period of time is not recommended. The dosage ranges, ordinarily using ghee or a medicated ghee, are the following: day 1, 25 grams; day 2, 50 grams; day 3, 75 grams; day 4, 100 grams; day 5, 125 grams; and day 6, 150 grams. The entire oleation process is accompanied by the frequent and daily ingestion of plain hot water. In general, one cup of hot water is taken every few hours while awake.

Oleation, especially by internal ingestion, serves two principal functions: (1) protection of retainable body tissues and (2) loosening and separating the vitiated *doshas* from the healthy retainable body tissues. Although some degree of oleation is therapeutically necessary, it is used with caution in those with strong *Kapha* dominance, obesity, and significantly reduced *Agni*.

Oleation, especially the internal ingestion of ghee, induces the tissues to give up their accumulation of toxins and vitiated *doshas*. It enhances secretions through which the *doshas* can transport residual toxins and wastes to the gastrointestinal tract for ultimate elimination. Oleation lubricates and protects bodily tissues from damage while *Ama* and vitiated *doshas* are being reduced. Oleation strongly pacifies and nourishes *Vata*. Finally, oleation contributes to the removal of obstructions and blockages in the *srotas* and channels of circulation throughout the body.

Swedhana: Sudation

The last step in the *purvakarma* process is sudation (*swedhana*). This sweating therapy, of one or two day's duration, usually involves the application of external heat in the form of steam applied on a daily basis after external oil massage. On occasion, some internally heating herbs, such as ginger, may be given to induce diaphoresis. There are numerous types of sudation techniques devised to achieve heating up of the body and a mild to moderate rise in temperature. Sensitive areas of the body such as the head and the genital areas are protected from excess heat. The two principal objectives of *swedhana* are (1) to dilate the channels of circulation (*srotas*) and (2) to liquefy the already loosened excess and vitiated *doshas* in the tissues so that they may begin their centripetal flow back into the more central areas of the body. Although some degree of sudation is therapeutically necessary before *Panchakarma,* it is not used or used with great caution in the following situations: *Vata*-dominant constitutions; *Pitta*-dominant constitutions; *Pitta dosha* aggravation and imbalances, especially bleeding disorders, pregnancy, menstruating women, chronic alcoholism, and diabetes.

In summary, *purvakarma*'s actions, therefore, include detoxifying the body of *Ama,* increasing the *Agni,* calming vitiated *doshas,* and separating the vitiated *doshas* from healthy bodily tissues. Subsequently, there is a dilatation of the channels that aids in facilitating the vitiated *doshas* in their return from the more peripheral tissues to the central part of the body in order to eventually be eliminated by *Panchakarma*. The means to achieve this includes specialized diet, herbs, oleation, and sudation. During this almost two-week process, the patient is advised to rest and refrain from exercise. This helps to decrease the activity of *Vata* and thus add to the overall calming effect of the treatments. A day before *Panchakarma,* the patient is given a more specialized provocative diet called *adhishyandi.* This is specifically geared to increase the targeted vitiated *dosha* to high levels on a temporary basis immediately before the radical *Panchakarma* procedures that will promote their total elimination.

II. *Panchakarma* Proper: *Shodhana* and the Elimination of *Ama*

The second major phase of classical *Panchakarma* is *Panchakarma* proper (five primary therapeutic actions) that constitutes the basis of Ayurveda's core therapeutic interventions. These five actions or procedures include a range of direct and indirect forms and variations of a number of procedures. They are (1) *vamana* (emesis); (2) *virechana* (purgation); (3) *basti* (enema), two types; (4) *nasya* (intranasal applications of herbs and oils); and (5) *RaktaMoksha* (blood purification). Charaka (c. 1000–760 B.C.) regarded the first four procedures as fundamental and subdivided *basti* into two types: (1) *niruha basti* (herbal decoction enema) and (2) *anuvasana basti* (oil enema). Thus, he described five procedures with no emphasis on *RaktaMoksha*. The later work of Sushruta (c. 660 B.C.), the great Ayurvedic physician who specialized in surgery, laid emphasis on the specialized technique of *RaktaMoksha* along with the other therapeutic *Panchakarma* measures.

Panchakarma is the basis of all purification (*shodhana*) protocols; its aim is an in-depth extirpation of the vitiated *doshas* contained in the channels (*srotas*), the tissues (*dhatus*), and at the cellular level. Before a more indepth discussion of the five principal *Panchakarma* procedures, some preliminary ideas about Ayurvedic Materia Medica or herbology and indications for *Panchakarma* are reviewed.

AYURVEDIC MATERIA MEDICA

The range of *Panchakarma* techniques, like those of *shamana* (therapeutic attenuation of imbalances), involves both physical bodily manipulations and the administration of herbal preparations. Ayurvedic Materia Medica (*Dravyaguna Shastra*) is a blend of pharmacology and pharmacognosy whose origins extend back thousands of years with developments up to the present time.

Since *Panchakarma, shamana,* and Ayurvedic Materia Medica are complex, intricate, and finely detailed, not only in theory but also in clinical application, the present text addresses only some of the major theoretical principles that underlie them. Aspects of technique and some examples of frequently used Ayurvedic herbs are mentioned. These represent only highlights and, of necessity, omit other central and significant procedures, nuances of treatment applications, as well as the extensive and broad range of Ayurvedic herbology that may be found in currently available English texts (Lele, Ranade, & Qutab, 1997).

Indications for *Panchakarma*

Panchakarma, Ayurveda's most radical purification treatment, is given only to those who are relatively strong, healthy, and whose age and constitutions are resilient and able to endure the rigors of such intensive procedures. The range of less intensive, palliative techniques known as *shamana* is a more suitable course of treatment in the following cases: childhood, older age, pregnancy, and severe disease states, that is, diabetes, hypertension, alcoholism, drug addiction, thyroid imbalances, malignancy, immune deficiency, as well as in postsurgical patients, to mention only some representative examples. Maintaining purity of the tissues is central in Ayurveda and is accomplished by both *shodhana* and *shamana* therapies.

The three most important indications for *Panchakarma* are (1) health maintenance, (2) treatment of acute disease and generalized systemic healing, and (3) preparation for rejuvenation therapy (*rasayana chikitsa*). In Ayurveda, health maintenance requires that the normally cumulative amounts of *Ama* be periodically reduced and eliminated from the body using strong eliminative *Panchakarma*. In addition, factors such as chronological age, changing seasons, and normal as well as inordinate life stressors contribute to producing *dosha* vitiation on a regular basis. *Doshas* inevitably undergo unfavorable exacerbation at the junctures of seasons, especially the fall and the spring. At these times, *Panchakarma* is particularly useful. Periodic *Panchakarma* helps cleanse the system of toxic accumulations of a variety of impurities and rids the body of excess *doshas* that contribute to imbalanced states. *Panchakarma* in its health maintenance aspect is considered one of the best available preventative programs to ensure optimal well-being. With increasing age, the quantity and quality of vitiated *doshas* and *Ama* in the tissues (*dhatus*) increases; these amalgamated *doshas* lodge in intricate ways. A *Panchakarma* treatment most often removes only a portion of the many layers of embedded impurities. Repeated *Panchakarma* treatments go progressively deeper to remove more obstinate impurities caused by both material imbalances and the *samskaras* (imprinted conditioning over time) that result from past psychological trauma and conflict.

Panchakarma as a disease or *dosha* imbalance treatment is useful in some acute disease states. An acute exacerbation of asthma is one example. Although treating some acute disease states is a classical theoretical indication, it is not customarily done since *Panchakarma* is a powerful and involved technique that requires preparation, professional expertise and application, and a definite period of time. In other words, acute conditions often arise in an unplanned manner, whereas *Panchakarma* is usually an elective and planned procedure. Its therapeutic actions, therefore, may result in healing that is nonspecific but broad in range.

The last major indication for *Panchakarma* is its being the preliminary cleansing procedure that precedes formal *rasayana* or Ayurvedic rejuvenation programs. The elimination of *Ama* and excess *doshas* from the body acts to clear the channels (*srotas*) and tissues (*dhatus*) and make them more receptive to the highly toning, enriching, and rejuvenative herbs and minerals that comprise the elements of rejuvenation therapy. *Rasayana chikitsa* (rejuvenation treatment) is a specialized form of supplementation therapy used in middle and older age to revitalize the tissues and retard the aging process.

THE FIVE PRINCIPAL PROCEDURES OF *PANCHAKARMA* PROPER

Formal (*pradhana*) *Panchakarma* commences only after adequate *Purvakarma* has properly prepared the patient. *Panchakarma* is *shodhana*, the elimination of *Ama*. Inordinate amounts of *Ama* should not be present in the system at this phase of treatment. Although *Ama* is always present to some degree in the body, excessive amounts should have been significantly reduced. Any "loose" *Ama* in the tissues (*dhatus*) and channels (*srotas*) and virtually all *Ama* in the gastrointestinal tract should have been burned up and eliminated. Vitiated *doshas* that had been embedded in the deep tissues (*shakha*) should now be mobile in order to facilitate their facile movement into the central parts of the body, particularly the entire gastrointestinal tract. In this state of readiness (*utkleshana*), the vitiated *doshas* become accessible and are prepared for subsequent elimination.

Vamana: Therapeutic Emesis

Vamana (therapeutic emesis or vomiting) is the first of the five principal purificatory procedures. It is administered generally on the second day after *swedhana*. Since it is targeted to eliminate vitiated *Kapha,* it is particularly useful in those with *Kapha*-dominant constitutions and in those with *Kapha*-dominant imbalances. The sites of vitiated *Kapha* accumulation are the stomach and the lungs. Such imbalances include but are not restricted to the following: asthma, upper respiratory infections, states of excess phlegm and mucus, that is, allergies, early stages of diabetes, obesity, migraine, sluggish metabolism, lack of taste sensitivity, and poor appetite. The optimal season for this procedure is spring when *Kapha* is normally provoked by the moist climate. *Vamana* is generally contraindicated in the following situations: *Vata*-dominant constitutions; *Vata* imbalances; those under 12 and over 65 years; patients who are emaciated, anorexic, or convalescent; those with upper gastrointestinal or respiratory bleeding, heart disease, ascites, dry cough, constipation, and acute fever.

Vamana is a one-day procedure. It is performed under qualified Ayurvedic supervision, as are all *Panchakarma* treatments. Foods that strongly elicit *Kapha,* such as rice, milk, and yogurt, along with extra salt and sweets are given on the previous day. This diet is called *adhishyandi* (moisture producing) and temporarily increases *Kapha* in the gastrointestinal tract. On the morning of the procedure, the patient is not to eat breakfast, although some hot beverage may be taken. Under supervision, he or she is given about 500 cc or 4 to 8 cups of liquid. This may consist of warm milk with sugar, or a tea of licorice, honey, and salt, or buttermilk, and is to be consumed in 15 to 30 minutes. At this point, an emetic herbal preparation that contains calamus, lobelia, or Madana phala (emetic nut) is administered. These are the most commonly used herbs, although others may be used depending on the specific situation. In about 45 minutes, vomiting naturally begins; if it does not, some judicious stimulation of the back of the throat with the fingers to activate the gag reflex may trigger vomiting. Vomiting is then guided under close supervision until completion usually within two hours.

The vomitus is expelled serially beginning with food substances, then *Kapha*-containing mucus, then yellow-green *Pitta* secretions, and finally *Vata* gases. Observations and measurement of the expelled contents are made. A quantitative range of the patient's *vamana* is determined. This includes (1) a minimum number (consisting of at least four) of emetic episodes amounting up to about 325 cc, (2) a moderate number (at least six) of emetic episodes amounting up to 650 cc, and (3) a maximum number (at least eight) resulting in a quantity of vomitus up to 1,300 cc.

Adequate or successful *vamana* is reflected by subjective and objective parameters. The patient reports feeling light, uncongested, and relieved; vomiting terminates easily; pre-*Vamana* symptoms are decreased; and the digestive power, experienced as normal appetite, is restored. Inadequate emesis occurs when there is an absence or a very slow onset of vomiting, when only the emetic fluids and herbs are expelled, when symptoms like a subjective sense of heaviness in the chest and abdomen and lethargy occurs, and when signs such as skin rashes appear. The physician supervising the case manages disturbed emetic treatment in a variety of ways.

A definite postemesis regimen is then begun. The basis of this is a very light, graduated food intake (*samsarjana krama*), which occurs over a three-day period. On day 1, other than intermittent warm and hot liquids such as herbal teas, food intake begins in the evening with *peya,* which is the hot liquid that some basmati rice has been cooked in without the addition of condiments. On day 2, the morning and afternoon meal consists of *vilepi,* which is a moderate amount of steamed, plain basmati rice. On the evening of day 2, *akrita yusha,* which is a basmati rice and yellow split mung dal soup without spices, is consumed. On day 3, the morning and afternoon meals consist of *krita yusha,* which is rice and mung dal soup to which mild spices have been added. On the evening of day 3, a regular diet, proper to the individual's constitutional type, is resumed. Along with the *samsarjana krama* diet, classical Ayurvedic texts recommend several days of rest and the avoidance of any excessive activity as well as exposure to cold both in food and environmentally. In addition, the smoking of medicated, herbal mixtures, devoid of regular tobacco, has been suggested. The *samsarjana krama* concept, in fact, may be the historical precedent for modern postoperative feeding protocols.

Virechana: Therapeutic Purgation

Virechana (therapeutic purgation) is the second of the five principal purificatory procedures. *Virechana* is performed about two to three days after *vamana.* Since it is targeted to eliminate primarily vitiated *Pitta* as well as some *Kapha,* it is particularly useful in those with *Pitta*-dominant constitutions and in those with *Pitta*-dominant imbalances. Vitiated *Pitta* comes out of the liver, the gallbladder, the spleen, and the small intestine and settles in the small intestine. Some *Pitta* imbalances include skin inflammation, allergic rash, acne, chronic fever, acute diarrhea, the range of hepatic disorders, general inflammatory diseases, and some hematological problems. The aforementioned may and usually do contain some *Kapha* component and *virechana* addresses this aspect as well. As with all *Panchakarma* procedures, *virechana* is used to treat average problems. In the United States, *Panchakarma* is not recommended or used to treat any life-threatening disease, cancer, immune deficiency problem, or terminal illness. The optimal season for *virechana* is summer when *Pitta dosha* is naturally provoked by the hot weather. *Virechana* is generally contraindicated in the following situation: *Vata*-dominant constitutions and *Vata* imbalances; those under 12 and over about 75 years; patients who are emaciated, weak, or who have significant lower gastrointestinal and rectal problems such as bleeding, fissures, chronic diarrhea, and prolapse; menstruating, pregnant, and postpartum women; significant cardiovascular disease; alcoholism; very low *Agni* (digestive capacity); and acute fever.

Virechana is a one-day procedure under Ayurvedic monitoring but able to be done at home outside of a clinic. It is usually performed about three days post-*vamana; virechana,* however, may be given as an individual or singular treatment as the case requires. After adequate preparatory oleation and sudation, one may begin *virechana.* Purgation-inducing substances are usually administered on an empty stomach the evening before. The selection of an appropriate purgative is varied depending on the individual's specific constitution and condition. Castor oil and senna compounds are commonly used since they are suitable for most situations. For those with *Vata* tendencies, warm milk with ginger or psyllium may be used; for *Pitta* situations, rhubarb, aloe, or psyllium are good choices; for those of *Kapha* constitution, rhubarb, aloe, or Epsom salts work well. Other Ayurvedic herbs and compounds include haritaki, triphala, trivrit, and katuki. Purgation usually begins the next morning and may last until noon. Several bowel movements yielding fecal matter, mucus, and some yellow-colored *Pitta* material are produced. The general character of these is observed and recorded for the physician to assess.

Adequate *virechana* is accompanied by a feeling of lightness in the body and a normal increase in appetite. Inadequate purgation is reflected in the absence or very little bowel movement, a continued sense of heaviness and discomfort in the abdomen, loss of appetite, and vomiting. In this event, the physician applies appropriate remediation to correct this condition. The post-*virechana* protocol is similar to that for post-*vamana*. It consists of *samsarjana krama* (graduated, light diet) for three days and rest; medicated herbal inhalation is not suggested.

Basti: Therapeutic Enema

Basti (therapeutic enema) is the third of the five principal purificatory procedures. It was hailed by Charaka as being the greatest and most efficacious of all treatments. It is useful for all *Vata* imbalances in all constitutional types. *Vata* imbalance manifests in three main areas: (1) neurological disorders, (2) skeletal disorders, and (3) mental disorders. In addition, *basti* is used for chronic constipation, chronic fever, and kidney and sexual disorders. The optimal season for *basti* is the fall wherein *Vata* is heavily provoked. Like *virechana, basti* may be done alone and not as part of a *Panchakarma* series. If it is done in series, about three days should elapse between the different procedures. *Basti,* considered the safest and simplest of the *Panchakarma* procedures, however, is generally contraindicated in the following: children under 12 years and the elderly over about 75 years; severe emaciation; diarrhea; diabetes; acute fever; anemia; asthma; vomiting; chronic poor digestion, especially accompanied by excess *Kapha* and *Ama* in the gastrointestinal tract; and liver disorders with ascites.

Basti occurs within a 24-hour period. It may be done at home or in a clinic under supervision. Preparation includes only external oleation, sudation, and no intake of food six hours before the procedure. There are many types and subtypes of *basti*. The two most common are (1) *niruha-asthapana* (herbal cleansing decoction) and (2) *anuvasana* (oil retention). The composition of the *niruha-asthapana basti* may vary considerably. A common formulation consists of about 200 cc of sesame oil, 250 cc of an herbal decoction that may include the dashmoola compound (ten Ayurvedic herbs), calamus, fennel, ginger, and some salt. This amounts to about 16 ounces or two cups of liquid. It is administered, per rectum, either early in the morning or in late afternoon and retained for at least 15 minutes and up to 50 minutes. It is then evacuated and the procedure is terminated. The *anuvasana basti,* unlike the *niruha-asthapana basti,* is less cleansing but more tonifying and nourishing. Its composition is made up primarily of sesame oil (2 to 4 ounces) with some warm water, salt, and, perhaps, a small amount of a mild decoction of toning herbs. The *anuvasana basti* is administered at bedtime, retained overnight, and then evacuated in the morning.

A relatively complete bowel evacuation, a sense of relief and well-being, and a normalized appetite follow adequate *basti*. Inadequate *basti* is an uncommon occurrence. A post-*basti* regimen is lenient and includes recommendations for rest and a light diet.

Nasya: Intranasal Therapy

Nasya (intranasal therapy) is one of the last of the five principal purificatory procedures. It is indicated in the treatment of any or all of the *doshas* that are situated in the head and neck region. In this way, it is less targeted and broader in range covering treatment of the five senses, including the throat, the nasal passages, and aspects of the brain or central nervous system. The importance of *nasya* therapy is reflected in the ancient saying: "*Nasa hi shiraso dwarum*" meaning the nose is the doorway to the contents of the head. This connotes the possibility of affecting the subtle or energetic dimensions of the individual including breathing, *Prana* (vital energy), mental functioning, and consciousness.

There are several types of *nasya*. Some of these include the following:

1. *Pradhamana-virechana nasya,* cleansing *nasya.* This is performed using dry herbal powders, such as Brahmi, ginger, sage, or calamus, which are inhaled. This cleansing treatment specifically reduces excess *Kapha* in the head area.

2. *Bruhana nasya,* nutritional *nasya.* This is performed using oils such as ghee or sesame with the addition of nourishing herbs such as ashwaghanda, shatavari, or tulsi. *Vata* imbalances in the head area, such as migraines, anxiety, and agitation, for example, are responsive to this treatment.

3. *Shamana nasya,* palliative *nasya.* Medicated oils and herbal decoctions are applied intranasally to reduce aggravated *Pitta* disorders as, for example, conjunctivitis, tinnitus, and even hair loss.

4. *Navana nasya,* oil and herbal decoction *nasya.* This is useful in mixed *Vata-Pitta* and in mixed *Kapha-Pitta* disorders.

5. *Marshya nasya,* strong purificatory *nasya.* This refers to a large quantity (8 to 32 drops) of medicinal substance applied intranasally.

6. *Pratimarshya,* mild palliative *nasya.* This refers to a very small (2 drops per nostril) amount of medicinal substance used intranasally. This form of *nasya* is recommended for everyone as an aid to daily health maintenance. It usually consists of a small amount of plain ghee or of plain or herbalized sesame oil put on the pinky finger and gently inserted in each nostril using a mild lubricating and massaging motion.

7. *Dhooma nasya,* inhalation or smoking of dry herbs. This *nasya* is used after *vamana* since it, like *vamana,* dispels *Kapha.* It is also part of the post-*Panchakarma* protocol. Herbs such as cloves, calamus, and bayberry are used. Tobacco is never used.

   Nasya can be used alone or as part of a classical *Panchakarma* routine in which case it would follow any of the other procedures with an interval of one to two days. Before and after *nasya,* mild oleation and sudation to the face, throat, and neck are recommended. At the completion of the procedure, a small amount of ghee is applied intranasally.

RaktaMoksha: Therapeutic Blood Purification

RaktaMoksha (therapeutic blood purification) is the last principal procedure of classical *Panchakarma*. As was mentioned earlier, it was devised in ancient times by the Ayurvedic surgeon Sushruta (c. 660 B.C.), who regarded it as highly efficacious. He laid such great emphasis on *rakta dhatu* (blood tissue) that he considered it to be the fourth *dosha*. The quality of blood, its purity and its impure states, is a leading concern in Ayurveda. Since *Pitta dosha* is the product of the breakdown of blood (*rakta mala*), blood and the condition of *Pitta* are closely intertwined. In addition, the body's digestive fire (*Agni*) uses *Pitta dosha* as its vehicle and modus operandi.

RaktaMoksha is a therapeutic intervention considered in some cases of *Pitta* and blood vitiation. Such conditions include the following: skin infections, skin inflammations, urticaria, rashes, acne, eczema, hives, gout, and some hematological, hepatic, and splenic disorders. Some major contraindications include anemia, severe emaciation, edema, menstruation, pregnancy, asthma, impotency, and in the very young (under 12 years) and the elderly (over 75 years).

Classical Ayurveda has distinguished several types of *RaktaMoksha*. Some of the most important are the following:

1. *Prachhana:* blood letting using quick, sharp incisions.
2. *Siravyadha:* removal of blood by syringe.
3. *Jalauka:* the use of topically applied leeches. This classical method is considered the mildest and one of the most effective. It, like the other bloodletting techniques, is still used in India under medical supervision.

Therapeutic bloodletting is not performed in the United States; other less invasive means have been devised to address what are considered impure or toxic blood conditions. These methods use herbal substances that specifically target impurities in the blood. Herbs that are primarily bitter and those with some characteristics, such as burdock root, katuki, turmeric, goldenseal, pomegranate, and neem have been used. These herbal interventions are coupled with restrictions of *Pitta*-aggravating dietary substances such as yogurt, salt, sour and fermented items (citrus and soy sauce), vinegar, and alcohol.

UTTARAKARMA: POST-PANCHAKARMA REGIMEN

When a course of *Panchakarma* is completed, *Uttarakarma,* also called *Paschatakarma* (follow-up actions), is prescribed. These include both dietary and lifestyle recommendations that facilitate the gradual reentry of the newly treated person back into a regular, daily routine. The intensity of the entire purificatory experience alters the intrinsic state of the tissues and the metabolism. Large amounts of *Ama* and vitiated *doshas* have thus been eliminated with an opening of the channels and cleansing of the tissues resulting from this physiological debridement. The tissues, therefore, are purified and in a state of enhanced receptivity. A mild and graduated diet, along with selected toning herbs, helps restore their nutrition and strength. In addition, clinical experience has demonstrated that the overall condition of the *Agni* is greatly reduced following the purificatory procedures. This temporarily lowered state must be clearly recognized and addressed with the *samsarjana krama* (graduated diet) suggestions. The classical dietary regimen is as follows:

1. *Manda:* rice water. This is the plain broth in which basmati rice has been cooked. A small amount of ghee and saindhava (Indian rock salt) or Indian black salt and ghee is added.
2. *Peya:* thin rice soup. This is a very thin mixture of basmati rice cooked in about eight parts of water with some salt and ghee.
3. *Vilepi:* thick rice soup. This is basmati rice cooked with about four parts of water to which a very small amount of salt, ghee, and mild herbs such as ginger, fennel, turmeric, cumin, and coriander has been added.
4. *Odana:* plain cooked rice.
5. *Yusha:* light soup. This is a mixture of basmati rice and a small amount of split yellow mung dal (lentils) cooked together in a manner similar to *vilepi.*
6. *Kichari:* This is a more substantial mixture of basmati rice and split yellow mung dal cooked with spices and vegetables.

Although the time frames may vary according to the constitution and condition of the individual patient, the above *samsarjana krama* is observed over the course of about three days. On day 1, only *manda* and *peya* are consumed; on day 2, *vilepi* and *odana;* and on day 3, *yusha* as the first meal and *kichari* as the evening meal. After this, a regular diet according to one's *prakruti* (constitutional body type) is resumed. Overeating is to be avoided at all times.

Daily routines should resume in a graduated fashion over the course of about one week. Inordinate physical activity and exposure to cold, both dietary and environmentally, should be avoided.

11

THE CULTIVATION OF CONSCIOUSNESS

Ekam sat vipra bahudha vadanti
Truth is one, many are its names

Rig-Veda CLXIV (46)
(c. 1500 B.C.)

THE *TANTRA* OF AYURVEDA: VISION, MISSION, AND METHODS

Ayurveda has strong Tantric features. *Tantra*, a Sanskrit term, is broadly defined as a system characterized by threads of multiply diverse techniques, methods, and practices used in special ways in order to achieve mental, physical, and spiritual change. It puts robust emphasis on psychological techniques to induce *BioPsychoSpiritual* development. *Tantra* is an effort to unite all opposites within experience; this is its ultimate vision and mission.

Tantra encompasses a dazzling fabric of complexly interwoven mechanisms that incorporate significant use of the power (*Kundalini*) of the life force (*Prana*) to promote integration and to achieve degrees of self-actualization. Charaka defines *tantra* as a garland or wreath of interconnected topics that adorn and display the Ayurvedic corpus. This "path that liberates from crudeness" implies a unified strategic base both ideologically and practically. An action modality such as this rather than a contemplative mode characterizes Ayurvedic practice. The precepts of Ayurveda are integrations both of principles of understanding and of rules of conduct. Putting health regimens into action is essential. Ayurvedic wisdom denotes the incorporation of its views and principles into the fabric of everyday living. Not only are the choices of specific activities of daily living more consciously selected, but their very enactment becomes an engagement that is more consciously savored.

All dimensions of consciousness—conscious awareness, preconscious subliminality, and unconscious (patala) mental life—participate in the process of integration when the goal of refining and cultivating consciousness becomes a conscious choice. The cultivation of consciousness, therefore, is achieved by practices that regulate and enhance both bodily health and mental functioning. This, in essence, is the aim of Ayurveda.

Ordinary or conventional experience is viewed as naturally tending to be faulty and as continually subjecting an individual to imbalanced states. This everyday state of mind is characterized by partiality, perceiving and conceiving only limited portions of the entire range that an experience provides. For example, focusing on a blade of grass, one forgets that it is only a single element within the larger perspective—lawn, forest, territory, country, planet, and so forth.

This partiality in understanding results, in large measure, from the fact that everyday consciousness, whether awake or asleep, is dynamically conditioned by the ever-changing qualities (*gunas*) and cognitive focal points that are experienced. Two factors contribute to this: (1) the binary information processing structure of the mind and (2) the ever-changing stimuli from the external environment. This constant state of psychodynamic flux reflects the impermanence of mind (*Manas*) on all its levels. Since this is seen as a regular and expectable occurrence, it is actively embraced with positive therapeutic enthusiasm. Rather than addressing man's imperfect states with an attitude of opposition, Ayurveda, in this way, becomes deeply involved with and initially accepting of these inconsistent and disordered conditions. Often, they instigate pain. Ayurveda takes note of the manner in which the mind relates to this pain, that is, in the experience of suffering.

Suffering, in this sense, may be considered to be a normative, natural phenomenon within the dynamic interplay of health maintenance. Great Nature provides both the gift of illness and the gift of wellness. Suffering understood in this way may act as a spur eliciting self-development and an advance in compassion and empathy, which connotes an extended social benefit. Seen in this light, suffering provides an opportunity rather than a misfortunate closure; man's will and his capacity for choice can thus be exercised. In addition, a consideration of the problem of evil, both natural and man-made, from this angle of perception, opportunity, and individual choice (free will), perhaps, may broaden insight into this vexing and often troubling phenomenon. Evil, in this sense, can be defined as the malignant destructiveness that adds to experiential suffering. Ultimately, the one who advertently and intentionally seeks to damage comes to suffer more than those upon whom evil is directed.

The original Vedic prescription for a balanced life stressed adherence to self-discipline through prescribed actions within mainstream society. Enacting dharmic responsibilities and obligations maintained the *bandhu* (harmonizing balance) between man and extended nature, the animate and inanimate environments. Man's purpose in life was and is considered to include active participation with Great Nature, *Prakriti,* in the ongoing dynamic processes of reparation and creation: healing, restoring balance, and bringing freshness to the self and to the world at large. Life, in this sense, was and is considered to be a moral task.

History, personal and social, to be sure, is the arena within which *Prakriti* grows, matures, and develops. God, in this sense, is immanent within, not split apart from, history and the world. God is not in a state of contraction removed from the world; on the contrary, man, in effect, is a contraction of God. Each man and woman is a centrated sphere of such an ineffable and vast majesty. If the meaning of *dharma* is understood to encompass aspects of one's inherent destiny, then it is conceivable to entertain the prospect that to discover human nature would be to discover human destiny. The purpose of man's life then would reside in the spirit of his nature, which is a reflection of the wisdom and meaning inherent in greater Nature. Uncovering this and aligning the two, microcosm and macrocosm, would contribute to the fulfillment of human destiny. In some sense, this may appear to be tautological; nonetheless, it is an idea worthy of further consideration. An essential aim of Ayurveda, then and now, continues to reside in the goal of transforming less refined into more refined states of experiential being by means of active adaptations to ongoing changes as, for example, those produced by chronological age, diurnal cycles, and seasonal shifts. Purity, in the Ayurvedic sense, is the ongoing effort to purify the *dhatus* (tissues) of accumulated impurities in order to make living both more comfortable and more optimal. The means and choices used to achieve these goals has been addressed in this book's discussion of dietary, lifestyle, and purification techniques. This chapter addresses how Ayurveda conceives of and works with the mind and consciousness.

Consistent with the *Rig-Veda*'s predominantly world-embracing view, Ayurveda's recognition, acceptance, and willing penetration into the material world continue to reflect those axiomatic values. Any efforts, advertent or inadvertent, to elude reality and to slip into fantasy are recognized as escapist. Such events cause pause and psychological reorientation. A strong sense of the sacredness of the body and of the physical world, including social agencies, gives Ayurveda a world-affirming quality and world-espousing tone by its ongoing efforts to transform naturally occurring imbalances into more *sattvic* (pure, harmonious) and balanced states. Ayurveda's health-oriented, antiritualistic, and antirigid stance renounces renunciation. The deep oneness underlying all apparently diverse manifestations within experience is emphasized, and the microcosmic and macrocosmic interplay within Nature is reverently acknowledged. Such a reconnection between individual consciousness and the consciousness within the extended environment is the experiential basis of *Moksha,* the attainment of freedom. It has been referred to as an awakening of the "Buddha mind." In Buddhism, it is termed *Vimukti.*

Ayurvedic care, in general, requires consultation, evaluation, guidance, and coaching from a highly qualified Ayurvedic practitioner or physician so that an appropriate dietary-, lifestyle-, and consciousness-enhancing program may be constructed. Active self-care is thus supported and augmented. All of this begins in one's native habitat. A thorough examination of the geography of the inner world of the mind and spiritual resources and the outer world of material realities and connectedness launches this journey.

SOTERIOLOGY: A CONTEMPORARY REAPPRAISAL AND CONTRIBUTION

Soteriology, the examination of paths and means to salvation, reconciliation, redemption, and enlightenment, has always been an important concern within the domain of visions of man, both Eastern and Western, that include the spiritual dimension (Anandamurti, 1993, 1994; Eliade, 1978, 1982; Forte, 1990; Gurdjieff, 1963; Lamm, 1986; Mead 1895, 1913; Osho, 1994, 1995, 1996; Steiner, 1964, 1968; Urbach, 1979; Yogananda, 1946; Zaehner, 1961). I align Soteriology with the cultivation, refinement, integration, and expansion of consciousness.

If we regard Ayurveda as being embedded within a worldview whose conception admits of the existence and reality of multiple experiential dimensions, particularly those of consciousness and spirit, then a consideration of the soteriological implications within it is important to explore. A theoretical framework outlining some major principles and practice guidelines will be given. All substantial work toward spiritual development and the refinement of consciousness, however, requires earnestness and dedication. The assistance of a qualified teacher or guide in the context of an appropriate setting over time is needed. This is not because the subject matter to be experienced is difficult, but because the individual subject, himself or herself, is overwhelmingly complex.

Individual choice, effort, and self-work are primary values. Choice must be conscious and be an experience that is unendingly recurring. In some systems of self-development, such a path has been referred to as one that is hidden, occult, and esoteric. To the extent that the experience of an individual who seeks substantial self-change is always deeply personal, subjective, idiosyncratic, and motivated by innumerable unconscious factors, it is a hidden or unrevealed phenomenon. This again highlights the profoundly personal, essentially mysterious, and multidetermined nature of the urge within the human heart toward psychological and spiritual development.

In the broadest sense, Ayurveda's *tantra* encompasses a range of activities that are imbued with powerful reparative aims and ends. The ancient Vedic seers (*rishis*) were keenly aware of man's spiritual origins, recurrent ills, pain, suffering, feelings of being incomplete, the problem of evil, the dark side of man's nature, the desire for freedom, and the need for an organized system of reparation both ideologically and technically. The *Vedas* provided dharmic mandates for the regular ordering of life through prescribed observances. Spirituality was thus integrated into daily life and expressed itself as a practical religion of social immersion in the world of everyday living. Goals, values, and purpose in life were applicable to all in general (*samanya*). Life's meaning was embodied in the acceptance and implementation of the four Vedic aspirations: *dharma* (duty), *artha* (material possessions), *kama* (pleasure in living), and *Moksha* (ultimate liberation or salvation). The Vedics, however, recognized that all individuals are born and develop in unique and differing ways; therefore, as individual *karmas* (actions and their consequences) vary, so do individual destinies. Individual choices as well as a number of extraindividual influences were believed to combine in unique ways to create one's particular path in life.

While all of the Vedic goals were considered opportunities for everyone, it was recognized that *Moksha,* a choice potentially available to all, may not be, and usually is not, universally chosen as an active pursuit. It required and still requires an essential and volitional impetus. This impulse may emerge, perhaps, out of an innate longing to know the truth of one's own being, a state of mind with cosmic connotations and existential ramifications. The nature of *Moksha* clearly is complex, both conceptually as well as experientially. It is certainly not a negligible sentiment for those who experience its stirrings. It has been loosely regarded as being a state of freedom, particularly from blind bondage to *Prakriti* (the manifest and material world), to the cycles of *samsara* (repetitive rebirth into the phenomenal world of impermanence), and to the driving forces of forgetfulness, object-seeking desire, unconscious envy, and ignorance that perpetuate these attachments. However true this understanding may be, it risks being incomplete without further examination.

One essential key to this initiation process into *Moksha* is a clearer recognition of the role and meaning of one's individuality within group culture. An individual is born as a "singularity" but existing and, in fact, embedded within a group context throughout life. The natural order of things, particularly survival, necessitates membership and participation in group existence. Infants ordinarily undergo socialization by learning and by adopting the habits, beliefs, values, and so forth of the social matrix into which they are born, raised, and enculturated. This deep embeddedness involves the assimilation of an infinite variety of elements in the experiential and interactional world. This makes for an individual's inevitable participation in "herd" or "pack" consciousness and stereotyped typical behaviors. Such virtually enslaved participation fosters habit and blindly enacted mental and behavioral rhythms.

This natural state of being born into a given social system, however, confers a multitude of apparent benefits. These include security, identity, group reliance, protection, support, a passive sense of comfort, acceptance by others, and membership within a perceived, accepted "normality." These benefits necessitate a significant degree of submissiveness, especially to the power and authority of the group. The constraints it imparts has been referred to as being "in the box." This perceived sense of protection, in fact, is partly illusory since within group culture there is an overriding expression of diffusion of responsibility; no one in the group usually thinks, behaves, or acts in a truly independent manner, especially in the face of existing rules, mores, and guidelines for established conduct. The degree to which this is rigidly adhered to, of course, varies from person to person. When an individual expresses individualized needs, often the group's responsiveness is excruciatingly and agonizingly slow. Following the pack in a monotonous and routine manner, adherence to habit, and resistance to adaptive change constitute the usual, conventional course for most group members. Blind adherence often becomes an unconscious habit, and it reinforces an ongoing, perpetual state of induced passivity. With this, intellectual acuity, especially an introspective sensitivity, is dulled.

The path of *Moksha,* of freedom, at first, demands a psychological individuation out of group mores, and an overcoming of the hypnotic pull of blind participation in mass existence. This phenomenon parallels the individual mind's own bondage to its endless and innumerable chatter, the inherent *vritti* of *Manas.* To accomplish this without feeling alienated, disloyal, or like a traitor is exceedingly difficult. It is virtually impossible to accomplish and to sustain because of the almost irresistible power (of virtual enslavement) demanded by the group to maintain conformity. In order to conform, the mind tends to intellectualize the nature of the self and then to assume a role of false sophistication, no matter what one's socioeconomic or educational level is. Conformity by members is also strengthened by the individual wish to avoid the fear of isolation, rejection, abandonment, and the loneliness that might result from challenging or leaving the group. Psychological individuation, however, is essential for self-development. This path, although arduous, is possible. It entails a renegotiation, a reintegration that aligns one's individuality with a new sense of interacting and sharing. It becomes the experience of intentional and balanced group communion. It then may be lived through as active and conscious participation, not as passive, slavish adherence.

The ancient Vedic corpus unfalteringly maintained the truth, reality, relevance, and necessity of man's immersion in society and in the material world. Ayurveda still holds this to be true. Using an epistemological perspective that is also consonant with Buddhist thought, a broad description of the processes of thinking will be given as a backdrop for an interpretive contribution to the meaning of the highest of these ancient values, that of attaining *Moksha.*

CONVENTIONAL, EVERYDAY LIVING: ACCOMMODATING TO THE DEFORMITY OF AN UNCONSIDERED LIFE

Why some choose to become aware of the possibility of *Moksha* and to strive for it remains a mystery. Ordinary man, with his given, mundane, everyday awareness, is described by Eastern and some Western traditions as being passive and machinelike. Ordinary men and women live on the circumference of life, particularly removed from the inner heart of their own lives. Attention remains only on the periphery, the outer boundary both of the self and of the things experienced in the world.

The individual's existence in a culture (family, social, geographical, and so forth) that is so heavily imbued with group living experiences for survival, a necessity to some extent, reinforces a dulling habituation to all experience both introspective and stimulated by the environment. Behavioral tolerance is the learned ability to compensate for the effects of a life in which creative meaning has not been self-generated. This promotes the mechanical repetition of habit-based cycles of perceived need and the desire to satisfy these needs.

The experience of "self" in this context comes to be felt as a fragmented, ephemeral aggregate of reflexive thoughts. For the most part, these thoughts are randomly evoked. They arise in automatic fashion by constantly changing conditions both internal and environmental. A profound and deeply experienced sense of passivity is synonymous with this given, conventional ordinary state of being. Stress and stress responses are inevitably linked with feelings of pain, that is, mental suffering resulting from experiencing continuous change and the need to adapt to it. Feeling incomplete, inadequate, and frightened produce low-grade dysphoria, dissatisfaction, and exacerbations of anxiety and depression. Such an unhappy state of mind typically has a base in primary, unconscious envy. It is the underlying feeling that senses life as an emergency.

This naturally occurring, default mental (*vyavaharika*) set is innately structured to perceive experience in the form of seeing "gaps" or missing parts. This takes shape interpersonally in the form of feeling both that something wonderful and needed is outside oneself and that another person unfairly possesses it. The mind then abruptly responds to this by trying to stop this unsettling feeling of envy through acts of vitiation. Vitiation spoils the perceived and unattainable ideal object by precariously trying to mitigate the cycle of desire. Feelings of greed, jealousy, and destructiveness, however, inevitably ensue and constantly recur.

TWO STATES OF CONSCIOUS AWARENESS: PARTIAL MIND AND COMPLETE MIND

Within the experiences of everyday life, man, interacting with and a participant in the social order, makes sense of the world initially using the ideational process termed *samvritti-satya* or conventional, relative, everyday thinking (*vyavaharika, sarva arthata*). It typically constitutes a partial apprehension of the superstratum of the world; the more complete field is inadvertently ignored. The quality of this mentation is complex in its detailed nuances. In a general sense, however, it includes sensation, perception, concept formation, logic, memory, and reasoning. Mental functioning in this sense is denoted by the broad term *Manas* in Sanskrit; within *Manas* is the capacity for *chetas,* the Sanskrit term that denotes logical thinking. This given mode of apparently rational thinking is that aspect of "mind" associated with the Eastern concept of *Maya,* the erroneous or incomplete recognition and interpretation of the meaning of reality. Nonetheless, it may be considered to be a relatively valid and necessary human faculty vital to successful adaptation. It is incomplete because it naturally tends to cover over or to falsely mask (*adhyaropa, adhyasa, vikshepa,* and *avarana*) that which is perceived by it. This state of conscious awareness is called "partial mind."

Amid the intricate layering that *Manas* erects within cognition is the spectrum of the feeling of certainty. Ordinary thinking and experience is accompanied by a need for clarity. This contributes to the mind's use of defense mechanisms. In addition, the process of thinking and its products are regarded in an overvalued way, often, at times, to regulate the unsettling experience of uncertainty, ambiguity, and doubt. Doubt (*shamshaya*), when excessive, stimulates anxiety and fear. The wide ranges of experience that contribute to an individual's psychological equilibrium, therefore, are manifold. They draw from the inextricable mix of thinking and feeling and how these contribute to stress responses and to the management of anxiety that result from perceiving the world in a limited way.

This reflects the intrinsic default tendency (*Prajna-aparadha*) within information processing. It is the mind's tendency for cognitive dualism (*dvandvas*). This denotes a twofold process: (1) the inability to grasp the entire truth of an experience and (2) the ability to believe (to misinterpret) that the partial and illusory interpretation of what is (merely partially) seen is true; that is, that it is the entire, complete, and only truth.

Maya is the compelling experiential sense of incompleteness. This encompasses not only the perception of the world but also the subjective experience of the inner world.

Perhaps the most profound understanding of *Maya* recognizes that the world, both inner and outer, is the real manifestation, in fact, of *Prakriti* (Great Nature), the creative base of reality that dynamically unfolds in the form of human life as well as in the objective reality of the extended universe. Material realities, therefore, although incomplete in themselves, are not, in fact, nonexistent, false, or artificial. The Western concept of "idolatry" (false objects of worship) reflects the Eastern idea of *Maya* and *Prajna-aparadha*. *Maya,* then, in this perspective, may be seen not as a deceiver but as the *Great Teacher,* a stern yet gracious entity offering repeated, diverse, and fresh opportunities and challenges in the course of one's life trajectory.

Samvritti-satya (conventional thinking), however, is the epistemological process that puts a ceiling on cognition and limits its range and the scope of its comprehension thereby truncating knowledge, reason, interpretation, and belief. It is *consciousness conditioned by dynamically changing and impermanent experiences.* This conditioning narrows the focus of understanding; in fact, it imparts only a provisional status to knowledge derived in this way. It is the epistemological superimposition of relativity (apprehension of dualisms or *dvandvas*) on the continuum of ontological unity. This is the meaning of the Vedic concept *Prajna-aparadha,* the mind's inherent cognitive fault that predisposes to errors in wisdom and to forgetting the essential unity underlying the fundamental integrity of the entire universe.

The chief modus operandi of conventional thinking and behavior is the automatic oscillation between the extremes of indulgence and those of denial.

This reflects the more mechanical, untrained, and ordinary states of human experience. Repressions are created and maintained and act as magnets that continue to attract and to reinforce unreflective, repetitive mental and behavioral patterns. Varying degrees of nonfully conscious awareness and of enslavement to habit, thereby, are perpetuated. Some contemporary examples of this include an unquestioning acceptance of and an automatic preoccupation with fads and trends such as the use of personal cell phones, beepers, electronic equipment, information technology, fashion, and so forth. Yet since *samvritti-satya* constitutes the commonsense cognition that contributes to the maintenance of basic survival, communal integration, and social order, it has natural value and is useful. It is the means well suited for achieving a preliminary understanding of and an initial adherence to the dictates of *dharma, artha,* and *kama.* In fact, since the natural world, particularly the social order, has "real" value, whatever position or walk of life one finds oneself occupying either psychologically, socially, or even geographically is the precise location where the journey toward *Moksha* naturally must begin.

The maturation and intentional development of partial mind, *samvritti-satya,* needs to be fostered to incorporate within it the deeper and broader level of awareness termed *paramartha-satya,* an awareness that includes an appreciation of the substratum of phenomena, the existence of the ultimate truth—consciousness—upon which *samvritti-satya* rests. This transformation brings about a more discriminating and comprehensive apprehension of reality; it is a cognition characterized by "complete mind." The broadening of partial mind and the experience of complete mind entail a process of dynamic change, the lifelong journey of cultivating and refining consciousness.

THE PSYCHOLOGICAL PREREQUISITES FOR CHANGE

The possibility of self-development, in fact an authentic self-creation beyond this mechanical and reflexive ordinary state of mind, is possible. It is achievable, especially since pain and suffering are conditions for creating opportunities for change on all levels. What must be reiterated, moreover, is that being born yields only an essential birthright, the fact of *opportunity;* in this case, the opportunity for the soteriological justification of suffering referred to here as enlightenment. Although degrees of this may be achieved by all, substantial advances are rare occurrences. They demand extraordinary and persistently conscious self-activity. In this sense, passivity is lame and ineffectual; personal change requires active self-work. The present endeavor of this book not only continues to advance and endorse this view, but also is an attempt to contemporize its recognition and to demonstrate its suitability for modern times.

Modern man has been said to experience inner states of existential loneliness. This profound sense of being incomplete may be universal and an inherent part of the nature of all men and all women of all times. The dysphoria, restlessness, and challenge that accompany feelings of incompleteness, if recognized, can act as opportunities to spur searching and self-exploration. In this context, the approaches presented in this book are truly pragmatic. They present timely, practical, and realistic problem-solving strategies for change. Profound movement, that is, life change, such as this, moreover, can come only from within. Self-care is key.

The proposed shift from being more passive to becoming more active requires radical change, intentionality, and sustained effort (*pranidhana*). Man's will to change must prevail. The transition to this new state often requires a mental shock to galvanize its organization. Daily, habitual routines must undergo profound disruptions. Things—emotional and material—in one's life must be shaken up. Outside events, as well as one's response to these, must be experienced as traumatic enough in intensity to instigate a penetrating and far-reaching life upheaval. Underneath this platform of disturbances, however, must lie the seeds of an innate talent that in order to become activated require conscious choice and deliberate effort.

This entails an initial recognition of one's utter helplessness in the face of enormous complexity and of the infinitely unknowable universe. A willing surrender (*prapatti*) to this is essential. Such an attitude may have its roots in the oceanic feeling of infantile oneness that accompanied the developmental fact of primal helplessness. To whatever extent this attitude of surrender is rooted in innate, human phylogenetic memories and in the most profound preverbal experiences of infancy as well as in earliest childhood is clearly acknowledged. These etiological conjectures, however, neither diminish the importance of this attitude nor make it less radically meaningful.

Faith, in this sense, is understood as nascent trust, confidence, and reliance on the intrinsic goodness of the self within nature, and a faithful adherence to the pursuit of self-development. Preeminent focus, nonetheless, must continue to rest on individual accountability and responsibility for personal advancement. Recognizing and pursuing *Moksha,* then, amounts to a voluntary covenant with sacred nature, a reality understood to be one in essence with self and with the extended universe. The dynamics of this voluntary choice constitute a self-election to the path of self-development. This evolves into a veritable self-creation that is actively renewed by conscious choosing at virtually every experiential moment. The distinguishing feature of free choice, then, is axiomatic to the pursuit of *Moksha* and to the path of enlightened consciousness.

Since the multidimensional roots of such a qualitative change are, in fact, beyond comprehension, one may only begin to launch the process of change by attempting to create conditions within which actual, substantive change, by means of its own inherent powers, will begin to consolidate. If change is viewed as being a dynamic process having an infinite spectrum of activity, then its first stages might aptly be described as "a getting ready for change." In this preparatory phase, the obstacles, barriers, and resistances that emerge might best be addressed through a loving engagement rather than a rejection. Acknowledging and gently courting apparent impasses, especially under the guidance of a qualified helper, can act, in a gradual manner, to dematerialize these inevitable stumbling blocks. Such therapeutic strategies, needless to say, are complex and require expert handling tailored to individual needs at each moment in the process. Ongoing, constant, daily engagement with this establishes maintenance and renewal.

Pursuing *Moksha,* therefore, must include intentional choice along with the emergence of other apparently nonspecific and seemingly random etiological factors. Implicit in this conception is a clear acknowledgment of the influence of the spiritual, the consciousness base of existence. The phrase *God's will,* in fact, may be related to, if not identical with, this consciousness-based, inherent intelligence within Nature. The incommensurability of this, of necessity, leads us to continue to lay exceedingly strong emphasis on whatever part *man's will,* his free will, plays in the mysterious processes underlying the pursuit of *Moksha.* The interplay and subtle concordance between these two fractal dimensions, however, must always be underscored.

TECHNIQUES WHOSE AIM IS TO REFINE THE EXPERIENCE OF CONSCIOUSNESS

In order to achieve degrees of *Moksha,* the present author submits *now,* as the sages had in the past, that *samvritti-satya* needs to be expanded to include the deeper and broader level of awareness termed *paramartha-satya,* an awareness of the existence of the ultimate truth upon which *samvritti-satya* rests. Recognizing that, within the created world, all human epistemological realizations have these superimpositions embedded within them is considered to be light on the path toward *Moksha.*

A wide range of dietary, lifestyle, and other practices, particularly meditation and quality psychotherapy (Chapter 12), are employed in the cultivation of consciousness. This chapter discusses both the Ayurvedic philosophy of mind and techniques for change as well as the meditative means aimed toward achieving an integration of consciousness.

Consciousness is cultivated by enhancing the subtle, energetic roots of the *doshas: Prana* (life force), *Tejas* (flame of intelligence), and *Ojas* (strength to endure). To do this, one must feed *Manas* (mind) with the subtle *Tanmatras: Shabda* (sound), *Sparsha* (touch), *Rupa* (vision), *Rasa* (taste), and *Gandha* (smell) in healthy ways. This promotes the refinement, integration, and expansion of consciousness. The aim of work on the self is not only to achieve health of the physical body, but, more notably, to achieve progressive degrees of personal transformation toward subtleness in body, mind, and spirit. Doing this creates conditions that substantially improve the quality of life.

Grasping ultimate truth encompasses a dynamic spectrum of varying degrees of deepening understanding. The attainment of right knowledge (*sama jnana*) was advocated early on in the vast body of Vedantic literature. The methodology described often included three basic processes. The first step, *shravana,* included serious study through a focused attention by means of reading, listening, and observing. The second step, *manana,* denoted a critical testing, analysis, and contemplation of the material observed through *shravana.* The third phase of this process, *nidi-dhyasana,* denoted the insights achieved by means of ongoing meditation in order for the studied and contemplated information to refine itself into a faculty capable of advanced discrimination (*viveka*) and clarity. The functioning of *Manas,* the mind, was gradually purified through these efforts.

All of this is arrived at in the first place by using the conventional thoughts and concepts within ordinary reasoning processes. With the cultivation of consciousness, conventional thinking begins to expand. Intuitive experience and insights emerge. The universe (*Prakriti*) is multifaceted and human cognition is unable to grasp any aspect of this "manifold" in its entirety at any one moment. The cultivation of consciousness, however, enables the mind to hold multiple views in a more integral fashion. Such states of expanded consciousness are fostered by developing the capacity to entertain this multiplicity of views. It includes looking at things from varied perspectives all at once. Multiple outlooks begin to be considered simultaneously. Acknowledging that reality is not one-sided (*anekanta*) necessitates recognizing that all language statements, in fact, really possess only provisional status (*naya*). This has been well known in Eastern traditions for millennia. It has been referred to by several names: *Syadvada* and *Anekantavada.*

Creation (*Prakriti*), to be sure, is an infinite series of innumerable possibilities. Human cognition, at any point in time, is able to grasp and to apprehend only a partial dimension of this intrinsically unified whole. "Cognitive momentariness" is the epistemological side of what is measured in real time. Time, change, and the human ego as *Ahamkara* coexist inseparably. They rest, however, within the ineffable eternity of changeless *Purusha. Moksha* is the path toward reconciliation, the restoration of experiential wholeness.

One of the groundwork techniques suggested here entails total immersion into the experience of conventional reality using astute perception and an exquisitely developed sensory receptivity. For example, a necessary and essential first step would be to curtail the activity of talking; speaking should occur only when truly necessary. This consequently would contribute to an enhancement of sensory perception, which would become increasingly receptive and thus play a greater role in cognition. This, in fact, also contributes to a normalization of any tendency toward experiential enchantment, that is, maintaining a fixed and typically idealized attitude that biases information processing in an unchanging direction.

Rather than bypassing and blurring the distinctions that are part of everyday thinking, one would begin to develop a keener awareness of an experiential universe filled with crisp and meaningful qualities and attributes, a virtually infinite array both of grosser and of more subtle nuances and meanings. Opening up all the sensory faculties and engaging awareness in a twofold manner with both environmental and internal perception creates a bridge of unity, a contact that is both nourishing and satisfying. To be sure, if done properly, one's boundaries in the ordinary or even a pathological sense of the word are not dissolved; the scope of inclusive experiential awareness is merely extended. Silence, and eventually "being," is restored and put back into experience. The silence used in the technique of meditative awareness not only is a means but also a large part of its end aim—personal synthesis.

The given, natural state of the undeveloped mind is likened in Eastern thought to an agglomeration of wild, unruly, and passion-driven impulses (*vikalpa*), a concept akin to the image of a mob of thugs. Hence, developing this more random condition into an experiential field with more detail and order must undergo an evolution that, of necessity, requires expansion over time. It does begin, however, with self-inquiry and within the very psychological and geographical space that one currently occupies. Ultimately, one's apprehension of oneself within the world is experienced in a more nonconceptual way. Discursive reasoning becomes supplanted over time by a burgeoning intuitive apprehension that is hallmarked by more immediacy and greater coherence.

It is worthwhile to state that no attempt is made here to contrast in detail Ayurvedic meditative techniques with Western psychotherapy, although their aims share similar features. The aims of meditation include personal integration and the refinement of consciousness. The aims of Western-based psychotherapies include the gradual development of useful insight, freedom from inordinate conflict, and more successful adaptation to daily living. While the aims of each share the goal of increasing one's quality of life, the techniques of each are different. However, both do share, to some degree, self-inquiry and self-change methodologies.

In Ayurveda and in Western psychotherapy, self-inquiry in some form is key. Self-inquiry (*aham tarka*) denotes a looking inward and self-examination. Working on the self, in this mode, may uncover the opportunity for a deeper analysis of self that could further delineate one's true nature, the fundamental *prakruti*. One's basic constitution and its vicissitudes over the course of a lifetime (*karma*), that is, temperament, habits, defense mechanisms, character, style, preferences, likes, dislikes, and so forth, would become increasingly more accessible. Leading questions that would emerge include the following: Am I willing to face hidden, unacceptable aspects of myself? What are these? Can I fully acknowledge and begin to accept these? To the extent that I am able to do this, what are strategies for change and improvement?

Such direct experiential states, moreover, may open one to the proposed idea of a transcendental unity immanent throughout reality. Meditative techniques such as described here can further enhance one's frame of mind. Meditation, therefore, acts to augment any currently held pursuit, worldview, or faith thus introducing more clarity, depth, and strength. In fact, one would be encouraged to remain, at least initially, in one's current life space and to attempt to maximize ongoing engagements in personal, social, and occupational activities of daily living in order to optimize these everyday interactions. Introspective, spiritual, and other contemplative pursuits, as well, would also become enriched.

The principal technical modality described here is that of meditation. This concept and its applied techniques, however, encompass a wide range of methodologies and strategies for implementation. Two broad categories include individual meditation and meditation in the company of another. I denote the latter as coming under the umbrella of *BioPsychoSpiritual* quality psychotherapy. It is discussed in depth in Chapter 12.

Individual meditation may use a variety of techniques, some formal, some informal. For example, in Buddhism, meditation on the breath is an often-used technique. In Hinduism and Yoga, for instance, individual meditation may consist of the use of the AUM as an idea, a sound, and as the subject matter of contemplative study. The importance of the meaning of AUM was explicated roughly 2,500 years ago in the *Mandukya Upanishad* as an addition to the *Atharva-Veda*. The teacher of the great sage Shankara (seventh century A.D.), named Gaudapada (eighth century A.D.), wrote a famous commentary on this *Upanishad* called *Karika Mandukya* in which he expounded the epistemological processes around ordinary thinking, meditation, and the refinement of the mind's capacity to appreciate the nuances of consciousness. Techniques used to refine consciousness have a long and revered history.

MEDITATIVE AWARENESS: THE PATH OF ALIGNMENT WITH *MOKSHA*

A more detailed elaboration of the aforementioned two cognitive-experiential processes (*samvritti-satya* and *paramartha-satya*) is beyond the scope of this book. Some relevant commentary, however, on the philosophy of meditative awareness follows. The spiritual path toward self-realization and the integrative refinement of consciousness highlights six basic psychological qualities. These prime mental states and processes are intentionally brought into awareness and worked on in terms of their relevance in everyday living. These are known as *Adhyatmika gunas*.

The *Adhyatmika gunas* are the following:

Buddhi: Spiritualized intellect; awakened consciousness;

Iccha: Desire;

Dvesha: Aversion;

Sukha: Happiness;

Duhkha: Suffering; and

Prayatna: Effort, motivation, persistence, and tenacity.

Paramartha-satya can be understood to be the discerning insight achieved initially by the various intellectual, emotional, and physical disciplines outlined in this book, which subsequently become restructured by the transcending influence of meditative awareness. The cognition marked by *paramartha-satya* becomes more complete and less partial in its faculties of apprehension. This is hallmarked by a state of contemplative receptivity, a silencing of "mind" in Eastern terms, which connotes a condition of experiential immediacy, a sense of being completely present in the here and now. This state has been described as one of being in the "eternal now," a feeling of timelessness, and, in fact, a state of virtual "mindlessness." The latter, it is believed, reflects more refined levels of consciousness and aspects of what in traditional Eastern thought is called "enlightenment," an experiential phenomenon that, in part, denotes the essence of *Moksha.*

Mentation, therefore, becomes augmented, purified, and refined by meditative awareness. The path of meditation establishes a deeper, more authentic contact with one's self, and this emerges as the experience of a more centrated focal point of autonomy and creativity. An innate intelligence (*buddhi*) is uncovered that brings profound wisdom (*prajna*) and compassionate empathy (*karuna*) to the fore. The clinging and acquisitive nature of desire and the spoiling nature of envy become attenuated. A deeper appreciation of and for the self and a more natural, ethical concern for others emerge. This profound experience of gratitude reflects the process of creative reparation throughout the breadth of one's being. Meditative awareness both develops and sustains states of mind (*Brahma-vihara*) characterized by kindness (*maitri*), compassion (*karuna*), joy for the good fortune of others (*mudita*), and mental equanimity (*upeksha*).

Moksha, then, becomes experienced as a gradually evolving state characterized by the satisfaction of a range of basic needs that includes the epistemophilic instinct for clearer understanding, the achievement of a sense of security and trust in the self and in extended nature, and an approaching feeling of serenity, peace of mind, and contentment. Repeated states of meditative awareness become a surrendering of one's mind in the limitless containment of meditation. Cognitive dissonance recedes. This comes to have a considerably normalizing effect on the natural instability, turbulence, fluctuations, unreliability, and propensity for intellectualization that characterize ordinary mental processes (*vritti*). One becomes more able to engage in the details and practical tasks of everyday living with a keener focus, absorption, enthusiasm, and sense of renewal. Cognitive functioning and its content undergo a transformation. Conventional knowledge becomes enriched by a deeper knowledge, one enlightened by an expanded, spiritualized consciousness. *Chitam and chitta* as limited and conditioned consciousness come closer to becoming *chit,* which is a more boundless and nondualistic state of consciousness. This, in turn, becomes further enhanced as it is imbued with degrees of the ultimate wisdom (*prajna*) that self-realization and self-actualization bring. *Prajna,* the wisdom that *Moksha* engenders, has been called "the ultimate medicine."

A deep purification is set in motion. This results in the defragmenting of disparate ideas and the organization of more stabilized thought patterns, which contribute to clearer thinking and mental equipoise. The Sanskrit term *anubhava* connotes the transition from an initial state of abstract, theoretical knowledge toward a more direct, authentic, almost intuitive, experiential awareness. It is a gradual yet inclusive penetration in meaning from surface to depth. In its entirety, it connotes the development of *prajna* (wisdom). The mind (*Manas*) influenced by such states becomes relaxed and finds it easier to transition to different levels of consciousness. Sentient awareness during waking hours and transitions into silent witnessing (*sakshat kara*) become more natural and regular. It is to be remembered, however, that these states are, in fact, ongoing dynamic experiential processes. They are relative, relational, and developmentally sensitive. They can be understood to be more attitudinal in nature rather than being final or terminal ends.

Psychological development from birth to death undergoes recognizable stages spurred on by physical growth, neurophysiological maturation, and psychological experience. Each stage provides differing cognitive and emotional faculties. The earlier stages absolutely require the care and guidance of a significantly perceived nurturing figure. This is an ideal time for caregivers to expose children and adolescents to the range of Ayurvedic lifestyle principles, especially those of *sadvritta* (values and ethical behavior). From adult life on, the individual becomes increasingly more self-reliant for basic and extended survival and self-care.

Envy management skills, a phrase and mental health strategy that I have developed in the course of my work on *envy theory,* offers one such practical example of effective and health-promoting parenting. In brief, this skill set may result from psychoeducation as well as from personal psychotherapy. It entails the following: Based on a review both of behaviors and of attitudes that interpret the meaning of behaviors, values, ambitions, interpersonal comparisons, and all the positive and negative feelings around these, a definition of the manner in which envy—impulses to destroy what is perceived as very good and ideal—manifests itself begins to emerge. Once the role of the more self-destructive aspects of envy is ascertained, a further examination of its roots is investigated. This analytic inspection, itself, is therapeutic and produces some degree of self-change. Over time, alternative options for perceiving arise. In turn, emotions marked by empathy, admiration, gratitude, and cooperativeness come to the fore. Behaviors that are less self-sabotaging, less cynical, and characterized by sharing and helpfulness emerge. When parents undergo such beneficial personal changes, the stage is set for them to integrate these into everyday family life and the raising of children. Children are especially sensitive and responsive to some of envy's most glaring manifestations, that is, in examples dealing with fairness and equality. Helping children to see the destructive elements in these contexts proves fruitful.

In this regard, an important stumbling block that adults often face on the journey from "partial mind" to "complete mind" also relates to unconscious envy. It is the insidious experience of envy's self-sabotaging effects. These most often appear in the form of a mental impasse marked by feelings of meaninglessness, doubt, and questioning the point of trying to achieve change in the face of such overwhelming resistance to change. Feelings of cynicism, skepticism, and distrust regarding the basic goodness of life may emerge. These warning signs reflect envy's operation on the self. Envy, itself, denotes resistance to change and must be looked for at every step.

The refinement of consciousness by meditative awareness in many ways parallels the developmental life cycle. Both are processes and can be viewed as a journey or a path. Meditation is the gradual process that transforms the experience of mental activity. At first, meditation requires the tutelage of a mentor or guide. Getting ready for change puts one in a position to focus on seeking help from others. Various techniques and practices then direct the meditator toward self-help and attaining an experiential state of witnessing rather than immediately identifying with each thought and feeling as it arises. The meditative trajectory begins with perceptual focus on an environmental object, then progresses its attention to the subjective chatter (*vritti*) of the mind (*Manas*) (*samprajnata-samadhi*) and finally rests within the empty spaces that had previously been filled with objects. It is an understanding of profound proportions without words.

This penultimate meditative achievement denotes emphasis on the psychological tasting of experience rather than an automatic identification with the objects of experience. In essence, meditation is the attempt to experience desire as desire, free of the objects of desire (*asamprajnata dhyana*). The journey of meditation begins with the preparatory suspension of discursive thought referred to as "witnessing" alluded to in the foregoing. The journey reaches completion when no mind is experienced (*asamprajnata-samadhi; nirvikalpa-samadhi*).

When this state of watching becomes sufficiently consolidated, the gaps between mental events widen. They are experienced as states of silence, a presence that prevails where mental activity once had been. This quietude is the state called "no mind" or in Chinese Buddhism *wu nien*. In Japanese Zen Buddhism, it is called *mushin,* the mind-set or state of awareness within which subject and object distinctions dissolve. It is the flowering of meditative awareness. Often, the stage of meditative witnessing in contrast to no mind is easier to understand and to attain. The state of no mind is perplexing and may never be achieved. One may, perhaps, have isolated glimpses of no mind as an experiential state of consciousness. The meditative paradox is that once "complete mind" is fully achieved, it is then experienced as no mind. Meditation proceeds from witnessing the object to witnessing the subject and then to experiential witnessing, in itself, virtually free of object and free of subject. This "emptiness" is the state of no mind.

The meditative achievement termed "no mind" does not mean that the mind has been destroyed. The state of no mind denotes that, through conscious self-work, the ordinary mind has been delicately refined and temporarily put to rest, that is, into a state of equipoise. It thus becomes a silent servant, a helpful assistant that can be marshalled when its functions of thinking, feeling, judgment, and communication are needed.

While the refinement of consciousness can occur to varying degrees at all stages, adult life is usually the time when the impulse for self-examination emerges on a more solid basis. This experiential capacity develops over time and, in part, is related to psychological maturity. Although aspects of this more refined state of mind can be present, to some extent, at any age, it is more commonly achieved later in life, usually after the 40s. The Zen concept of enlightenment and self-realization termed *kensho* aptly connotes this state of developing awareness that gradually deepens over time. In Chinese traditions, it has been referred to as the path of the *Tao.*

Meditative awareness may begin with isolated periods of meditation. Traditionally, this has been called "sitting meditation" (*satipatthana; zazen*) and consists of discrete periods of time set aside specifically for the meditative process. Attention to and using breathing to settle the body and to organize disconnected thought processes is often useful. This has been variously called *pranayama* (Hindu) and *anapanasati* (Buddhist). Each system is different in its modality. The preliminary stages of meditation involve conscious and intentional practice, sometimes referred to as *samatha,* a meditative concentration that promotes mental equanimity and tranquility. This may eventually lead to the attainment of *vipassana,* more naturally enduring states of insight.

Eventually, these sacred moments of meditative mindfulness may develop in fuller ways to become more pervasive and more enduring. This meaning (*bhavana, smriti,* and *vipassana*) of meditation (*Dhyana, sati*) denotes the 24 hours a day, daily, continuous state of experiential awareness that is optimal for, and is, in fact, real self-development. It becomes a state of mind incorporated, at first, into a part of one's daily routine and then eventually imbues all parts of every waking moment; meditative awareness becomes the very act of living life to its fullest. It can be understood, in fact, to be a developmentally progressive spirituality by means of sublimations.

Sama sati, satipatthana, sadhana, and *sakshat kara* are Eastern terms and concepts that connote right mindfulness, right awareness, watching the watcher, witnessing the witnesser, and self-remembering. This state of mental equanimity (*samatva* and *upeksha*) brings with it the return of silence within one's experience. It is a hovering in the middle between extremes.

It would not be incorrect to understand meditative awareness using the Western concept of prayer in the sense of its being "prayer of the heart." The techniques used to expand one's range of consciousness and to achieve a steady state of meditative awareness are arduous. They require dedication, perseverance, and self-discipline. Yet, success in these pursuits not only requires, but also necessitates, an attitude of lightness that is both playful and evocative of a sense of joy. As meditative awareness becomes a more regular state of mind, its spontaneity is felt as natural, a natural expression of one's nature. The literature left by great masters of the Buddhist and Hindu traditions is replete with descriptions of *samadhi* (meditative absorption) and *Nirvana* (profound identification with the Absolute) that suggest experiential states that are amusing, cheerful, awe filled, wondrous, and having childlike qualities. The fulfillment of *dharma,* then, becomes an experience characterized by naturalness, spontaneity, and a sense of adventure.

ELEMENTS ON THE PATH TO *MOKSHA*

The broad means used to achieve varying degrees of *Moksha,* therefore, encompass an active striving to include wholesomeness (*satmya* and *kushala*) in all aspects of living: diet, daily routine, exercise, recreational activity, work, study and learning, meditation, and interpersonal and social relations. Incorporating Ayurvedic principles and practices into one's life enhances all aspects of daily living and raises the qualitative caliber of *optimal engagement in the world.* In other words, meditative awareness is much more than an isolated, contemplative state of mind. It must include ongoing concrete action, responsiveness, and renewed activity. These means of striving for ongoing purification, balance, and optimal living may initially require enormous determination and so be experienced as requiring ongoing "superefforts." One's primary focus is on self-development, avoiding interpersonal control and unnecessary interference in other people's lives. Compassionate sharing becomes the norm. The insights perceived through meditative awareness foster magnanimity, an attitude of generosity and forgiveness both toward the self and toward others. In other words, a character that is noble, not petty, arises. As a result of this self-work, however, previously built-up *karma* is deconstructed. This brings about dissolution of the accretions, knots, and layers of concealment (*samskaras*) incurred over time. Corruptions in the experience of the authenticity and of the purity of the self are detoxified. A reparative and a creative restructuring is set into motion.

The processes of sensation and perception gain more clarity; the repertoire of thinking becomes less rigidly constricted by the characterological defense mechanisms erected by past traumas. In effect, mood and affective demeanor become more stable. The unhealthy splitting processes characteristic of *Manas* or mind, including the impoverishing effects of the envy dynamic, diminish, and this softens the proverbial contrasts between dogma versus deed and faith versus reason. The adamantine chains (*samsara*) of past habitual, repetitive, volatile, and unwholesome modes of experience and behavior (*samskara*) fueled by inordinate desire and envy are loosened.

As these roots slowly dissolve, feelings of admiration and gratitude emerge. These newly developed attitudes are then reflected in behaviors characterized by helpfulness. In fact, one becomes more helpful both to one's self as well as to others.

Not only does this increase in psychological integration make the experience of the ineffable meaning of the self more majestic, but it enhances a less egocentric attitude toward others, one that is more kindly, respectful, and tolerant, if not enthusiastic, in regard to perceived differences. The roots of bias and of interpersonal hatred have fear and envy at their base. When sufficient work on every aspect of the aggregation of dissociated experience (unorganized self-awareness) occurs, transforming states of more integrated self-awareness are set in motion. The constraints that fear, anxiety, and envy impose begin to dissolve. It is at this moment that what has been called the *bodhichitta* emerges. This experiential state comprises the *BioPsychoSpiritual* position both of personal and transpersonal intentionality that drives the awakened mind toward attaining *Moksha*. It is living in the world with naturalness and spontaneity (*wu wei*). It is the ability to live with others in noninterference. A life of immersion in this attitude of nonviolence minimizes self-abuse and molestation toward others and so lightens the karmic load.

Self-inquiry and self-development contribute to the progressive refinement of the coarser elements within human nature, to the enhancement of consciousness, and to the path toward *Moksha*. These act as medicines to heal malignant emotional states and as nourishment to vitalize moral consciousness. *Prajna* as wisdom and *karuna* as compassion suffuse one's life. The use of concepts that deal with sorrow, remorse, regret, and guilt traditionally contained in terms such as contrition, repentance, and atonement are more abundant within the spiritual traditions of Western religions. Their meaningfulness within an Ayurvedic worldview emerges from the recognition of imbalanced states emerging both by commission and by omission, a personal sense of distress, and the individual resolve to restore harmony.

Over the course of time, previously experienced intentionality in efforts aimed at achieving this newly created disposition toward wholesomeness gradually transforms. An experiential state begins to emerge that is characterized by increasing receptivity, acceptance, and ease. More relaxed, effortless action comes about and a natural spontaneity (*wu wei*) emerges from this more integrated advance. A *BioPsychoSpiritual* galvanization is gradually produced that uncovers the engendered awareness of a personal foundation (*atman*) of absolute purity (*Purusha*). This newfound self-realization, then, becomes an integral part of everyday living and ushers in a higher overall quality of life that is experienced more consistently over time. As the natural and limitless breadth of consciousness is felt with increasing conviction, perceived helplessness in all its guises—inordinate arousal, anxiety, fear, envy, and the defensive sense of danger—reconfigures. One becomes grounded in the safety, simplicity, and wonder of experiential witnessing. Mental equanimity (*samatva*) is restored as silence is put back into one's overall experiential states. An inner security is felt as a sovereign presence.

MOKSHA

Although words can only meagerly describe the elusive and virtually unfathomable meaning of *Moksha,* it can be thought of as the zero point experience termed *Avyakta* (beyond being and nonbeing). In Buddhism, it is the achievement of *Vimukti,* liberation from defilements, suffering, and desire. It is Emptiness. In Chinese Taoism, it is *Wu* or the Void. Equally as true, one could call it the positive realization of identity with infinite potentiality or *Brahman* (the Absolute). *Moksha,* then, appears as the felt and sustainable experience that one has always been *Brahman.*

Awareness promotes this concrescence and reveals an alignment that, in fact, has always had substantive reality. The meaning of this awareness approximates the achievement of a unity that somehow reflects the very witnessing of awareness, itself. This state of being is beyond the ordinary condition of the very act of experiencing, itself. The Sanskrit expression *Tat Tvam Asi* (Thou art That), found in one of the oldest *Upanishads,* the Chandogya (c. 500 B.C.), denotes this fundamental Vedic maxim. *Tat* is a very ancient Sanskrit term literally meaning "that" but implying the unknowable principle constituting the foundation of the entire universe, that is, the Absolute.

Moksha, thus, is the direct, intuitive, and nonconceptual sense of identity with the transcendental Absolute experienced as pure consciousness yet commensurate with an individual's level of *BioPsychoSpiritual* development. It is not an ontological change, but a personal psychological breakthrough. This is termed the state of *Chaitanya-Purusha,* the consciousness of unity within multiplicity. It is a *Sahaja-samadhi* and a *Jivan-mukti,* a state of liberation while being alive. One's personality becomes purified and one's attitude takes on an innocence. The quality and character of this experiential dynamic may be understood to be a developmentally progressive (not regressive), healthy advance. This mastery (*prajnaparamita*) is the gain achieved by sublimations that result from conscious and intentional self-work. Its virtue and value are ensured by the underlying reparative and creative impulses that add to the enrichment (*vibhuti*) of the breadth, depth, and scope of one's consciousness. This insight, it is suggested, is the mutative element within the root meaning of *Moksha.* Crossing over into this state is true *prajnaparamita,* a lived state of insight into emptiness (*shunyata*) or what I have called *Zephirum.* The broad scope of Ayurveda with its engaging presence provides a robust means of achieving both physical well-being and the liberating, spiritual advancement referred to as *Moksha.*

12

THE *BioPsychoSpiritual* PERSPECTIVE IN CONTEMPORARY CLINICAL PSYCHIATRY

Modern Psychiatry is the subspecialty within contemporary medicine that deals with a focused consideration of psychological phenomena and the diagnosis and treatment of mental disorders. *Bhutavidya* is the branch within Ayurveda that corresponds to the study of the mind. In an attempt to draw the best from these two fields, a novel approach—the *BioPsychoSpiritual* perspective—is introduced and discussed. It is a consciousness-based, phenomenological model. Some theoretical considerations regarding human psychology, the nature of mental disorders and emotional suffering, and psychotherapeutic technique are offered.

The *BioPsychoSpiritual* (Ninivaggi, 2001, 2005a, 2005b) perspective is an integrative approach that may have a place within contemporary psychiatry. It provides a comprehensive understanding of human psychology in health and in disorder. Its propositions rest both on Western Psychiatry and on the principles of Ayurveda. Splitting, self-integration, envy, greed, loneliness, aloneness, meaningful survival, empathy, and compassion as they play out in the mind are themes. The refinement of consciousness, a primary aim, is cultivated by means of attention to and work on the mind (*Manas*).

The *BioPsychoSpiritual* perspective in its largest scope is a worldview with philosophical and psychological features. It is a consciousness-based and phenomenological model in its epistemology and its ontology. The core paradigm rests on the proposition that experience, witnessing (or silent observation), and understanding are key human values. Human existence as personalized individuality in the world is viewed in a particular way. Each individual is regarded as an experiencer who simultaneously participates both in the experience and in the experienced. In other words, the self, the process of knowing the other, and the other are virtually inseparable. All are seen to have a share in a unified continuum both of experience (epistemological reality) and of being/existing (ontological reality). This entire conception of "knowing" is predicated on systems-based information processing. The microcosmic unit of body-mind-spirit reverberates both within and as an integral dimension of the extended macrocosmic environment. The phenomenology of experience here denotes more than sensation, perception, and conception. It includes these but goes beyond them. It taps direct experiential consciousness, which implies intuition and insight. It is more than ordinary, conventional cognition.

The essential unity within the perception of real experiential diversity is held to reflect a truer apprehension of reality, its ontological status. This touches on the age-old philosophical problem of "the one and the many": Is reality essentially a unified whole, or is it a disparate agglomeration of distinct and unrelated entities?

The *BioPsychoSpiritual* view sees distinctions as real. The perception of distinctions is a natural part of the manner in which human cognition operates. The *BioPsychoSpiritual* perspective brings forward, however, a mobilization of the healthy synthetic impulses within both intellectual and emotional cognition. This broadening of cognition achieved through the cultivation of consciousness ultimately permits an appreciation of the essential unity that exists both within the self and within the self's relation to all else.

Suffering is universal and has existed since the dawn of humankind. Two primary motivations at the base of this mental and physical discontent are the intrinsic need for survival and the innate desire to survive in a meaningful way. The *BioPsychoSpiritual* perspective attributes the cause of suffering to the natural default state of human cognition. This is termed *Prajna-aparadha*. It has a twofold denotation: (1) the ability to experience the world as split and (2) the inability to experience the world in its essential unity.

Throughout the prehistoric and extended course of civilization, all sectors of human culture have strived not only to secure survival but also to attain a good quality of life. Hence, the incarnation of a vast spectrum of methods, techniques, even rituals aimed toward achieving meaning, reinforcing hopefulness, and alleviating stress and suffering. A major branch within traditional Ayurveda—*Bhutavidya*—is roughly akin to what we now know as the contemporary medical subspecialty of Psychiatry. Bringing the two together in a creative marriage can engender insights hitherto untapped. Recognizing the consciousness-based, spiritual, and existential dimensions that energize and give meaning to all life's activities is a challenge in today's world of science and high technology. A serious consideration of this consciousness-based *BioPsychoSpiritual* view, however, may offer such an opportunity.

The material presented here admittedly simplifies highly complex realities. With this in mind, a conceptual and methodological approach, the *BioPsychoSpiritual,* is introduced. It is a further elaboration of the *BioPsychoSpiritual* concept, which was first introduced earlier (Ninivaggi, 2001). It is more a perspective, a mind-set, and a point of exploratory departure rather than a series of definitive statements or formulaic techniques. It does not replace standard, mainstream psychiatric theory and practice; it is complementary to them.

The cumulative insights of generations cannot be dismissed entirely with an anti-non-scientific bias, which might regard such worldviews and their powerful implications as having inferior evidential value. Rather, this qualitative approach to health and health imbalances may function as an orienting background to enhance and to complement other therapeutic modalities and clinical strategies. This encompasses practices within Ayurveda, Psychiatry, psychotherapy, as well as in other healing traditions.

THE BASIC PERSPECTIVE

BioPsychoSpiritual Self

To focus on the essential qualities of the subject under consideration, definitions are used, but they can be limiting. They omit a fuller appreciation of the extended realities toward which they point. Although the written word employs the verbal and conceptual capacities of the mind in an effort to communicate, the broader existential-experiential arena of human life is ultimately what is being addressed. This vast field transcends language and also goes beyond what conventional thinking typically apprehends. With this proviso, the *BioPsychoSpiritual* self is defined in the following way.

The *BioPsychoSpiritual* self is the entire life spectrum of an individual: a unified life that has three broad dimensions, the physical, the psychological, and the spiritual. These three aspects reflect different perspectives of one intrinsically unified presence, the living, dynamic entity called the "*BioPsychoSpiritual* self." It is a continuously growing, maturing, developing, and actively communicating sentient being. It creatively emerges anew at all points in time. I have termed this constant self-evolution *self-signature updating.* Its unity, integration, abilities, skills, and subjective awareness differ among individuals. Its fluid nature continuously restructures itself, especially in interpersonal engagements.

This "self," a centrated sphere of experiential awareness, is what each person calls home in the ultimate scheme of things. The self, in fact, maintains a seamless unity with all else. This idea is echoed in one of the most important precepts (*mahavakyas*) of the *Vedanta* contained in the *Chandogya-Upanishad,* the second oldest of the *Upanishads* belonging to the *Sama-Veda* (Ganapati, 1992) The revered statement *Tat Tvam Asi* points to the fact that the Absolute is, in essence, one with the individually experienced self.

The primary dynamic impulse within the self, it is proposed, is the drive or creative principle toward ever more refined levels of integration. This self-integration is experienced as "meaningful survival." The very term "Ayurveda" has often been translated into English as "the knowledge and the science of life." As previously suggested (Ninivaggi, 2001), its deeper meaning denotes "life wisdom." This living experience of life's meaningful wisdom is contained in the history and practice of all that Ayurveda has to offer.

Ayurveda and Yoga have traditionally described the makeup of an individual in terms of an esoteric anatomy. In this view, five sheaths surround but do not touch the *atman* or pure spirit. Each sheath is a progressively increasing material densification of primal consciousness from which everything in the created world emerges. These five layers are termed the physical, the prana, the mind, the wisdom, and the bliss dimensions. The *BioPsychoSpiritual* perspective accepts this and also employs a tripartite descriptive variation.

The three dimensions of the *BioPsychoSpiritual* self are the physical body, the mind, and consciousness. Consciousness is the spiritual base of the body-mind or *biomental* complex.

The material, psychological, and spiritual significance of the physical body, the gross aspect of the self, cannot be underestimated. The body remains the most obvious and palpable base of human being. Identification with the body is continually reinforced by others who recognize an individual's physical self as being who the individual is. Looking in the mirror also reinforces an individual's identification with the physical form. Realizing the potential value of the physical aspect of the self adds to acknowledging the fullness of one's tangible presence in the world and hence contributes to a sense of emotional security.

Sensation, perception, and feeling are materially based in the very flesh and blood of the body's central nervous system. Feeling the flesh is one of the primary purposes of human existence. Not only is the physical body a given fact; it also functions as an opportunity to foster increased psychological awareness. Since feelings are dynamically being pulled into and out of the very flesh of the body, these affective experiences or emotions are more poignant than thoughts. Their exquisitely sensitive pleasure-pain reactivity, however, makes them easy prey for suppression, denial, and repression. The rawness and brilliance of the biopsychological awareness of felt emotions is continually being dulled by the mind. This is both a defensive as well as a protective measure. It assuages the sense of being overwhelmed, even traumatized by such affective overload.

How the physical dimension of the self, that is, the "body image," is regarded always needs to be taken seriously. Its status repeatedly impacts the mind and is, itself, partially reflective of one's entire being. In fact, in Eastern psychology, the physical body is regarded as the "exterior mind," while the psychological mind is regarded as being the "interior body."

The psychological aspect of the self includes the mind whose function is to experience and to process emotions and thoughts, that is, objects in the mind. The mind is a measuring instrument. It is the center of cognition that uses reason, logic, sequential processing, and memory. Speech and language—including the written word—closely reflect how the mind functions. Excessive intellectualization or overthinking reflects imbalanced cognition. In Ayurveda, the term *Manas* refers to the mind in the sense described here.

In the *BioPsychoSpiritual* perspective, mind and body are intimately identified. They constitute a *biomental corporeality*. Since body and mind are two sides of the same coin, what occurs in the flesh always is experienced mentally. As previously mentioned, emotions have a strong body-based experiential dimension. Thoughts, concepts, and their formal architecture, however, tend to be more mind based. The mind is more energetically structured while the body is more an organism of gross matter. This subtle differentiation, in fact, is merely academic since the two are experientially indivisible.

Both body and mind are included in the concept of *Ahamkara*. *Ahamkara* is defined as one's individualized sense of being a separate entity within the extended universe. *Ahamkara* is the individual ego clinging to its belief that it is separate and that its sole identity coincides with its body and its mind.

The function of emotions is to impart to consciousness, instantaneous signals, and information relating to survival. In addition, emotions offer continuous opportunities to maintain *BioPsychoSpiritual* homeostasis and ongoing self-regulation. Healthy responses facilitate thinking processes that interpret these messages more correctly and so enhance successful adaptation. The mind, however, naturally tends toward a state of imbalance, typically in the form of extremes of feeling and appraisals. Wrong diet, life-style, and the changing seasons contribute to this. The emotional imprints derived from early parent-child relations and current interpersonal relationships collude with the aforementioned and result in this tendency toward confused thinking and misapprehensions in memory. Hence, biomental pain and suffering—anxiety, fear, insecurity, depression, hopelessness, envy, and malcontent—become established as part of everyday experiences.

The mind when in a state of imbalance has the capacity to intensify the experience of suffering. Imbalance or mental vitiation occurs when inordinate splitting processes in thinking and feeling occur. The experience of suffering is always an experience filled with extremes. These take the form of intense attractions and intense repulsions. The extremes of indulgence versus renunciation/denial/repression arise from the mind's innate binary default ways of processing information. Leading examples include an intense preoccupation with avoiding, ignoring, or denying the fearful, hostile, and negative tendencies that appear within one's impulses, feelings, and thoughts.

Equally as unproductive are obsessively pressured preoccupations with striving for that which is considered positive: love, kindness, spirituality, even God. These extremes constitute indulgences that blur the acceptance and proper management of the usually more prominent inescapable negative aspects perceived in one's life. Any thought, feeling, or overvalued set of ideas, in fact, limits one's full range of consciousness. So-called positive affirmations signal that negativity and suffering are present. They often act to reinforce these disturbances by a reflexive, unhealthy resorting to their polar extremes. When balance is achieved through practices that awaken self-awareness and self-understanding, the mind (*Manas*) relaxes and is less driven to extremes either of overindulgence or renunciation. It is then able to rest for longer periods in states of equilibrium and in equipoise. The range of consciousness and of self-awareness becomes broadened. Silently witnessing one's experiences assuages the tendency to identify with any one aspect whether it be felt as positive or negative.

On the one hand, traditional psychiatric perspectives have focused on these mental processes in highly scientific ways. The biopsycho*social* approach, an integral, foundational perspective in modern Psychiatry, for example, takes into consideration measurable behaviors, classifiable disorders, and environmental stressors when making diagnoses and formulating treatment. The *BioPsychoSpiritual* approach, on the other hand, assumes a much wider perspective in its understanding and treatment of the whole person—body, mind, and consciousness. The health and care of the body, emotions, and mind as well as attention to right awareness are all part of the Ayurvedic tradition. Both perspectives are not only valid, but they can also be complementary.

The spiritual self indicates an individual's share in the experience of consciousness, which includes self-awareness and a sense of the sacred. It is to be remembered that the *BioPsychoSpiritual* perspective denotes consciousness in a broad manner. Consciousness as contained within the experiential mind (*Manas, Buddhi,* and *Ahamkara*) pulls its content from three sources: conscious awareness, preconscious subliminality, and the dynamic unconscious. The cultivation of consciousness, which results from intentional work on the self (body, mind, and spirit), is a lifelong process that continuously integrates that which is more nonconscious into more conscious awareness. The sense of the sacred is a reflection of the self's awe-inspiring yet feeble awareness of the ineffable ground of consciousness, that is, its superlative refinement, the immaterial ground of all, being as well as non-being. The spiritual dimension of self is imbued with meaning. Consciousness in its most intimate, human, and spiritualized action maintains an endless love affair with both body and mind.

Consciousness as meaningfully oriented self-awareness, moreover, may be the most subtle and under-recognized aspect of being human. This intimate, sacred, and sensitively responsive dimension may also be the most undernourished, especially since it is not really matter or energy. Although the measurable world of matter and energy emerge out of consciousness, it transcends them. In a sense, consciousness exists "in the world, but is not of the world."

Thus, the trinity of body, mind, and spirit constitutes each individual's share both in the perceived material and in the spiritual aspects of nature, existence in its entirety.

To the extent that balance, coherence, and unity are experienced, the *BioPsychoSpiritual* self has access to a cognition that is imbued with *Buddhi,* which is an individual's personal share in *Mahat,* the transcendent intelligence inherent in *Prakriti,* the created world. Self-integration thus acts to awaken clearer perception, understanding, and an appreciation of the unity underlying all experience. One's reality sense is thus enhanced. In other contexts, I have referred to this as the *epistemophilia within the self.*

PSYCHOTHERAPY AS ART AND SCIENCE

The Aims of Therapy

Just as there is material food for the physical body and mental "food for thought," so too there can be sacraments and offerings for the spiritual self. Historically, religions have traditionally been the primary vehicle for this. Today, this spiritual nourishment can also exist outside of organized faith traditions. Spiritual hunger is existential loneliness. The cultures of today experience a general malaise, which reflects a hankering for something more than is ordinarily experienced. Humanistic and compassionate psychotherapies comprise one such form of this nourishment. This is not an "other worldly" phenomenon. Used conscientiously and diligently, therapy may act to foster an authentic *BioPsychoSpiritual* engagement, which is therapeutic in the here and now, in everyday living. This can be restorative, growth promoting, and life enhancing.

The broad aim of any psychotherapeutic process is an increase in the integral quality of life—subjectively and behaviorally. This includes a greater experience of the sense of well-being, both personally and interpersonally. Fear, anxiety, insecurity, dysphoria, and suffering are lessened. One's sense of self and one's more successful adaptation to the tasks and joys of living are thereby improved.

In the context of the *BioPsychoSpiritual* perspective, aiming toward—not reaching—an integration of this more complete state of wholeness is foremost. It is a dynamic, ongoing journey rather than a final destination. Reaching a final target is not the objective. Maintaining an active awareness (right mindfulness, *sama sati*) of the process, itself, on a moment-to-moment basis is the primary aim. It constitutes the journey from a split sense of self toward a more unified experiential self-awareness. Ultimately, this *BioPsychoSpiritual* integration becomes experienced as a simultaneous, unified living in the body, mind, and consciousness spheres of experience with as alert an awareness as possible. Cognition, in this sense, connotes wisdom (*prajna* and *chit*), and all emotion becomes imbued with compassion (*kushala*).

From a Western psychological perspective, this manner of psychotherapy could be termed "cognitive-adaptive therapy" (CAT). It is a method currently being developed within the *BioPsychoSpiritual* field of Psychiatry. Its ultimate outcome in the real world affords pragmatic adaptation to everyday living. It specifically targets the mobilization of what I have termed *adaptive intelligence.* This is understood to be the central plexus subtending the wide range of abilities underlying ease of effective responsiveness to change. This hub of all abilities is activated specifically by techniques that foster *instinctive resourcefulness,* the repository of silent aptitudes that are the learning-sensitive mediators between intellectual and emotional abilities and their timely and successful implementation as problem-solving behavioral skills (Ninivaggi, 2005c).

Splitting and Self-Integration

Two fundamental issues must be addressed in order to understand and utilize *BioPsychoSpiritual* interventions. They are the theoretical concepts of splitting and self-integration, and the clinical experiences of loneliness and aloneness.

Sigmund Freud (1938a, 1938b), Melanie Klein (1946), and Wilfred R. Bion (1959), distinguished pioneers in establishing psychoanalytic theory and its therapeutic applications, introduced the notions of splitting—of the ego and of the object. Since this realization emerged late in Freud's work, he had little time to adequately develop it. Klein and Bion, however, developed this idea and continued to regard it as axiomatic, as do their contemporary followers.

The phenomenon of splitting is understood to be one of the primary functions of "mind" both in everyday life and in clinical disorders. Splitting is the force that keeps things apart, as, for example, idea and idea, idea and emotion, ideation and behavior, and that which is conscious from that which is latent and unconscious.

The psychological mechanism of splitting results in the mind's processing information in a binary manner, that is, dualistically. This is the mind's initial approach in its journey toward further more accurate cognitive processing. When balanced and healthy, cognition becomes more synthetic and integrative.

While normal splitting is healthy, excessive splitting drives unintegration, disconnectedness, and impaired adaptation. These imbalances underlie the experiential condition of suffering. They are reflected in feelings of fear, anxiety, dysphoria, discontent, and estrangement.

In Ayurveda, the concept of *Prajna-aparadha* (also spelled *pragya-aparah*) reflects the mind's inherent tendency toward splitting. *Prajna-aparadha* is the ordinary experience of forgetting the underlying unity of all existence. The real diversity within creation and in great Nature, that is, in *Prakriti,* is not wrong, incorrect, or evil in any way. The mind's inherent fault sees and interprets *Prakriti*'s interconnected diversity, however, as being vastly unconnected, split apart, and seemingly incoherent.

The reparative trend toward integration of the self is an outcome of successful therapy. It brings about creative links between all the aforementioned mental and behavioral events. In a way, one might say that increases in self-integration contribute to the healthy buildup of psychological immunity, which enhances emotional resistance to stressful life events, anxiety, and impaired functioning.

Integration, in this sense, can be seen in a metaphorical manner as the grand architect that builds and designs unity and coherence into experiential self-awareness. The greater the integration, the greater is the experience of being more fully awake. One becomes more aware of and awake to an internal sense of completeness and to a feeling of kinship, affiliation, and cooperative partnership with others. Living in the real world, then, is experienced as a joint interpersonal adventure.

Loneliness and Unconscious Envy

Emotional suffering is usually accompanied by loneliness—the pain of feeling separate and of feeling disconnected. Loneliness, in fact, is a deeply conflicted sense of the fear that one's perceived inextricable attachments to others are being pulled, split apart, or are absent in some way. Loneliness reflects a state of bondage and excessive attachment. It is the agonizing sense of feeling incomplete, insecure, and ungrounded. Loneliness emanates from the mind's intrinsic default tendency toward excessive splitting, that is, *Prajna-aparadha.*

The manifestations of unconscious envy and of conscious greed in everyday life may be the most common expressions of loneliness. They are the emotional articulations of a feeling of absence, feelings that may be quelled only by strivings toward acquisitiveness. Consequently, loneliness results in the feverish pursuit of clinging to persons and of the acquisition of inanimate material objects. It is the feeling that life is an emergency in need of immediate action.

Envy is more nuclear and malignant than greed. It arises from deeply unconscious sources. It is rooted in splitting processes, which fuel dualistically driven experience on all levels. Primary envy, an inherent force within human nature, goes hand in hand with *Prajna-aparadha,* its experiential state of mind. Its aim is the destructive spoiling of what is sensed to be exceedingly good and ideal, yet unattainable. Envy is the deepest source of vitiation on all experiential levels; spoiling the envied object results in the envier feeling traumatized. *Projective identification* is the unconscious mechanism that the mind employs to aggressively control conflictual elements within itself. This typically involves projecting these outward, away from the experienced self, as it were. This constitutes a pathological attempt to vitiate all sources that instigate envy and desire. *Projective identification* ultimately becomes autodestructive and causes an autoerosion, which, in turn, leads to states of fragmentation and isolation. Greed, by contrast, is more akin to feelings related to jealousy. Greed is more benign than envy. It is characterized by unsettling feelings of gnawing dissatisfaction, of never having enough. Jealousy is a passionate feeling of disappointment and exclusion. Jealousy, unlike envy, is based on more loving and affectionate feelings.

The state of painful loneliness is often accompanied by perceptions that are excessively directed to persons and to objects outside the self. This is reflected in the often seen attempts of the lonely person to behave as if all his or her needs could be and must be satisfied only by that which comes from the external environment rather than from more internal resources.

Since loneliness is a feeling of being isolated, unconnected, insecure, estranged, alienated, and empty, the natural defense of clinging and of grasping is automatically elicited. It is experienced as an endless series of repetitive, temporary arrangements of the self clinging to another person or, for example, holding on to inanimate possessions such as money, property, video games, toys, power, or a no longer vital and adaptive ideology. The clinical extremes of schizoid isolation and of manic expansiveness also reflect inner states of perceived emptiness. Temporary attachments to material objects are attempts to negate feelings of loneliness and of incompleteness and to restore a sense of wholeness. They prove futile over the long run. This ultimately leads to adaptive collapse.

Aloneness

Aloneness (*Kevalam, Kaivalya*) is different from loneliness. Aloneness is regarded in the *BioPsychoSpiritual* perspective as a healthy state of mind characterized by feelings of trust, security, and relative completeness. A beautiful exposition of this is found in the *Kaivalya Upanishad* within the *Atharva-Veda* (Whitney & Lanman, 1996).

Effective psychotherapy, as understood in this perspective, creates conditions whereby the patient's splitting processes diminish and self-integration is enhanced. Feelings of loneliness are restructured and a greater sense of comfortableness of the self with the self is established. This entails a brutally clear acceptance of oneself in the present moment, in the "now" of the experiential present. In existential and also in Buddhist terms, it means the authentic acceptance of the experience of being in the here and now and of the emerging realization of being essentially free and alone, "on your own" so to speak, within the vastness of existence. It is putting silence back into one's experience.

Alone in this sense includes being related to others—but not emotionally fused. This state of *interdependence* may appear paradoxical in that it describes experiencing one's being in simultaneity: both as a single individuality and simultaneously as an integral part of one's family and social context. Healthy interdependent aloneness, in effect, is a psychological state of *communicative, inner silence.*

Certainly, this view of aloneness manifests very differently at each chronological age and at different developmental stages. Degrees of wholesome aloneness may be present in healthy children alone at play and also in the secure presence of a caregiving parent. It is only in mature adult life, however, that its fullness can flower in a more conscious way.

THE *BIOPSYCHOSPIRITUAL* PERSPECTIVE IN CLINICAL PRACTICE

The *BioPsychoSpiritual* perspective encompasses a comprehensive theoretical culture that translates into practical action (*abhyasa*) in many ways.

One major application is in psychotherapeutic practice. Quality psycho-therapy may be considered a *sadhana,* a means toward self-development and self-realization. The practical implementation of its propositions, values, and aims may be termed the *praxis* of effective treatment. Praxis here denotes several features: a therapeutic interaction that does not follow a preconceived plan, a reflective deliberation in a situational context shaped by an intimate interpersonal dialogue, and a yield of creative insights that emerge within a lived experience. Both therapist and client/patient participate in this praxis of "action—reflection—action" in differing ways.

Since action (*karma*) is a powerful activity, especially for the initiator of such an interpersonal process, the concept of *naish-karmya-karman* is impor-tant to understand. It denotes formulating therapeutic intentions and their implemented actions in a manner that is least controlling, manipulative, and interfering. It emphasizes the ideal of "action transcendence," that is, a truly empathetic and compassionate sharing of guidance for the benefit of the other with the least amount of directiveness.

The roots of such a therapeutic interaction go back several thousand years and can be found in the methods that the ancient sages used in the *Upanisha-dic* period (c. 600 B.C.) in ancient India. *Upanishad* literally means "sitting down near to." This deeply interpersonal dialogue denoted the physical, men-tal, and consciousness-based proximity that the guru/teacher/therapist/guide jointly created in relationship with the disciple/client/patient. In the twenty-first century, quality psychotherapy using the *BioPsychoSpiritual* model car-ries this connotation of a shared dialogue.

Quality psychotherapy is a clinical, psychologically hands-on therapy that is experience-near. In the métier of Eastern meditative techniques, it can be called a *sadhana,* a means to self-development. By analogy (*upamana*), this *sadhana* harkens back to the *Upanishads* (c. 600 B.C.) and to their ancient and time-honored techniques. These include a one-to-one, deeply interper-sonal dialogue, which generates motivational heat (*tapas*). A *vedi,* a psycho-logical altar of fire, is established as a process within which change is forged both analytically and synthetically. In the heat of this flame, there is an articu-lated emphasis on the metabolism (*Agni*) of the *Tanmatras,* primal matter, that is, experiential hearing, emotional touching, insightful seeing, and emo-tional tasting and smelling. An intimate and guided tour that helps develop discriminatory (*viveka*) experience of the self and of the self in relationship to others is created and witnessed by both participants.

This type of quality psychotherapy facilitates conditions that experien-tially demonstrate a method of knowing reality. It is not directive instruction. Quality psychotherapy results in the acquisition of real-world self-study skills through a kind of mutual meditation. Little by little over time, multiple layers of the superimpositions (*adhyasa*) of *samskaras,* habits and misperceptions, are dissolved. Various degrees of *darshana,* the experience of insight, emerge.

The *BioPsychoSpiritual* perspective puts heavy weight on cultivating the self-qualities of responsibility, accountability, leadership, and self-directedness. Patients or clients choosing to participate in psychotherapies have the best chances of success if these choices are voluntary, intentional, consciously planned, and motivated. The decision to work on the self must involve a recurring series of moment-to-moment experiential choices.

The *BioPsychoSpiritual* perspective emphasizes artful and creative psychotherapeutic skills. The person and function of the therapist is viewed as a "humanized therapeutic instrument."

"Humanized" here means empathetic and compassionate. "Instrument" connotes precision and expertise in applied skillful and efficacious techniques of diagnosis and treatment. The therapist is the humanized instrument who—through empathy and compassion—in conjunction with the patient, facilitates meaningful personal change. Excessive emphasis on diagnoses is avoided. A much broader vista goes beyond conventional classifications. It positions the patient in the larger scheme of things so that all interventions remain as balanced as possible.

With this mind-set, erroneous views that reduce and marginalize patients merely to a series of measurements, diagnoses, or chemically imbalanced arrangements of neurotransmitters are avoided. The therapist, as well, needs to be cognizant of the natural tendency to overly intellectualize in the therapeutic engagement. Overintellectualization always signals excessive splitting processes, which degrade understanding and disrupt the flow of the therapeutic moment.

This concept of balance has two technical emphases: (1) a mindfully rational treatment approach that is duly comprehensive and not one-sided in any direction and (2) a moment-to-moment awareness of the essential and changing uniqueness of the individual. This denotes a literal "being with the patient" on all levels—physically, emotionally, cognitively, and existentially. It means being present and available to the patient's suffering.

Psychotherapeutic technique endeavors to examine and to elicit a restructuring in the patient's *perception* of the *meaning* of his and her own experience. All levels of communication—from those on the rational surface through their preconscious and unconscious underpinnings—are selectively addressed. Since one's interpretive perceptions arise automatically from implicit values and beliefs, some examples of these include how one experiences life and its meaning, the world around, family, school experience, job/occupation/career, earning money as well as decisions about what to hold on to, buy, and possess, and whether or not and how to be with others.

THERAPEUTIC GUIDELINES

Flexible, dynamic therapeutic guidelines support the framework of the *BioPsychoSpiritual* technique. A rigid cookbooklike, standardized, and manualization approach is disadvantageous to this.

The therapist's psychological position and technique are characterized by several important factors. They are as follows:

1. An authentic presence that is conscientious and responsive. The *BioPsychoSpiritual* approach requires that each therapeutic encounter be given adequate, unpressured time. The therapist's astute attention and sensitive listening provide a frame around each session. This includes an open recognition of negative and disturbing thoughts and feelings without any attempt to dispel them. Tapping onto one's therapeutic sensitivity and an appropriate quality of naturally spontaneous humor are essential to this.

2. The absence of memory and desire. This means minimizing feelings of wanting, expecting, and desiring that something *specific* should happen. Such a highly focused, targeted, and expectant attitude cuts the roots that ground the living therapeutic engagement that is born within the present experiential moment. In the *BioPsychoSpiritual* perspective, it is only in the present moment—the witnessing of experience—that enduring insights and change can emerge in an optimal way.

3. The therapist's silent, receptive listening; and a therapeutic voice. The role of sensitively measured therapeutic silence is a cardinal feature of quality psychotherapy. In addition, when other communicational vehicles are used, for example, facial expression, gesture, and language, the form of their delivery can have a strong therapeutic impact. Tone, melody, prosody, and intonation carry many nonconscious messages. Their role in information exchange requires careful attention.

4. The presence of empathy and compassion. This receptivity and expressivity connotes caring. It facilitates emergent understandability, which acts to gradually organize and link the patient's seemingly incongruent communications into meaningful realizations. Understanding—achieving progressively emerging levels of *understandability*—rather than using other pointedly didactic interventions is the premier mechanism facilitating change. The use of unconsidered reassurance, especially when it acts to deny and not face significant issues of negativity and other problem areas, is particularly unproductive. Understanding achieved through empathy and compassion restructures suffering and activates a subliminal undercurrent of hopefulness. In this way, unconscious envy then begins to undergo a healthy maturation. Lived goodness expresses itself in the emergence of attitudes of caring and the performance of helpfulness both to the self and to others.

5. The therapist and patient's collaboratively developed identification of conscious and unconscious processes, which includes an ongoing discussion both of innate subliminal feelings and of rote thinking patterns. This collaborative effort is a sharing, one that is a delicate balance of action and reflection. The concept of *karma* as action connotes avoiding forceful control and unnecessary interference. Special awareness of all the subtle aspects of unconscious envy is key.

6. Proper attention to the physical body—its constitution, needs, strengths, weaknesses, and requirements to restore balance and maintain health; and

7. Respect for a measure of therapeutic silence.

The above are techniques that create conditions for the growth, maturation, and development of self-awareness. It is particularly important to highlight that this methodology is one in which the therapist relates to the patient in a profoundly intimate psychological and spiritual way. It is chiefly accomplished by the therapist's focus on empathy, compassion, and shaping understandability. It is minimally directive and generally avoids the use of techniques such as, for example, positive affirmations and homework assignments.

The therapist shares with the patient the skills that naturally facilitate non-judgmental observation and experiential witnessing. There is no directive to the patient to dismiss any thought or feeling as, for example, with a strong action word such as "stop," or "be gone." Furthermore, there is no suggestion to use substitute thoughts or feelings such as inspiring affirmations. In fact, meditative masters, when giving the aspirant a concrete *mantra* to use as a tool upon which to initially ground a meditative practice, often have used a nonsense term or merely a word with a distinctive sound in order to minimize its having too concrete, directive, or distracting a content.

When the client is instructed to actively dismiss an experience, this, in fact, acts to increase defensive mechanisms, which then artificially and ineffectively attempt to negate some perceived mental event. "Logic therapy" and psychoeducational techniques tap onto and use the conscious and rational aspects of the mind's capacity to direct itself. The ill-considered use of apparently conscious and rational choices advocated in such therapies, however, fails to take into account that the bulk of mental functioning is unconscious. Much of it, moreover, is hardwired in almost impermeably unfathomable (let alone controllable) ways. In fact, the unconscious dimensions of the mind behave as rogue entities. They are much wider in scope than the consciously accessible features of awareness. They possess considerably more breadth and more power over everyday thinking, feeling, and behavior. Attempts to rationally guide the profoundly complex autonomy of the mind, therefore, are fraught with inevitable failure. Any therapist or client who resorts to such methodologies may be motivated by the perceived threats or challenges that perpetually assault one's perceived identity as a conscious, rational being who wishes to be in control.

Struggling to maintain such a precarious and perceived self-control is, in itself, conflictual. It reflects the real state of a self who is actually not in control. It is only by first recognizing that one is helpless that real work can begin. After such an acknowledgment, surrender (*prapatti*) to the inexorable power of the complexities of being human emerge.

While the *BioPsychoSpiritual* perspective fully acknowledges one's capacity to change, it duly recognizes the enormity of this undertaking. It advises that more than a modicum of humility, even surrender, be considered as a prerequisite to change. In other words, it is best for one to tackle, in a gentle yet firm manner, the illusion of having to be in absolute control. Control issues are dealt with by softening and restructuring them so that they may become experienced more in the form of self-management skills and as self-guidance directives.

Effective meditation and effective psychotherapy encourage reflection, observation, and experiential witnessing (*sakshin*). Unnecessary control and directiveness are minimized. Emphasis is on self-development in the context of balance and poised neutrality in mental functioning. This is a difficult and time-consuming endeavor. There are no shortcuts. Dedication is essential. Mutual motivation needs to be continuously generated; only then will the inner heat (*tapas*) unleashed continue to drive the process forward. Yet, both must be able to access what is natural and spontaneous, even childlike in perspective. The idea of being genuinely present in the experiential moment most characterizes the framework of this path of endeavor.

Embracing suffering in this way, moreover, acknowledges it as one of life's major opportunities to discover meanings that were previously unborn. Close examination of feelings, thoughts, and their meanings can ultimately lead to greater affect regulation and clearer, less unruly thinking. Over time, this process also brings to light the articulation of previously unrecognized alternative views of issues, conflicts, problems, and the development of adaptive skills and strategies. In particular, the role of unconscious envy becomes a central focus. Its examination over time is essential. Mental health is reflected in attitudes of admiration, appreciation, and gratitude. These, in turn, are reflected in behaviors marked by helpfulness, a helpfulness both to self and to others. The mind, therefore, is given the opportunity to stabilize and to recalibrate itself toward balance and toward equipoise (*samatva*).

The material proper for therapeutic discussion is anything and everything the patient presents, even if by its conspicuous absence. The apparently mundane is the gift wrap, so to speak, within which one discovers the sublime. In fact, both the patient's obvious communications along with his or her hidden "presents" are sublimely meaningful.

The material that the patient presents is ordinarily a description of his or her everyday life experiences with particular reference to significant interpersonal relationships. Conflicts and distressing emotional and behavioral problems of various sorts unfold. For the experienced and psychodynamically trained therapist, however, the phenomenon of the "transference" is key to identify and to tactfully interpret. Transference denotes the concept that the patient's entire presentation, in some almost inscrutable manner, recreates via unconscious mechanisms early infantile and childhood experience with significant persons, most notably mother. The "unconscious phantasies" or scenarios containing anxieties, conflicts, and unresolved dilemmas that contain this unconscious content are transferred into the relationship with the therapist. They are thus played out in the therapeutic relationship so that they may be recognized and gradually worked through. A further delineation of the concept of transference and its crucial role in effective treatment is beyond the scope of this chapter.

Using this approach, the therapist offers the therapeutic partner a perceptual taste of the beauty and the power of secure aloneness. To the extent that
this *BioPsychoSpiritual* psychotherapy is effective, this awakening acts to
engender an empowerment, which is driven by a gradually emerging recognition of self-completeness and self-fullness.

While life's inevitable pains do not entirely disappear, they are experienced as being more manageable. A newfound mental equanimity accompanies greater degrees of self-regulation and of impulse control. This
experience of internal stability becomes reinforcing and consequently permits activities of daily living to take on greater meaningfulness. *Adaptive
intelligence* becomes activated. This then enhances one's *instinctive
resourcefulness,* the capacity to adaptively respond to change in successful
and health-promoting ways in everyday living.

Each child, adolescent, and adult then personalizes this increase in the
quality of *felt* meaning in a variety of concrete ways (Ninivaggi, 2005c).
Signs of it can be seen, for example, in a smile, in what in ordinary terms is
called good and cooperative behavior, and, by extension, in other more subtle
ways that, in turn, reflect a fresh sense of meaning, hope, as well as a greater
modicum of gratitude and of helpfulness to others.

CONCLUSION

The *BioPsychoSpiritual* perspective is an attempt to uncover the commen-
surability or consonance between modern science and spirituality. A range
of scientifically based paradigms over the last two millennia in the West
have formulated clinical questions and problems, provided a scientific language, and determined what constitutes valid solutions. The truth claims of
what is scientific fact, according to the logical positivist school, rests on the
perceived objectivity resulting from experimentation using the hypothetico-
deductive method. This method, thereby, is purported to discover evidence-
based facts that are reproducible and also have predictive value. In general,
this continues to be the currently accepted paradigm in scientific circles
today.

The *BioPsychoSpiritual* perspective introduces another lexicon. It consists
of the language, laws, and insights of generations of truth seekers, especially
those coming from civilization's humanistic, philosophical, and spiritual traditions. Human culture today has arrived at a point where multiple paradigms
and lexicons attempting to explain and to understand reality exist simultaneously. By recognizing and drawing from this expanded scope and knowledge
base, our wisdom grasp in this context-specific environment has the ability to
uniquely empower our grasp of reality with untapped potential.

A leading premise of the *BioPsychoSpiritual* perspective has been an
examination of the creative and synthetic impulses within human nature.
What we now recognize as the potential for self-awareness of and for self-
integration within our nature, if conscientiously developed with empathy

and with compassion, may be a principal vehicle toward the cultivation of consciousness and the improvement of quality of life. Once unconscious envy in all its guises is recognized, at least in part, its gradual mitigation may uncover a variety of newfound attitudes, especially admiration, appreciation, gratitude, and helpfulness. These are personally reparative and also extend benefits to others. Meaningfulness increases more as a lived experience in everyday life. The mind becomes more capable of resting in equanimity (*samatva*). Restorative silence is reestablished. Quality of life and lived goodness go hand in hand.

EPILOGUE

The primary aim of this book has been to introduce the elements of Ayurveda and its practices to a contemporary Western audience in as original a form as is possible. The author suggests that the term "original" connotes a share in the authentic historical spirit of Ayurveda's traditions plus the modern conception of the way in which its present-day adherents grasp and implement it. The modern Western reader may question whether Ayurveda, Traditional Indian Medicine, has archaic, dogmatic, rigid, and static characteristics that remain outside of or even impervious to the sphere of scientific investigation, which comprises such a large part of Western technomedicine.

In his favorable review of *An Elementary Textbook of Ayurveda: Medicine with a Six Thousand Year Old Tradition,* Andrew Stoll, M.D., director of the psychopharmacology research laboratory at McLean Hospital, an affiliate of Harvard, raised the question: Are there modern developments and new research within Ayurveda? He optimistically stated that it was his hope that this book would inspire others "to design and carry out scientific studies to confirm or refute the utility of Ayurvedic treatments" (Stoll, 2002).

As described in Chapter 1, tradition states that Ayurveda was received in its entirety by the ancient sages thousands of years ago. This suggests a "revelation" with primary authenticity and with essential completeness. Far from encapsulating Ayurveda in a closed system, the spirit of Ayurveda has prompted its adherents to actively develop and expand its practical range. While it may be true that the Ayurvedic corpus has remained fairly constant as codified in the works of Charaka, Sushruta, and Vagbhata, it is also true that the last 20 years have seen the proliferation of more peer-reviewed scientific research in Ayurveda than ever before.

While a comprehensive survey of such studies is beyond the scope of the epilogue, some representative work includes the following. The roles of hormonal shifts, stress, and Ayurvedically oriented meditation have demonstrated positive, beneficial findings (*Journal of Behavioral Medicine* 15

(4):327–341, 1992). Early work on Ayurvedic herbs and murine neuroblastoma cell cultures has shown promise in cancer treatments (*Neuropharmacology* 31:599–607, 1992). Improvements in cardiovascular risk factors produced through Ayurvedic *Panchakarma* treatments have shown positive results (*Journal of Research and Education in Indian Medicine* 12(4):2–13, 1993). The *Journal of Ethnopharmacology,* January 2007, recently devoted a large section to Indian medicinal plants as a source of antimycobacterial agents. This shows great promise for the treatment of tuberculosis and HIV. A comprehensive discussion of integrated approaches toward modern drug development derived from Ayurveda is elaborated in the *Journal of Ethnopharmacology,* 2006, Volume 103, pp. 25–35. The principles of Ayurveda have also been used in agriculture for centuries. Renewed interest and current research investigations have arisen with the publication of a text believed to have been written around the seventh to tenth century A.D. (Sadhale, N. [translator]. 1996. *Surapala's Vrikshayurveda, The Science of Plant Life.* Secunderbad, India: Asian Agri-History Foundation). A major compendium, *Scientific Basis for Ayurvedic Therapies,* edited by L.C. Mishra (2004), introduces the work of a broad number of Western and Indian physicians and researchers using standard scientific methodogy; hence, it is an important addition to the evidence-based foundation of Ayurvedic practices.

Yamini Tripathi, Ph.D, Professor and Head of the Department of Medicinal Chemistry at the Institute of Medical Sciences, Banaras Hindu University in Varanasi, India, has worked extensively with Ayurvedic plants for over 22 years. His work involves herbal biotechnology and the scientifically recognized standardization of plant substances used in Ayurveda. His research has produced drug patents (2002) for the prevention of radiation hazards and carcinomas. Some of his current work has been reviewed in the Ayurvedic journal *Elements,* vol. 2, no. 1, 2004 (ISSN#1557-0592).

Rajendra Badgaiyan, M.D., Assistant Professor of Radiology at Harvard Medical School and Associate Neuroscientist at Massachusetts General Hospital in Boston, has published extensively on the interface between consciousness and brain processing using a variety of imaging techniques and including event-related potentials (ERPs) and positron emission tomography (PET) (*International Journal of Psychophysiology* 55:257–262, 2005; *Human Brain Mapping* 10:197–203, 2000).

A new class of what appears to be a novel, endogenous neurotransmitter system, the endocannabinoid, has only recently been discovered. One of the main cell-based ligands is N-arachidonoylethanolamine. The medicinal and psychotropic use of Cannabis or marijuana has a long history in the East. Interestingly enough, the body's own ligand has been named *anandamide,* which is derived from the Hindu word *Ananda* meaning bliss or joy. Anandamides have been found to lower intraocular pressure, decrease activity level, and relieve pain. A high concentration in the thalamus suggests a relationship to anxiety, fear, and other emotional states (Siegel, Albers, Brady, and Price,

2006). Evidence-based medicine is now uncovering the scientific details of traditional practices.

In 1998, the United States government established the National Center for Complementary Medicine and Alternative Medicine (NCCAM) within the National Institutes of Health (NIH). Many scientifically based clinical trials at NIH and academic research institutions are currently investigating the potential benefits of herbs as well as other practices. In addition to advancing scientific research, NCCAM trains complementary and alternative medicine researchers, disseminates timely and accurate information, and supports the integration of proven complementary therapies.

A new generation of adherents to Ayurvedic medicine, many having Western training in mainstream scientific methodologies, has arisen both in India and in the United States. Ayurveda continues to remain a living body of knowledge, theory, treatment, and health maintenance. It can be seen to be evolving and adaptively responding to the demands of evidence-based medicine; at this juncture in history, Ayurveda is science in a context of discovery. This adds contemporary validity to its apt justification as a science of life, life wisdom.

Appendix 1

AYURVEDIC ORAL AND WRITTEN TRADITION TIMELINE

These works have only approximate dates of origin and many are not available in English translation.

Pre-1000 B.C.: Vedic *rishis* receive and transmit the Ayurvedic conception as an oral tradition that only later becomes explicitly codified in the four Vedic texts, *Rig-Veda, Sama-Veda, Yajur-Veda,* and especially the *Atharva-Veda.*

c. 760 B.C.: *Charaka Samhita* of Charaka. This is the axiomatic, foundational text, broadest in scope, that delineates Ayurvedic medicine.

c. 660 B.C.: *Sushruta Samhita* of Sushruta. This is the next fundamental medical text but with a strong emphasis on the structure, functioning, and treatment of blood tissue and on surgery.

c. A.D. 100: Nāgārjuna's texts on Materia Medica with original contributions of iatrochemistry, the medicinal preparation of minerals.

c. A.D. seventh century: *Asthanga Sagraha* and *Asthanga Hridaya* of Vagbhata of Sind: texts that are a summary of the previous works of Charaka and Sushruta.

c. 1331: *Madhava Nidana* of Madhava (Vidyaraya) of Kishkindha, southern India. This is the most comprehensive text that delineates Ayurvedic diagnosis and the classification of disease.

c. fourteenth century: *Sarangadhara Samhita.* Ayurvedic pulse diagnosis presented in detail.

c. 1483: *Rasapradipa* by Vashaldeva. This text describes the medicinal use of purified mercury preparations.

c. 1495: *Rasamrita* by Pandit Vaidya Kendra. This work describes the pharmacology of mineral and metal medicinal substances.

c. 1550: *Bhavaprakasha* by Bhava Mishra of Madra Desha near Benares in northwest India. This is held to be the most important summary of the scope of all Ayurvedic medicine to date with special attention to dietary and rejuvenative treatment innovations.

c. 1633: *Yogaratnakara* by Nayanashekara, a Jain priest. This text elaborates the art of compounding medicinal preparations.

c. 1734: *Ayurveda Prakasha* by Madhava of Benares. This is a work on Materia Medica.

c. 1751: *Yogatarangini* by Trimulla Bhatta: a nosology of Ayurvedic Materia Medica.

c. 1794: *Jvaraparajaya* by Jayaravi: a work on the nature of fever.

c. 1859: *Hastamalka* by Bavabhai. This is an updated consideration of the preparation of mineral-based medicinal preparations.

c. 1867: *Nighantaratnakara* by Vishnu Vasudeva Godbole. The body of this work constitutes additional notes on Ayurvedic medicine and pharmacology.

Appendix 2

DISEASES CAUSED BY THE *DOSHAS*

Disorders Caused by *Vata*

1. *Aksepaka* (clonic convulsion)
2. *Aksibheda* (eye pain)
3. *Aksisula* (pinching pain in eye)
4. *Aksivyudasa* (ptosis of eyeball)
5. *Anavasthitacittatva* (mental disorder and agitation)
6. *Arasajnata* (impairment of taste)
7. *Ardita* (facial paralysis)
8. *Asabdasravana* (tinnitus and partial hearing loss)
9. *Asvapna* or *Asapna* (insomnia)
10. *Atipralapa* (delirium)
11. *Badhirya* (deafness)
12. *Bahusosa* (atrophy of arm)
13. *Bhrama* (giddiness or dizziness)
14. *Bhruvyudasa* (ptosis of eyebrow)
15. *Dandaka* (tonic convulsion)
16. *Dantabheda* (toothache or tooth loss)
17. *Dantasathilya* (loose teeth)
18. *Ekangaroga* (monoplegia)
19. *Ghrananasa* (impairment of smell)
20. *Gridhrasi* (sciatica)
21. *Grivastambha* (stiffness of neck)
22. *Gudabhramsa* (prolapsed rectum)
23. *Gudarti* (tenesmus or rectal ulceration)
24. *Gulphagraha* (stiff and painful ankle)
25. *Hanubheda* (jaw pain, dislocation of face bones)
26. *Hikka* (hiccup)

27. *Hriddrava* (tachycardia)
28. *Hrinmoha* (bradycardia)
29. *Janubheda* (bow legs)
30. *Januvislesa* (knock knees)
31. *Jirmbha* (yawning)
32. *Kanthoddhvamsa* (hoarseness)
33. *Karnasula* (earache)
34. *Kasayasyata* (Astringent taste in mouth)
35. *Kesabhumisphutana* (dandruff or scalp sores)
36. *Khanjatva* (ambulation disorder)
37. *Kubjatva* (kyphosis)
38. *Lalatabheda* (pain or fracture in frontal skull bone)
39. *Manyastambha* (torticollis)
40. *Mukatva* (aphasia)
41. *Mukhasosa* (dry mouth)
42. *Nakhabheda* (cracking of nails)
43. *Osthabheda* (lip pain)
44. *Padabhramsa* (peroneal nerve palsy)
45. *Padasula* (pain in foot)
46. *Padasuptata* (numbness of foot)
47. *Paksavadha* (hemiplegia)
48. *Pangulya* (paraplegia)
49. *Parsvavamarda* (pain in chest or flanks)
50. *Pindikodvestana* (calf cramps)
51. *Pristhagraha* (stiffness and pain in the back)
52. *Rauksa Parusya* (dryness and hardness)
53. *Sankhabheda* (pain fracture in temporal skull bone)
54. *Sarvangaroga* (polyplegia)
55. *Sephastambha* (stiffness of penis)
56. *Siroruk* (headache)
57. *Sronibheda* or *Conitabheda* (pain, possibly bleeding, around the pelvic girdle)
58. *Syavarunavabhasata* (dusky red complexion)
59. *Tama* (severe fatigue or fainting)
60. *Timira* (cataract)
61. *Trikagraha* (arthritis of sacroiliac joint)
62. *Uccaihsriti* (hard of hearing)
63. *Udaravesta* (spasmodic abdominal pain)

64. *Udavarta* (peristaltic dysfunction)
65. *Urusada* (thigh pain and weakness)
66. *Urustambha* (stiffness, arthritis, or paralysis of thigh)
67. *Vaksanga* (hesitant, stammering speech)
68. *Vaksastoda* (stabbing pain in chest)
69. *Vaksa Uddharsa* (dull chest pain felt as coming from inside)
70. *Vaksa Uparodha* (impairment of thoracic movement felt as imposed from outside)
71. *Vamanatva* (dwarfism)
72. *Vanksananaha* (pain and tenseness in groin)
73. *Vartmasankoca* (eyelid inversion)
74. *Vartmastambha* (ptosis or paralysis of eyelid)
75. *Vatakhuddata* (club and painful foot)
76. *Vidbheda* (diarrhea)
77. *Vipadika* (cracking, sores, or blisters of feet)
78. *Visada* (asthenia)
79. *Vrisanaksepa* (pain or hernia in scrotum)
80. *Yepathu* (tremor)

Disorders Caused by *Pitta*

1. *Aksipaka* (conjunctivitis)
2. *Amlaka* (acid eructation)
3. *Amsadaha* (burning sensation in shoulders)
4. *Angagandha* (unpleasant body odor)
5. *Angavadarana* (cracking pain or sores on the body)
6. *Antardaha* (burning sensation in the chest)
7. *Asyavipaka* (stomatitis)
8. *Atisveda* (excessive perspiration)
9. *Atripti* (inability to feel satiated)
10. *Carmadalana* (itching of the skin)
11. *Daha* (sensation of burning)
12. *Davathu* (sensation of boiling)
13. *Dhumaka* (sensation of fuming)
14. *Galapaka* (pharyngitis)
15. *Gudapaka* (proctitis)
16. *Haridratva* (yellow tinge to the skin)
17. *Haritaharida netra muttra varcastva* (greenish and yellowish coloration of eyes, urine, and feces).

18. *Haritatva* (green tinge to the skin)
19. *Jivadana* (bloody stools)
20. *Kaksa* (herpes or skin abcesses)
21. *Kamala* (jaundice)
22. *Lohitagandhasyata* (smell of blood from the mouth)
23. *Mamsakleda* (muscular disorder)
24. *Medhrapaka* (inflammation of the penis)
25. *Nilika* (blue or black skin moles)
26. *Osa* (sensation of inordinate body heat)
27. *Plosa* (sensation of body being scorched by fire)
28. *Putimukhata* (halitosis)
29. *Raktakostha* (urticaria)
30. *Raktamandala* (red wheals)
31. *Raktapitta* (bleeding tendency)
32. *Raktavisphota* (red vesicles)
33. *Sonitakleda* (hematological disorder)
34. *Tamahpravesa* (delirium and fainting)
35. *Tvagavadarana* (cracking of the skin)
36. *Tvagdaha* (burning sensation of the skin)
37. *Tiktasyata* (Bitter taste in mouth)
38. *Trisnadhikya* (excessive thirst)
39. *Usmadhikya* (increased temperature)
40. *Vidaha* (burning sensation in chest)

Disorders Caused by *Kapha*

1. *Alasya* (lethargy)
2. *Apakti* (inability to digest food)
3. *Atisthaulya* (obesity)
4. *Balasada* (severe loss of strength)
5. *Dhamanipraticaya* (hardening of vessels)
6. *Galaganda* (goiter)
7. *Gurugatrata* (heaviness of the body)
8. *Hridayopalepa* (fluid buildup in cardiac region)
9. *Kanthopalepa* (phlegm adhering to throat)
10. *Maladhikya* (excessive excretion of bodily wastes)
11. *Mukhamadhurya* (Sweet taste in mouth)
12. *Mukhasrava* (salivation)
13. *Nidradhikya* (excessive sleep)

14. *Sitagnitva* (suppression of digestive power and loss of appetite)
15. *Slesmodgirana* (mucous expectoration)
16. *Staimitya* (timidity)
17. *Svetavabhasata* and *Svetamutranetravarcastva* (pallor and whiteness of urine, eye, and feces).
18. *Tandra* (drowsiness)
19. *Tripti* (the sense of feeling full without having eaten)
20. *Udarda* (uticaria or erysipelas)

Appendix 3

CLINICAL CASE EXAMPLES

The following is a representative sampling of some common disorders. The views of Western medicine and those of Ayurveda are compared. Standard medical treatments of disease and Ayurvedic approaches toward balancing vitiated *doshas* are presented. The perspective put forth here is one of offering treatment choices and, perhaps, mutually enhancing complementary treatment strategies. Illness manifestations are unique in each patient. In Ayurveda, the orienting principles of assessment and management rest on the detailed analysis of *Vata, Pitta,* and *Kapha.* The careful evaluation of *prakruti* (individual constitution) is given punctilious attention. Nuances of the manifold qualities and attributes of the *doshas,* and the specific circumstances of timing, life-cycle stage, and the seasons, play a significant role in the inception and manifestation of the disease process, all of which impacts the quality of the patient's life. A rational approach to any disorder would include an appropriate examination by a qualified medical doctor in order to secure a sound diagnosis and treatment plan. This then provides one with a rational basis for the selection of appropriate and reasonable treatment choices. The following examples of Ayurvedically based care represent commonly seen, broad clinical presentations and are submitted, in general terms, only to suggest general management guidelines. Therapies that are more specific must be individualized by the medical doctor or the Ayurvedic practitioner depending on the particular manifestations of a disorder as it emerges at a particular time in the life of a patient. An important therapeutic issue and difference between Western medicine and Ayurvedic approaches is that Ayurveda addresses developing trends (imbalances of the *doshas*) that, if left unchecked, may develop into fully manifested disorders. In addition, Ayurveda always takes into consideration the complete *BioPsychoSpiritual* person when assessing and recommending balancing approaches. The comprehensive nature of Ayurvedic evaluation and care incorporating both physical and psychological aspects (*umada*) can even be found in the writings of Charaka over 2,000 years ago (Haldipur, 1984, 1989).

PREMENSTRUAL SYNDROME

Premenstrual syndrome (PMS) is a recurrent condition that affects about 35 percent of menstruating women with peak occurrences in their 30s and 40s. The clinical presentation manifests about 7 to 14 days before the onset of menstruation. While the signs and symptoms may be varied, the following are often present: decreased energy level, irritability, mood sensitivity, tension, general malaise, dysphoria, altered libido, breast pain, backache, abdominal bloating, and edematous swelling of hands and ankles. The biological mechanisms responsible for PMS are complex. Some major features, however, include relatively high estrogen and relatively low progesterone levels with an increased ratio of estrogen to progesterone; corpus luteum insufficiency with increased prolactin levels; and possibly lowered thyroid function and elevated cortisol levels.

While Western medicine recognizes the occurrence of this syndrome, there is no consensus regarding formal and standardized treatment. Symptoms such as pain are treated with analgesic medications, depression with antidepressants, and edema with antidiuretic drugs, for example. Ayurveda approaches the treatment of PMS by first examining the individual patient to establish the basic *prakruti* (constitutional type) and then the *vikruti* (current state of *dosha* imbalance within the *prakruti*). Although all three *doshas* (*Vata, Pitta,* and *Kapha*) may be vitiated, *Vata* is usually the primary *dosha* with *Pitta* and *Kapha* being secondarily affected.

Treatment strategies address each *dosha. Kapha* is usually increased due to excess *Ama* (toxins). This results in edema, sluggishness, and lowered energy level. Dietary recommendations would include a lighter than average diet and the avoidance of all cold foods and dairy products. Hot tea and ample amounts of dry and fresh ginger in tea and foods would act to reduce excess *Kapha* and *Ama*. This, in turn, would reduce the associated signs and symptoms. The vitiated *Pitta* aspects of PMS show as irritability, mood sensitivity, sensations of heat, skin irritation, and irregular menstrual blood flow. To the extent that this may be the dominant clinical presentation, one would recommend an anti-*Pitta* diet that would exclude meat, nuts, alcohol, sour fruits, fermented foods, hot spices, and include more cooling foods like small amounts of dairy products, ghee, vegetables, and salads. Herbs such as aloe vera, turmeric, coriander, fennel, and saffron could be added to foods. The *Vata* aspect of PMS presents as anxiety, depression, insomnia, constipation, and cramping. To the extent that these symptoms predominate, one would recommend a diet that is warm, moderately oily, and regular as opposed to light or heavy. Herbs that balance *Vata* include shatavari, cinnamon, licorice, asafetida, and nutmeg. *Abhyanga* (oil massage) with warm sesame oil is particularly beneficial to pacify vitiated *Vata* and reduce dysphoria and agitation; the use of warm castor oil packs on the lower abdomen may also be soothing.

ATTENTION-DEFICIT/HYPERACTIVITY DISORDER

Attention-Deficit/Hyperactivity Disorder (ADHD) is a disruptive behavior disorder usually beginning in childhood before age 7 (Ninivaggi, 1999). Poor attention and concentration, motoric overactivity, and impulsivity characterize its presentation. Poor organizational skills, academic difficulties, low self-esteem, and behavioral problems often accompany this symptom constellation and manifest both at home and at school. Up to 5 percent of the school-age population is affected, with a preponderance of boys. ADHD usually occurs in conjunction with other psychiatric disorders and may be a secondary feature of or may disguise a primary problem such as a major mood disorder or a posttraumatic stress experience. There are no medically established causes responsible for producing this condition. Psychiatry considers it a clinical diagnosis with a variety of mixed contributing etiologies.

Western medicine treats ADHD with combined psychopharmacological and psychosocial interventions. Often, the psychostimulant drugs, such as methylphenidate, dextroamphetamine, and Adderall, are used. These substances are tightly controlled by the Drug Enforcement Agency of the federal government because of their abuse potential, tolerance, and withdrawal liabilities. As with all medications, there may be undesirable adverse drug effects. Other medications may be used, especially to address the other target symptoms that often accompany ADHD. The range of psychotherapies includes individual, group, and family therapy as well as a variety of behavior management strategies. Specialized educational programming is always necessary. Since the condition is usually chronic, treatments may go on for years.

Ayurveda considers ADHD to be a primary disorder of *Vata*. Treatment, therefore, includes a strict *Vata*-pacifying protocol. Some important features of this are the following: In general, nurturing, warming, moistening, calming, and grounding qualities should characterize all interventions. Dietary guidelines would stress a substantive, nutritive, and wholesome diet that predominates in tastes that are Sweet, Sour, and Salty. Since food allergies play some role in health and disease, a diet that minimizes dairy and wheat products and emphasizes rice, oats, fish, chicken, eggs, nuts, seeds, cooked vegetables, sweet and some citrus fruits, and oils is recommended. Most beans, raw vegetables, dry fruits, dry light snacks such as popcorn, and soda should be avoided. Food spices that are moderate in nature, such as ginger, fennel, cardamom, and cinnamon, may be used to optimize digestion. There are a variety of herbal tonics, such as ashwaghanda, shatavari, jatamansi, gotu kola, and basil, for example, that may be used depending on the needs of the patient. Modified *abhyanga* (oil massage) is of great benefit. Small amounts of oils such as sesame and almond may be gently massaged on parts of the head and feet before bed. Lifestyle suggestions would include early rising by 7 to 8 A.M., going to sleep about 10 P.M., and the reduction and significant moderation of highly stimulating activities such as listening to loud music, excessive watching of TV and movies, and excessive physical exercise.

A program of guided quiet time, i.e., meditation and breathing regulation (*pranayama*), should be structured into the child's daily routine by a responsible adult. As mentioned in Chapter 9, aspects of Yoga techniques, especially those directed to self-regulation of the body (*Hatha* Yoga) and the mind (*dhyana*) may contribute to increased attention and concentration. The quality time that a parent spends with a child may be viewed as therapeutic in the broadest sense; its therapeutic value is inestimable. One would consider, of course, the mutually enhancing interventions of the appropriate psychotherapies and solid educational programming to complement Ayurvedic care.

ASTHMA

Asthma is a disease of the respiratory airways characterized by inflammation, increased responsiveness of the tracheobronchial tree to a multiplicity of stimuli, neuronal activation, changes in vascular permeability, and increased mucus production. Signs and symptoms of narrowing of the air passages include paroxysms of shortness of breath, cough, and wheezing. This takes an episodic course with acute exacerbations being interspersed with periods of remission.

Western medicine regards the etiology of the spectrum of asthmatic presentations as heterogeneous and ambiguous at this time, although the inflammatory process is central. Subtypes are classified by the principal stimuli that trigger a flare-up. This distinction is regarded as artificial, in part, since specific causative factors and clear-cut disease states continue to be under investigation in order to refine current views. Three broad subtypes are recognized: (1) extrinsic or atopic asthma that has an allergic component characterized by elevated levels of serum IgE, the allergic antibody, and a personal or family history of asthma; (2) intrinsic or idiosyncratic asthma that appears not to be due to allergy and not having a family history, but rather the result of factors such as toxic chemicals, infection, exercise, cold air, and emotional stressors; and (3) mixed group asthma that has features of both the aforementioned types. Approximately 4 to 5 percent of the U.S. population is affected, and children under 10 constitute about 50 percent of cases. A commonly used four-step classification of asthma severity is based on clinical features before treatment. Step 1 is mild and intermittent asthma; step 2 is mild and persistent; step 3 is moderate and persistent; step 4 is severe and persistent.

Since an asthmatic attack may become a medical emergency, only a qualified medical doctor should evaluate and treat this potentially life-threatening circumstance. Routine care, according to Western medicine, includes attempts at removing known and suspected environmental causes, e.g., allergens, house dust, mold, fungi, and smoke, as well as using additional preventative desensitization or immunotherapy. Drug treatments are commonly used to control asthma. Chronic management includes (1) drugs that inhibit smooth muscle contraction, i.e., specific inhaler bronchodilators, especially for acute exacerbations; (2) agents that prevent or reverse inflammation, such as glucocorticoids and mast cell-stabilizing agents, especially for chronic maintenance; and (3) drugs that have antihistaminic and decongestant properties only as medically prescribed according to the needs of the particular condition. Ongoing medical monitoring care is mandatory.

Svasa roga or asthma is a condition that has been recognized in Ayurveda for thousands of years. Five types have been classified: (1) *maha svasa,* or great asthma, is the most severe and may include what in the West is called "status asthmaticus"; (2) *urdhva svasa,* or upwards asthma, a serious condition characterized by great difficulty in inhalation; (3) *chinna svasa,* or broken asthma, characterized by very irregular breathing that periodically halts, distension of the abdomen, and possible hemorrhaging in the head area; (4) *tamaka svasa,* or allergic asthma, characterized by pain, dryness, and wheezing; and (5) *ksudra svasa,* or minor asthma, characterized by minor and transient asthmatic symptomatology.

In Ayurvedic theory, all asthma components originate in the stomach, then pass though the channels carrying *rasa* (plasma) until they finally localize in the lungs. After comprehensive evaluation and assessment to determine the specifics of the particular case, intervention always begins by correcting the *Kapha* imbalances in the stomach. Since acute exacerbations may be life threatening, they should be treated by conventional medical techniques. Preventative care, i.e., between attacks, is conducive to Ayurvedic prophylaxis.

To prevent and reduce inordinate production of mucus, a *Kapha*-pacifying diet would include avoidance of all dairy products, no cold foods, and the inclusion of a light diet of cooked vegetables with as many pungent food spices (black pepper, red pepper, sage, ginger, etc.) as is possible to consume comfortably. Yogurt and bananas are to be avoided since they strongly increase *Kapha.* The therapeutic herb pippali is very useful in resolving vitiated *Kapha*conditions. When *Pitta* vitiation, evidenced by the production of yellow mucus, inflammation, and irritation, is prominent, then *Pitta*-pacifying herbs are added. These may include coriander, gotu kola, and turmeric. In addition to *Kapha* and *Pitta* factors, there is always a disturbance of *Vata* manifest by increased motoric activity and agitation. When this is an outstanding feature of the clinical presentation, a *Vata*-pacifying diet, recommendations for a slower paced life-style, and herbs such as haritaki, asafetida, and a mineral-based preparation of mica called *abhraka bhasma* are given. Respiratory distress is aggravated by the improper upward movement of *Apana Vata;* the aforementioned diet, herbs, and minerals tend to normalize this. In addition, moist heat with aromatic herbs and oils such as eucalyptus and menthol applied to the chest helps to liquefy excess *Kapha* and aid in relaxing and opening bronchial airways.

GLOSSARY

Abhaya: Fearless.

Abhinivesha: Instinctive craving for life.

Abhraka bhasma: Ayurvedically prepared mineral-based medicine with mica as the principal ingredient.

Abhyanga: Whole body oil massage.

Abhyasa: Practice; practical application and implementation.

Abyantar: Therapeutic internal oleation treatment.

Achintya: Unpredictable; beyond intellectual reasoning.

Achit: Nonconsciousness.

Acrid: Sharp and irritating, in the sense of Bitter taste.

Adana: Plain cooked rice. Also denotes receiving.

Adana Kala: The hot and dry time of the year, generally summer in the United States; see *Agneya.*

Adhibhautika: Causes of a disease that originate in the external environment.

Adhidaivika: Causes of a disease that have more esoteric origins, i.e., *karma,* fate, etc.

Adhishyandi: Therapeutic and moistening diet used to increase vitiated *doshas* on a temporary basis.

Adhyaropa: False cover, false interpretation, masking.

Adhyasa: According to Shankara, all subject-object knowledge is distorted by *adhyasa* or the superimposition that falsifies knowledge in such a way that the subject is unable to find objective truth.

Adhyatmika: Causes of a disease that originate from within the physical body: (1) *adhibala* (genetic), (2) *janmaja* (congenital), and (3) *dosaja* (due to *doshas*).

Adhyatmika gunas: The six psychological qualities to be highlighted on the path to self-realization and the refinement of consciousness. They are *Buddhi, Iccha, Dvesha, Sukha, Duhkha,* and *Prayatna.*

Adivasis: Peoples who were indigenous to ancient India; the first inhabitants; or the tribal groups within India.

Advaita: Nonduality; akin to the Western philosophical idea of monism.

Advaita-Vedanta: The *darshana* or worldview made explicit by Shankara (ninth century A.D.) stressing the absolute unity of all reality; also called *Utarra Mimamsa*.

Agadatantra: Toxicology, one of the eight branches of Ayurveda.

Agantu: Exogenous causes of disease.

Agneya: The warm and hot time of the year; in the United States, usually spring and summer.

Agni: Fire. In the *Vedas: Agni* is personified as a deity; both the deity and the physical, externally real fire that is the centerpiece of the most sacred ritual observance. In Ayurveda, *Agni* is the internal digestive fire responsible for nutrient transformation and tissue and cellular assimilation.

Agnimandya: Impaired *Agni*.

Agniyashaya: Pancreas.

Ahamkara: The individualized ego or circumscribed identity of any biological being.

Aham tarka: Self-inquiry, looking inward; self-examination aimed at achieving insight.

Ahara: Dietary food intake.

Ahara rasa: The preliminary state of the nutritive fluid just after ingestion and in the process of primary digestion; it is nonhomologous and as yet biologically unassimilable.

Aharayogin: Spices.

Ahimsa: Nonviolence.

Ahita: Improper, incompatible, unwholesome.

Ajativada: A Sanskrit word that refers to a concept found in some branches of Hinduism, in Buddhism, and in Jainism that creation as such is a non-event.

Ajna Chakra: The sixth energy node along the *sushumna* or central energy channel located in the area of the brain between the eyes; correlates with insight and enlightenment.

Akasha: The Ether or Space great Element.

Akrita yusha: Mixture of rice and mung lentils in a mild soup base.

Alaya: The unconscious foundation of the mind.

Alochaka Pitta: The subdosha of *Pitta* associated with vision in the eyes.

Ama: The toxic metabolic end product resulting from improper digestion; one of several factors that contributes to disease.

Amalaki: Amla fruit (*Emblica officinalis*); also called *Dhatri;* best for *Pitta* and rejuvenation.

Amashaya: Stomach.

Amaya: Disease.

Ambu: Water.

Amla: Sour taste; *Amla* medicinal fruit (*Phyllanthus Emblica; Emblica officinalis*); sometimes called emblic myrobalan. *Amla* was described in superlative terms by Charaka.

Amrit: Nectar.

Anabolism: The metabolic phase of cellular and tissue buildup.

Anahata Chakra: The energy node located in the region of the heart; associated with OM/AUM.

Ananda: Bliss; state of experiential joy; effortless relaxation; also translated as "love."

Anandamaya Kosha: The bliss sheath; the last of five layers or sheaths that compose the individual human being.

Anapanasati: Buddhist concept of meditation using mindfulness of breath and breathing.

Anekantavada: The philosophical perspective that connotes multiplicity within unity; the world as manifold, an ever-changing reality perceived by an infinite spectrum of viewpoints that differ depending on time, place, and the state of the perceiver or knower in relation to the perceived or that which is known. A Jain axiom.

Anguli pramana: Bodily proportions.

Anna: Food.

Annamaya Kosha: The food sheath; the gross, physical body; the first of five layers or sheaths and the most material dimension comprising the complete individual.

Annapanavidhi: Nutrition.

Annavaha Srotas: The digestive system, alimentary canal, or gastrointestinal tract.

Antahkarana: The inner organ or instrument of cognition and feeling; also *Antarindriya:* includes *Buddhi, Ahamkara, Manas,* and *Chitta(m).*

Antarindriya: *Antahkarana.*

Antharmarga: The Inner Disease Pathway that includes the gastrointestinal tract and the plasma tissue.

Anu: Ancient Indian term roughly akin to the modern concept of subatomic particle or atom; theory first formulated by the Indian Kanada (c. 600 B.C.).

Anubhava: Awareness that develops experientially from a surface understanding toward a more direct, intuitive, and profound apprehension.

Anuloma: Proper flow, especially of *Vata.*

Anumana: Reasoning based on inference.

Anuvasana Basti: Therapeutic enema of oil and herbs.

Ap: One of the Five Great Gross Elements, Water; also *Jala, Apas.*

Apana Vata: The downward moving subdosha of *Vata* primarily located in the colon.

Aparigraha: Nonoverindulgence and detachment; this is the counter attitude to desire, craving, hankering, lust, envy, greed, and jealousy.

Apas: The Element of Water; also called *Jala, Ap.*

Apauruseya: Not man-made, but of divine origin; denotes *sruti.*

Apta: The inspired and authoritative wisdom of sages (*rishis*).

Aptopadesha/Shabda: Information from texts, authoritative literature, and interviews.

Apurva: A concept used in *Mimamsa darshana* to denote the results of one's obedience to the Vedic mandates to perform rituals, and so make it more likely to accumulate the necessary grace (*apurva*) in one's lifetime to merit heaven (*svarga*) upon death.

Aranyakas: Texts of the *Vedas* composed in the forests and that consist of mystical interpretations of the chronologically earlier Vedic teachings.

Ardhashakti: Point in time after the initiation of exercise at which metabolic rate is increased as reflected in increased sweating, temperature, heart rate, pulse, and respiration; generally about 20 minutes; reflects an individual's *mamsa bala* (muscle strength) and *Agni bala* (strength of metabolic functioning).

Aristha: Herbal wine; connotation of an omen, sign, or symptom with a negative prognosis.

Arogya: Health.

Artav: Menstrual fluid; also spelled *artava.*

Artavavaha Srotas: The menstrual system.

Artav Beej: Maternal genetic material.

Artha: Necessary and appropriate material wealth; the Vedic life goal of securing appropriate wealth and possessions; also meaning the objects possessed by the five senses.

Arunasayava: Skin discolorations.

Arya: Noble, virtuous, honorable.

Arya Satya: The Four Noble Truths that constitute the foundation of Buddhism: (1) *Duhkha,* suffering exists; (2) *Trishna,* desire is the cause of suffering; (3) *Nirodha,* there is a method to attenuate and heal suffering; (4) *Asthanga Marga,* an Eightfold Path delineating the method to manage suffering.

Aryavarta: Ancient Vedic name for present-day India.

Asadhya: Disease with an unfavorable prognosis.

Asafetida: Spice (*Ferula asafoetida*).

Asamprajnata-samadhi: In Classical Yoga, the ultimate, "no-mind" state of consciousness wherein experience, paradoxically, is devoid of subject and object.

Asamskara: Unprocessed.

Asana: Yoga posture; seat.

Asantarpana: The difficult and arduous psychological sense that one experiences when undergoing *langhana* or reducing therapies that require abstinence.

Asatmya: Unwholesome.

Asatmyendriyartha Samyoga: The unwholesome and incompatible contact of the sense organs with their objects; this can range from no contact to excessive contact; a fundamental factor in the universal etiology of all disorders.

Ashaya: Hollow viscera; organ.

Ashtavidha Pariksha: The diagnostic examination of a patient using eight parameters.

Ashwaghanda: Herbal root (*Withania somnifera*).

Asmita: Unhealthy egoism; egotistical narcissism; inordinate self-preoccupation.

Asrama The Vedic delineation of four stages of life: student, family life, self-inquiry, and active pursuit of *Moksha*.

Asteya: Nonstealing.

Asthanga: Eight limbs.

Asthanga Ayurveda: The eight branches of Ayurvedic medicine: (1) internal medicine; (2) surgery; (3) otolaryngology and ophthalmology; (4) obstetrics, gynecology, and pediatrics; (5) toxicology; (6) psychiatry; (7) antiaging medicine; and (8) reproductive and aphrodisiac medicine.

Asthanga Hridaya: Ayurvedic text written by Ayurvedic surgeon Vagbhata (c. seventh century A.D.).

Asthanga Marga: The Eightfold Path of Buddhism; the methods used to manage human suffering caused by desire.

Asthanga Yoga: The eight steps of *Raja Yoga;* the path of self-regulation and the refinement of consciousness whose achievement is *Samadhi, Nirvana,* or *Moksha.*

Asthayi: Unprocessed, immature, unstable; similar to *poshya* and *posaya.*

Asthi: Bone tissue.

Asthidhara kala: The membrane of bone; also the membrane of the colon.

Asthivaha Srotas: The channels of circulation of bone tissue.

Astika darshana: Any orthodox worldview based on the primary authority of the *Vedas.*

Atapa-sevana: Therapeutic sun bathing.

Atharva-Veda: One of the four primary *Vedas,* considered the last one compiled, that is composed of 731 hymns whose content includes atonement ceremonies, maledictions, marriage and burial songs, and medical formulas.

Ati: Excessive, outermost, peripheral, reaching the highest levels.

Atipravrutti: Excessive flow.

Atiyoga: Excessive use or excessive contact.

Atman: The real, immortal Self or spirit of an individual; the microcosmic correlate of *Brahman.* In Buddhism, its meaning is approximated by terms such as Buddha-*dhatu,* Buddha-nature, and Buddha-Self. In Chinese contexts, it is the *Dharmakaya.*

AUM: This is a designation, sound, syllable, word, and symbol that refers to several things. It derives from the Devanagari alphabet descended from Brahmi script (2000 B.C.–500 B.C.) sometime around the eleventh century A.D. , originally developed to write Sanskrit but eventually used to write other Indian languages such as Hindi, Pali, Marathi, and Sindhi, for example. As a symbol form, it reflects the visible and concrete manifestation of Absolute Truth: consciousness pervading the universe. The worlds of the physical, mental, and unconscious are represented in the letters of the syllable AUM by the three curves that make it up. As a syllable or sound, it reflects the spiritual power within the consciousness that is the rock bottom of the entire universe. It is a sound used in meditation and in rituals. It also appears in *Vajrayana* Buddhism. AUM is the ordinary Hindu spelling; in Buddhism, it is also spelled OM. It is also denoted by the term *"Pranava,"* the soundless sound, sacred primordial Word, or Logos that attended the launching of creation. Discussions of AUM are found in the Chandogya, Mandukya, and Taittirya *Upanishads.*

Aura: The subtle energy field emanating from the body.

Aushadha: Herb or drug; also *oshadhi.*

Avalambaka Kapha: The subdosha of *Kapha* providing lubrication in the chest and spine.

Avaleha: Herbal formula with the consistency of a jelly or jam.

Avarana: Concealing.

Avastha: State of a thing, as, for example, a state of consciousness.

Avasthamabhana: Support, especially of the colon provided by the feces.

Avasthapaka: Primary digestion; also *Prapaka.*

Avidya: Ignorance.

Avyakta: Pure existence in its unmanifest state.

Ayana: Flow; circulation; pathway.

Ayoga: Negligible or deficient contact.

Ayurveda: The knowledge, science, and wisdom of life and longevity; an *Upaveda* or accessory *Veda* to the *Atharva-Veda.*

Ayu: Life.

Ayus: Life; a period or measure of life; see *Ayu.*

Ayushah pramana: Lifespan as the quantitative measure of an individual's duration of life.

Bahir: External.

Bahya: Therapeutic external oil massage.

Bala: Strength or power in the body; childhood; the herb *Sida cordifolia.*

Bandha: Bondage to or dependence on the material world that is mediated by the sensory faculties.

Bandhu: The correspondence or harmonizing, meaningful link between ritual, lifestyle choices and routines, and the cosmic order.

Basil: Herb (*Ocinum* spp.).

Basti: Ayurvedic therapeutic enema.

Bayhamarga: The Outer, Peripheral Disease Pathway leading into the limbs and the deeper compact tissues.

Bhagavad Gita: The sixth book of the Indian national epic poem, *Mahabharata,* composed between the fifth century B.C. and the second century A.D. that presents a spiritual gospel of values, ethics, devotion, and principles of self-development toward the goal of enlightenment and liberation (*Moksha*).

Bhakti Yoga: The Yoga of devotion.

Bharata: India.

Bhasma: Ayurvedic medicinal incinerated mineral, metal ash, or oxide.

Bhastrika: A therapeutic form of intense breathing resembling the action of a bellows.

Bhasyas: Commentaries on more primary writings.

Bhava: Becoming.

Bhavana: The process of transformation and production that has several connotations. In a material sense, sometimes using a mortar and pestle, *bhavana* is used to enhance or improve the qualities of a substance. In a spiritual sense, it is meditation. In a psychological sense, it includes techniques of self-development.

Bhavaprakasha: Sixteenth century Ayurvedic text delineating a range of medical treatments.

Bhaya: Fear.

Bheda: Piercing; existing in a state of divisions; the phase of pathogenesis that is the stage of differentiation.

Bhishak: Ayurvedic physician.

Bhrajaka Pitta: The subdosha of *Pitta* giving color and warmth to the skin.

Bhujangasana: The Yoga posture (cobralike) beneficial for *Tarpaka Kapha.*

Bhumi: Level or stage of maturation.

Bhuta: One of the Five Great Gross Elements that compose all physical matter: Ether, Air, Fire, Water, and Earth.

Bhutagni: The digestive fire residing in the liver that processes the unhomologous Elements of *Ahara Rasa* into homologous, biologically available, and humanly assimilable Elements, especially for the nutrition of the tissues (*dhatus*) and the sensory organs (*jnanendriya*).

Bhutavidya: Psychiatry, one of the eight branches of Ayurveda.

Bibhitake: Medicinal fruit (*Terminalia belerica*).

Black Pepper: Spice (*Piper nigrum).*

Bodhaka Kapha: The subdosha of *Kapha* associated with taste and contained in saliva.

Bodhichitta: The awakened mind whose firm resolve is to attain liberated enlightenment not only for the self but also for the welfare of all others.

Brahma: The first god of the Hindu trinity; god as creator of the universe.

Brahmacharya: The appropriate control and regulation of sexual energy and functioning.

Brahman: God as Absolute transcendence; the term for the One Ultimate Reality as described in the *Vedanta.*

Brahmanas: Texts of the ancient *Vedas* that are chiefly concerned with details of the ritual sacrifices performed by the ancient Brahmins.

Brahmanda: The macrocosm; the manifest universe.

Brahma-vihara: States of mind created by meditative awareness that one becomes able to maintain on an increasingly regular basis as part of everyday consciousness.

Brahmin: A Hindu priest; a member of the first caste of Vedic society, the Brahmin class consisting of priests, scholars, philosophers, and spiritual devotees.

Brhadaranyaka: The earliest known *Upanishad* (eighth century B.C.) describing Yoga practice and meditation.

Brihat: Enormous, vast.

Brimhana: Toning, strengthening, and supplementation therapy; one of the two broad classes of Ayurvedic therapies; see *Langhana.*

Buddhi: The faculty of intelligent discrimination emanating from pure consciousness that is potentially accessible to all individuals to enhance cognition and, therefore, to widen the range of available consciousness.

Cardamom: Spice (*Elettaria cardamomum*).

Castor oil: Medicinal oil (*Ricinus communis*).

Catabolism: The metabolic breakdown of cellular and tissue substance.

Cayenne: Red pepper (*Capsicum spp*).

Chaitanya: An aware state of consciousness; the *atman*; the individual soul or spirit, and also the universal matrix of consciousness.

Chaitanya-Purusha: The achievement of an aware state of consciousness of the *Purusha,* a lived sense of the experience of the essential unity within multiplicity.

Chakra: A subtle energy center located along the spinal canal and brain (*sushumna*); *Prana* and *Kundalini* are concentrated here; major nodes at which spirit interpenetrates with matter in the body.

Chakshu: Eyes.

Chala: Agitated, mobile.

Ch'an: Chinese Buddhism.

Charaka: One of the most famous of Ayurvedic physicians (c. seventh century B.C.) and author of foundational text by the same name.

Charaka Samhita: The textbook of Ayurvedic medicine compiled by the school of Charaka in the first millennium B.C. in Kashmir at the University of Taxila.

Chaya: Compexion.

Chela: Student, pupil, or spiritual disciple; also *shishya.*

Chetas: Rational, logical thinking.

Chetasah samprasadah: Mental repose.

Chi: The life force; *Prana;* also *Qi.*

Chikitsa: Therapy, treatment.

Chit: Absolute consciousness; cannot be known, only realized; also spelled *cit.*

Chitam: A technical term denoting the range of differing levels of consciousness, that is, unconscious, conventionally conscious, awake, or alert, and superconscious.

Chitta: The aspect of mind that regulates perception, thinking, and memory and is virtually identical to *Manas;* it denotes conditioned and dualistically oriented consciousness; thought; also spelled *citta; chitta* is the preferred term for mind in Classical Yoga.

Chyavanaprash: Herbomineral jam with tonifying and rejuvenating properties.

Cinnamon: Spice (*Cinnamomum zeylanicum*).

Cit: Absolute consciousness; also spelled *chit.*

Coriander: Spice (*Coriandrum sativum*).

Cumin: Spice (*Cuminum cyminum*).

Daiva: Spiritual.

Daiva Chikitsa: Spiritual therapy.

Damani: Pulsatile vessels; arteries.

Dandelion: Food and herb (*Taraxacum officinale*).

Danta: Teeth.

Darshana: Vision, viewpoint, philosophy, ideological system, and worldview.

Dashavidha Pariksha: The clinical examination of a patient using ten diagnostic parameters.

Deha: The physical body that is well nourished but is catabolically burning up.

Deha prakruti: The constitution or body type developed and stabilized at maturity.

Devi: Deity companion of Shiva; also known as *Shakti.*

Dhamani: Pulsatile vessels; arteries; also spelled *damani.*

Dhanvantari: Vedic deity, regarded as the father of Ayurveda.

Dhara kala: The embracing membrane sheaths specific to each of the seven bodily tissues that has nutritive, metabolic/digestive, protective, and structural functions.

Dharana: Focused concentration; mental stabilization; contemplation; support, supportive.

Dharma: The lawful order within the universe; one's values, ethics, morals, destiny, fate, duty, or obligations.

Dhatri: Wet nurse or nurturer.

Dhatu: The substantive root or source of a tissue; the tissue, itself; the physical body is composed of seven *dhatus* or tissues: (1) *rasa* (plasma), (2) *rakta* (blood), (3) *mamsa* (muscle), (4) *asthi* (bone), (5) *meda* (fat), (6) *majja* (nerve-marrow), and (7) *shukra* (reproductive).

Dhatuagni: The metabolic or digestive tissue fire that processes *asthayi,* immature tissue elements, into *sthayi,* mature tissue elements; it is secondary and tissue metabolism.

Dhatu kashaya: Tissue loss.

Dhauti: Yoga procedure to cleanse the stomach.

Dhi: Wisdom, understanding, and knowledge.

Dhooma: Therapeutic smoking of herbal preparations.

Dhruti: Patience, perseverance, steadfastness, impulse control, courage, and will power; also spelled "*dhriti.*"

Dhusti: Impairment or disturbance of *dosha* or of tissue, for example; sometimes spelled *dooshti;* also *Dushti.*

Dhushtyas: diseased tissues; also *Dhushya, Dushya.*

Dhuta: Shaking off and becoming free of bondage to desire and to the inordinate attachment to material possessions.

Dhyana: Meditation.

Dig: Direction.

Dinacharya: The daily routine of personal hygiene.

Dipana: Techniques and herbs used to stimulate the digestive fire, the *Agni.*

Doosha: Vitiated and damaged tissues, organs, or channels; also spelled *dusha* and sometimes as *dushya.*

Dosha: A fundamental bioenergetic principle and substance that regulates homeostasis in biological organisms; *doshas,* by nature, are dynamic and protective, and constantly become vitiated or stressed; there are three *doshas:* (1) *Vata,* (2) *Pitta,* and (3) *Kapha.*

Dosha dushti: *Dosha* vitiation.

Drashtri: Patanjali's term for witnessing or the seer who observes the mind (*Manas, Chitta*); *drashtri* participates in *Purusha* consciousness.

Drava: Liquid.

Dravya: Substance; particle of matter; a container housing qualities and actions.

Dravyaguna Shastra: Indian Materia Medica, pharmacognosy, and pharmacology; Ayurvedic medicine.

Dridhikarana: Hardening.

Drishti: Gaze; focusing the eyes on something to assist concentration.

Duhkha: Suffering and pain.

Dushika: Sclerotic fluid of the eyes.

Dushti: A qualitative disturbance; an impairment or abnormality; vitiation.

Dushya: Tissues, organs, and channels affected by vitiated *doshas;* also spelled *dusha;* see *Doosha.*

Dvandvas: The automatic trend toward dualism in perception and in conception.

Dvesha: Repulsion; aversion for unpleasant things.

Dynamic: The impermanent, ever-changing state of flux that *gunas* (qualities that condition) impart to all created reality on all levels; forces in active collision.

Ekagrata (Ekagra): The state of mind that is singularly focused.

Emmenagogue: Medicinal substance that promotes menstrual blood circulation.

Envy: Unconscious envy is intimately akin to the Buddhist conception of Desire. Primary envy is a principal function of *Manas* (psychological functioning). Envy is rapacious desire for objects along with sensing their unattainability. Subsequently, massive cognitive and emotional spoiling of the entire mental dynamic occurs in order to temporarily mute the intolerable anxiety produced. It is the emotional and cognitive underpinning of *Prajna-aparadha,* which is the mind's inability to experience the underlying unity within existence.

Fennel: Spice (*Foeniculum vulgans*).

Flaxseed: Medicinal oil (*Linum usitatissimum*).

Gandha: Smell, aroma; a *Tanmatra.*

Ganesha: The divine son of Shiva; the deity of wisdom and the remover of obstacles.

Garbhashaya: Womb.

Gati: The particular quality of a movement.

Ghee: Clarified butter.

Ghritam: Ghee in Sanskrit; meaning to shine.

Ginger: Medicinal herbal root (*Zingiber officinale*).

Gorasa: Dairy products.

Gotu Kola: Herb (*Hydrocotyle asiatica*).

Grahana: Nose.

Grahani: The small intestine, particularly the duodenum.

Guduchi: Herb (*Tinospora cordifolia*).

Guggulu: Resin (*Commiphora mukul*).

Guna: Attribute or quality that acts to dynamically condition an ever-changing arrangement within creation; adjectival description of the physical and chemical properties of a substance; all material substances can be characterized by *gunas* or attributes and qualities; ten pairs are described: (1) cold/hot; (2) wet/dry; (3) heavy/light; (4) gross/subtle; (5) dense/liquid; (6) stable/mobile; (7) dull/sharp; (8) soft/hard; (9) smooth/rough; (10) cloudy/clear; also referred to as *gurvadi gunas.*

Guru: Heavy; teacher, guide.

Gurvadi gunas: The attributes and qualities that are associated with material substances; see *Guna.*

Halasana: The Yogic plow posture.

Hamsagati: Pulse movements that are swanlike, and characteristic of *Kapha prakruti.*

Haritaki: Medicinal fruit (*Terminalia chebula*).

Harita varga: Raw vegetables.

Hatha Yoga: The Yoga of physical postures (*asanas*) and breath control (*pranayama*).

Hetu: Cause.

Hima: Cold.

Hita: Good; a distribution channel (*nadi*) coming off *nadis*.

Homa: Sacrificial offering put into a ritual fire; also *yajna*.

Hridaya: Heart; the connotation of heart as a center of power.

Humor: An older term denoting the concept of *dosha,* a primary bioenergetic regulatory principle and substance in the body.

Iccha: Desire.

Iksuvikara: Sugars.

Indriyas: The five sense organs (ears, skin, eyes, tongue, and nose) and the five motor organs of action (mouth, hands, feet, penis, and anus).

Irshya: Jealousy.

Ishvara: The manifestation of God or the Absolute having personalized characteristics.

Isthapaka: *Vipaka.*

Itihasa: The Great Epics: *Ramayana* and the *MahaBharata*.

Jagat: The universe or manifest world.

Jagrat: The state of waking consciousness; see *Vaishvanara*.

Jala: Water.

Jalauka: Therapeutic bloodletting using medically supervised applications of leeches.

Janma prakruti: The constitutional conformation or constitution present at birth.

Japa: Repetition.

Jatamansi: Herb (*Nardostachys spp*).

Jathara: Abdomen.

Jatharagni: The primary digestive fire centered in the stomach and small intestine; it is the *Agni* of primary digestion that transforms *ahara rasa* into *asthayi dhatu; virya* or the potent energy of a food or drug substance pulls some of its strength from the *Jatharagni*.

Jihva: Tongue.

Jing: A fundamental principle in Chinese medicine connoting the primary Essence of the body, the fundamental substance of organic life that underlies all vital development.

Jiva: The spirit or soul as the embodied individual self that identifies with the body and the mind.

Jivan-mukti: A state of liberation while still being alive; also *Sahaja-samadhi*.

Jivana: The invigorating function of blood via its delivery of both oxygen and *Prana* to cells and tissues.

Jnana Yoga: The Yoga of knowledge.

Jnanendriya: The five sensory organs of perception: ears, skin, eyes, mouth/tongue, and nose.

Jyotish: Vedic Astrology.

Kaivalya: Liberation from material existence as the ultimate *samadhi* of Yoga practice.

Kala: Time; sometimes used as a synonym for death; may also denote tissue membrane.

Kala-Parinama: The effects that the passage of time (age, aging, seasons, etc.) produces in the natural world.

Kale Kapota: The "land and pigeon" theory that explains the process of bodily tissue formation.

Kali: Black; the fierce and ominous appearing female deity; the companion of Shiva who, like him, acts as a destroyer, often with positive connotations, i.e., destroyer of ignorance.

Kama: Ordinarily connotes sensual desire or pleasure; in the *Rig-Veda, kama* is the first impulse that initiated primal creation; in the *Atharva-Veda, kama* is elevated to divine status and is the impulse toward creating good.

Kampa: Tremor.

Kandara: Fascia; tendons.

Kapha: The bioenergetic Water *dosha;* one of the body's three fundamental regulatory principles whose main function is that of providing cohesion, binding, and containment.

Kaphaja: That which causes vitiation by *Kapha.*

Kara: Rough.

Karana: Entirely spiritual; pre-energetic, causal, seed, magnetic, or soul dimension of created reality.

Karma: Mental or physical action and/or its consequences.

Karma Yoga: The Yoga of action and service.

Karmendriya: The five motor organs of action: mouth/speech, hand, feet, genitals, and anus.

Karuna: Compassion.

Kashaya: The Astringent taste; the residue left in consciousness by sensual pleasure; also spelled *kasaya.*

Katha Upanishad: An early *Upanishad* that is believed to be the first formal text to use the term *Yoga.*

Kathina: Hard.

Katu: The Pungent or spicy taste.

Kaumarabhritya: The Obstetric, Gynecologic, and Pediatric branch of Ayurveda.

Kaya: The physical body that actively transforms and assimilates nutrition; the *Agni* transformative body.

Kayachikitsa: Internal Medicine, one of the eight branches of Ayurveda.

Kaya Kalpa: Rejuvenation of the body; a specialty treatment within Ayurveda.

Kedara Kula: The channel irrigation theory that explains the mechanisms of bodily tissue formation.

Kensho: The Zen Buddhist understanding of self-realization and enlightenment as a gradually evolving process that deepens over time.

Kervaigunya: A weak or pathological area in a tissue or channel that may become the ground for or site of disease; also spelled *khavaigunya*.

Kesha: Hair.

Keshika: Capillaries.

Kevalam: The achievement of enlightenment, freedom, and state of healthy aloneness.

Khamalas: Wastes produced as by-products of muscle tissue formation.

Khara: Rough.

Khust: Dietary restrictions.

Kichari: Wholesome, balance, and cleansing meal specifically consisting of basmati rice, yellow split mung lentils, vegetables, and light spices.

Kleda: Nonspecific, subtle waste products that result from the formation of the seven primary bodily tissues (*dhatus*).

Kledaka Kapha: The subdosha of *Kapha* that aids digestion in the stomach.

Kledana: Moistening.

Kloman: Pancreas; also called *agnisaya, agniyashaya*.

Kopana: That which aggravates a *dosha*.

Kosha: Sheath or covering; one of the five sheaths comprising the individual and having *atman* at its core.

Koshta: Hollow spaces in the body, particularly the central gastrointestinal tract.

Koshta Marga: The gastrointestinal tract.

Krimi: Germs, bacteria, viruses, fungi, parasites, and other infectious organisms.

Kritanna: Cooked food preparations.

Krodha: Anger.

Kshalana: Cleansing action.

Kshatriya: The second caste of Vedic society composed of warriors, politicians, nobility, and royalty.

Kshaya: Decrease, diminishment; also spelled *kashaya*.

Ksheera Dadhi: The direct, transformative sequence theory that explains the formation of bodily tissues.

Ksheta: Field; womb.

Kundalini: Spiritual energy, related to the power of consciousness, figuratively depicted as the serpent power sleeping at the base of the spine available to travel upward through the *sushumna* and energize the *chakras* thereby further awakening consciousness.

Kushala: The Buddhist notion of wholesomeness that includes aspects of working through and dissolving one's *karma;* see *Satmya.*

Laghu: Light.

Lakshana: Signs.

Lakshmi: The deity of fortune and companion of Vishnu.

Langhana: Reduction therapy; one of the two broad classes of Ayurvedic treatments; see *Brimhana.*

Lashika: Intercellular tissue fluid; lumph; also spelled *lasika.*

Lasika: Intercellular tissue fluid; lymph.

Lavana: The Salty taste.

Laya Yoga: The Yoga of intense veneration using the vehicle of meditatively activating the *Kundalini* energies to bring about dissolution of *karma* and merging with the Absolute.

Lekhana: Scraping action.

Lepana: Adhering and binding action.

Licorice: Herbal root (*Glycyrrhiza glabra*).

Lila: Play or drama that unfolds as *Prakriti* manifests itself.

Lobha: Greed.

Madhava Nidana: Ayurvedic text (c. A.D. 700–1100) delineating the diagnosis of disease types.

Madhura: The Sweet taste.

Madhuvinashini: Herb (*Gymnema sylvestre*).

Madhya: Adulthood from adolescence through middle age.

Madhyamamarga: The Middle Pathway within the body through which diseases travel as they penetrate into the deeper tissues and vital organs.

Madya: Wines and spirits.

Mahabhutanis: The Five Great Gross Elements; also spelled *Mahabhuta(s)*; see *Bhuta.*

Maha gunas: *Sattva, Rajas,* and *Tamas;* these are the three fundamental, highly rarefied potentials within *Prakriti* (created nature) whose magnitude in any substance determines its specific nature, tendencies, and actions; some combination of *Maha gunas* are present in all dimensions of human life ranging from the biological through the psychological to the spiritual.

Maha Srotas: The gastrointestinal tract.

Mahat: The first and enduring manifestation of cosmic intelligence in the universe.

Mahayana Buddhism: The branch of Buddhism, arising in the first century A.D., that emphasizes the attainment of enlightenment for the sake of the welfare of all beings; developing wisdom (*prajna*) and compassion (*karuna*) through ethical behavior constitute fundamental values.

Maithuna: Sexual intercourse.

Maitri: Kindness.

Majja: Bone marrow and nerve tissue.

Majjadhara kala: The membranes of the nervous system.

Majjavaha Srotas: The nervous system.

Mala: Waste material of the body; also *malas;* Hindu prayer beads.

Mamsa: Muscle tissue.

Mamsadhara kala: The membrane sheaths of the muscles.

Mamsavaha Srotas: The channels of circulation of the muscles.

Manana: The second stage of attaining right knowledge by means of ongoing contemplation and pondering of observed information according to *Vedanta.*

Manas: That aspect of the inner cognitive organ (*Antahkarana*) roughly equated with mind as the faculty of the thinking apparatus; the conditioned, sensate, and thinking mind; mentation; mind as an organ of desire that is attracted to and that attracts objects. *Manas,* the preferred term for mind in Classical *Sankhya* is equivalent in meaning to *chitta,* the preferred term in Classical Yoga.

Manasa: Relating to the mind; psychological; bodily illness due to psychological causes.

Manda: Slow, dull; rice water.

Mandagni: The pathologically lowered state of the digestive fire or *Agni.*

Mandukagati: Pulse movements with froglike qualities that are characteristic of *Pitta.*

Manipura Chakra: The energy node located in the region of the navel.

Manomaya Kosha: The mental and emotional sheath; the third of five layers or sheaths that compose the individual human being.

Manovaha Srotas: The channels of circulation associated with mental processes.

Mantra: Originally, a sacred sound or word used to enhance meditation; a power-laden syllable or series of syllables used to imbue an action with auspicious transformative qualities.

Mantra Yoga: The Yoga that uses *japa* or repetition of a mantra as a primary self-development technique.

Mara: Passion, desire, murder, destruction.

Marana: A passing away or qualitative change such as death; an Ayurvedic mineral preparation.

Marga: A specific pathway or tract.

Marma: A vital, energetic area located near the surface of the body.

Marut: Another name for *Vayu* or the Air Element; the name of the Vedic storm god.

Maruta-sevana: Therapeutic windbathing.

Mat: Thought, doctrine.

Matsarya: Envy.

Mauna: Silence.

Maya: The conventional and erroneous experience of believing that first impressions or appearances constitute the entire nature of a thing; the mind's subjective deception or illusory beliefs, especially when cognition fails to recognize that consciousness is at the base of reality and that unity rather than diversity pervades the universe.

Medas: The fat tissue; also spelled *Meda.*

Medavaha Srotas: The channels of circulation of adipose tissue.

Medodhara kala: The membranes around fat tissue.

Misra: Ancient Vedic name for present-day Egypt.

Mithya yoga: Perverted or distorted contact.

Moha: Greedy bond, attachment, delusion.

Moksha: The state of liberation from bondage to attachments and to the experience of desire; freedom from *karma* and *samsara;* freedom that arises initially from conscious choice; the highest goal of life; not a cognitive process but a recovered realization.

Mridu (Mrudu): Soft.

Mudita: Joy for the good fortune of others.

Muladhara Chakra: The base or foundational energy node located between the root of the genitals and the anus.

Mushin: Zen Buddhist concept referring to "no mind," a state of awareness wherein subject-object distinctions are absent.

Mutra: Urine.

Mutravaha Srotas: The urinary system.

Nadi: Distribution channel, tube, vessel, canal; sometimes means artery; Ayurvedic term for the pulse.

Nadi Pariksha: Ayurvedic technique of examining the pulse.

Naish-karmya-karman: Formulating intentions and their implemented actions in a manner that is least controlling, manipulative, and interfering; the emphasis is the ideal of action transcendence, that is, a truly empathetic and compassionate sharing of guidance for the benefit of the other.

Nakha: Nails.

Nanatmaja: A disease state characterized by the involvement of one vitiated *dosha.*

Nastika darshana: Any worldview that does not recognize the *Vedas* as lawful and authoritative; observant Hindus consider such viewpoints as unorthodox.

Nasya: Administration of medicinals via the nasal canal.

Natha: Lord or ruler.

Neem: Herb (*Azadirachta indica*).

Nidana: Etiology; cause; link; and diagnosis.

Nidi-dhyasana: The third and last stage of attaining right knowledge by means of meditation according to *Vedanta.*

Nija: Endogenous causes of disease.

Nirama: The state of *doshas* that are free of *Ama.*

Nirguna: Without attributes or qualities.

Nirodha: Cessation, dissolution, and destruction in the sense of managing and attempting to extinguish the heat of desire, passion, and envy; may also connote *Nirvana* and *Moksha.*

Niruha Basti: Ayurvedic enema therapy primarily containing herbal water decoctions.

Nirvana: In many Eastern *darshanas* or worldviews, the highest goal to be achieved by an individual, especially by using spiritual practices, for example, meditation; degrees of extinction of bondage to the impermanent and the transitory; extinction of suffering; recognition of one's pure identity or oneness with the Absolute.

Nirvikalpa-samadhi: In *Vedanta,* it is the most refined state of consciousness in which no duality remains; see *Asamprajnata-samadhi.*

Niyama: In Yoga, devotedness to study, to correct or right actions, and to *personal observances (practices)* in order to achieve self-realization and expanded consciousness.

Nutmeg: Spice (*Myristica fragrans*).

Nyaya: One of the six orthodox Hindu philosophical systems that uses reason, logic, and analytic thinking to pursue knowledge.

Ojas: The bioenergetic bodily material that contains the life force (*Prana*) and serves the vital functions that maintain the body's energy reserve and proper immune status.

Oleation: Term that includes both the ingestion of oils and fats such as ghee (*antar* oleation), and the external application of oils to the body as in massage (*bahir* oleation).

OM: see *AUM.*

Oshadhi: Plant; herb; also *aushadhi.*

Pachaka Pitta: The subdosha of *Pitta* or the *Agni* that resides in the stomach and small intestine and helps regulate primary digestion.

Pachana: Techniques and herbs that digest and reduce *Ama* and toxins.

Pad: Feet.

Padmasana: Yoga posture, the lotus pose.

Paka: Digestion.

Pali: An Indian dialect derived from Sanskrit in which the canonical Buddhist texts, especially those of *Theravada* Buddhism, are composed.

Pancha: Five.

Panchakarma: The five primary cleansing actions of Ayurvedic purification therapy: *vamana, virechana, basti, nasya,* and *RaktaMoksha.*

Pancha Mahabhutani: The Five Great Gross Elements: Ether, Air, Fire, Water, and Earth.

Pancha Tanmatras: The five subtle essences energizing and a part of the Five Great Gross Elements

Pancha Tattvas: The causal, soul, seed, magnetic, and most spiritual level of the origin of the Five Great Gross Elements and the sensory organs.

Pani: Hands.

Parada: Mercury.

Paramanu: Ancient Indian term roughly akin to the modern concept of the atom.

Paramartha-satya: Ultimate and absolute truth; the realization of the unity underlying the apparent diversity that characterizes the ordinary experience of the phenomenal world; "complete mind."

Pariksha: Examination; diagnosis.

Parinama: Evolution and involution/devolution.

Parpams: The *bhasmas* used in Siddha medicine.

Paschatakarma: The final techniques used after formal *Panchakarma* is completed.

Pasupati: Lord of the animals; name for Shiva; a seal so named dating from the Indus Valley Culture (c. 3300–1500 B.C.).

Patala: Unconscious mind.

Patanjali: The codifier of one of the six major orthodox Hindu philosophical systems, Classical Yoga (c. second century B.C. to second century A.D.).

Pathya: Proper and wholesome diet and life-style.

Payu: Anus.

Peppermint: Herb (*Mentha piperita*).

Peya: Thin rice soup.

Phala: Fruit.

Picchila: Cloudy, sticky, and slimy.

Pilu: Cell, cell membrane; related to the theory of the "atom" first formulated by Kanada (c. 600 B.C.) in ancient India; he was the founder of *Vaisheshika darshana.*

Pinda: The microcosm; the individual.

Pippali: Herb (*Piper longum*).

Pithara: Nucleus of cell, nuclear membrane; in general means the combination of *pilus* into larger groupings called molecules.

Pitta: The bioenergetic Fire *dosha;* one of the body's three fundamental regulatory principles whose main function is that of transformation, penetrating heat production, and digestion.

Pittaja: That which is caused by vitiated *Pitta.*

Poshaka: The unstable, immature, inferior, and homologous precursor or nourisher/nourishing material (*asthayi dhatu*) that, when acted upon by the respective *dhatu Agni,* becomes stable tissue (*sthayi dhatu*); also spelled *posada, poshada,* and *posaka.*

Poshya: The fully formed, mature, superior, final, stable tissue (*sthayi dhatu*); also spelled *posaya, posya,* and *poshaya.*

Prabha: Bodily luster.

Prabhava: The special action of an herb that goes beyond the expectable effects of its taste, attributes, and actions.

Prachhana: Therapeutic blood letting using sharp instruments.

Pradhana: In *Sankhya*, it refers to material that is yet to be developed; roughly akin to *Prakriti.*

Prajalpa: Talkativeness.

Prajna: The innate wisdom that emanates from pure consciousness; see *Chit.*

Prajna-aparadha: The natural and intrinsic tendency for human consciousness and wisdom to be in error especially when the underlying unity of reality is forgotten; the influence of *Manas* (ordinary mental processes) on overall cognition; akin to the psychodynamic concept of splitting in Western psychology.

Prajnaparamita: The wisdom achieved through the cultivation of consciousness.

Prakashana: Luminous; also spelled *Prakasha* and *Prakshana;* see *Prakashika.*

Prakashika: Luminous, radiant, splendorous, clear, light as opposed to dark, clarity, and illumination; a prime feature of *Sattva:* see *Prakashana.*

Prakopa: The aggravated and excited state of a vitiated *dosha;* connotes severity.

Prakhya: Luminous.

Prakriti: Primordial Nature or Matter that is initially undifferentiated but then gradually organizes to become energetic and manifest as a multiplicity of substances composed of energy and matter; also Great Nature; creation.

Prakruti: The individual body type or constitution of a person; the structural and functional expression of the individual's genetic code.

Prakruti Pariksha: The process of evaluating the specific *prakruti* of an individual.

Prakshana: Luminous.

Prakupita: The action of vitiated *Vata* that pathologically propels *Ama* and toxins into the body's deep tissue structures.

Pralaya: The dissolution of a process out of manifestation and into unmanifestation.

Pramana: Any reliable and trustworthy technique for ascertaining knowledge; this includes both epistemological methods such as those deriving from the functions of *Manas* and *Antahkarana*, as well as the given data from authoritative sources as, for example, from the *Vedas;* connotes measurement and scale.

Prana: The life force, *chi* or *Qi;* the life force along with its vehicle, the breath. It also refers to the subdosha and main directive form of *Vata* associated with inhalation. *Prana* connotes direction, attention, and intake. *Prana* both holds together and animates the physical body, the mind, and consciousness. *Prana* and blood are inextricably intertwined.

Prana-agni-hotra: The emphasis in the *Upanishads* on the internal sacrifice of the *Agni* of the individual self and the Absolute, *Brahman.*

Pranamaya Kosha: The breath sheath containing *Prana;* the etheric body; the second of five layers or sheaths that compose the individual human being.

Pranava: See *AUM.*

Pranavaha Srotas: The respiratory system; the channels of circulation of *Prana.*

Pranayama: The technique of regulating the breathing process; a primary phase of Yoga exercises.

Pranidhana: Firm resolution and strong attentiveness to attain enlightenment for self and others.

Prapaka: Primary digestion; also *avasthapaka.*

Prapatti: Surrender to spiritual life.

Prasad: Food that is blessed, purified, and used in ritual offerings; grace or blessing received.

Prasadana: Solidifying and becoming dense.

Prasanna: Satisfied.

Prasara: Spreading.

Prash: Ayurvedic herbal jam or jelly.

Prashama: Alleviation or pacification of previously excited *doshas.*

Prashna: Contemplative exercises in the form of questions pondering the meaning of life and the nature of reality.

Pratiloma: The abnormal direction of flow within a channel of circulation, especially refers to the unruly and abnormal flow of *Vata.*

Pratimarshya: The intranasal administration of small amounts of therapeutic oil.

Pratyahara: The practice of attempting to withdraw the attention that emanates from the senses away from objects in the external world in order to discipline the mind; an advanced stage in Yoga.

Pratyaksha: The direct sensory perception, using the five senses, of objects in the external world; evidence from the senses.

Pravritti: Activity; the onset of a process into creation and manifestation.

Prayatna: Effort, motivation, persistence, and tenacity.

Prerana: Stimulating.

Prinana: A function of the plasma tissue that results in a sense of satisfaction and well-being following proper nutrition.

Prithvi: The Earth Element.

Pudgala: The embodied person; the individual as body, mind, and spirit. In Buddhism and Zen, it is roughly akin to the individual as composed of the five *skandhas:* body, senses, perception, mind, and *chitta* or consciousness.

Pungent: Burning, hot, and caustic in the sense of the Pungent taste.

Punya: The merit resulting from good attitudes and actions; opposite is *papa,* negative karmic consequences.

Purana: Contentment, filling.

Puranas: The body of Puranic literature; ancient, devotional stories referring to legends concerning the gods, Brahma, Vishnu, and Shiva, but including some royal genealogies, dating from about A.D. 320–520 through the Middle Ages.

Purgation: Strong laxative action; one of the Ayurvedic *Panchakarma* treatments; *virechana.*

Purisha: The bodily waste product of feces.

Purishadhara kala: The special membranes of the colon.

Purishavaha Srotas: The fecal elimination system.

Purusha: In the orthodox *Sankhya* worldview, absolute and unlimited consciousness and pure spirit characterized as completely immaterial and unmanifest.

Purushartha: According to the *Vedas,* the four prime goals toward which each individual has the opportunity to strive: *dharma, artha, kama,* and *Moksha.*

Purva: Preceding; premonitory; prodromal.

Purvakarma: The preparatory techniques used before formal *Panchakarma* is begun.

Purva-Mimamsa: One of the six orthodox Hindu *darshanas* or worldviews that emphasizes the meaningfulness of the words of the Vedic scriptures and their prescribed ritual obligations.

Purva Rupa: Prodromal signs and symptoms of a disease.

Qi: The life force; *Prana;* also *chi.*

Raga: The qualities of passion that evoke a sense of attraction.

Raja: Royal or best; menstrual fluid.

Rajas: One of the three *Maha gunas*; the highly rarefied principle of energetic transformation, transmutation, and turbulence.

Rajasic: Having the attribute of *Rajas.*

Rakta: The blood tissue.

Raktadhara kala: The special membranes of the circulatory system; includes endothelial lining of blood vessels.

RaktaMoksha: Therapeutic blood letting; therapeutic blood purification; one of the Ayurvedic *Panchakarma* procedures.

Raktavaha Srotas: The blood circulatory system.

Ranjaka Pitta: The subdosha of *Pitta* associated with erythrocyte formation and transformations within the liver.

Rasa: Plasma; taste of a substance perceived by the tongue; essence; spiritual enjoyment; in a more abstract sense, it can connote the emotional charm felt in the experience of beauty as, for example, in poetry and art; *Rasa* as tasting is also a *Tanmatra.*

Rasavaha Srotas: The channels of circulation of the *rasa.*

Rasayana: Antiaging and rejuvenation, one of the eight branches of Ayurveda; also a rejuvenative herbomineral preparation.

Rasayana Chikitsa: Rejuvenation treatment.

Retas: Semen.

Rig: Hymn; also spelled *rik*.

Rig-Veda: The preeminent and most ancient compilation of the four primary *Vedas* of the Hindus from which Ayurveda is derived in part; its origins are prehistoric; it contains 1,028 hymns that are the basis for all orthodox Hindu worldviews.

Rishi: An inspired seer originally one of many to whom the ancient *Vedas* were revealed.

Ritam: The innate law and order of the universe.

Ritu: Season.

Ritucharya: Lifestyle regimen adjusted according to the specific season in order to maintain proper doshic balance.

Roga: Disease.

Roga Pariksha: The examination of disease.

Ropana: Healing action.

Ruksha: Dry.

Rukshana: Therapeutic drying therapies that reduce bodily fluids and tissue substance.

Rupa: Symptom; seeing, vision, sight; a *Tanmatra*.

Sabda: Sound; hearing; teaching, scholarly testimony; also spelled *shabda*.

Sadhaka Pitta: The subdosha of *Pitta* located in the heart and the brain.

Sadhana: Spiritual and psychological practices used as a means to achieve self-development; Tibetan Buddhist meditational practices involving visualization.

Sadvritta: Ethical regimens that guide daily living.

Saguna: Having attributes and qualities (*gunas*).

Sahaja: Spontaneity; naturalness; innocence; that which is inherited.

Sahaja-samadhi: A state of liberation, a degree of *Moksha*, attained while still being alive in the world.

Sahasrara Chakra: The crown energy node located above the top of the head.

Saka: Vegetables.

Sakshat kara: Witnessing; direct experience of being-in-itself.

Sakshin: Witnessing; the atmanic self as observer; the ultimate, unblemished state of consciousness that, in repose, witnesses the play of *Maya* including *Manas* in the manifest world, *Prakriti*.

Sam: Same.

Sama: Balanced, healthily coherent; perfectly integrated; sometimes spelled *samyak*. It is spelled *samma* in the Pali dialect. *Sama doshas* may also refer to the state of the *doshas* when contaminated with *Ama*.

Sama Agni: The digestive fire or *Agni* in its balanced and optimal state.

Samadhi: The refined state of consciousness marked by degrees of freedom from illusion, error, and dualistic experience.

Saman: Songs and melodies; especially those found in the *Vedas* (*Sama-Veda*), used to transmit the hymns of the *Rig-Veda*.

Samana Vata: The subdosha of *Vata* associated with peristalsis and digestion in the gastrointestinal tract.

Samanya: Like increases like; one of two basic principles of Ayurvedic treatment; universal applicability; general feature; common feature, property, or quality; see also *Vishesha*.

Samanyaja: A disease state characterized by the involvement of two vitiated *doshas*.

Samatha: Meditative concentration and tranquility; a Buddhist concept in the Pali dialect.

Samatva: Mental equanimity; experiential hovering in the middle between extremes; the Hindu term for meditative tranquility.

Samavaya: Integration of different features within a substance (*Dravya*) that act in consonance, in a unified fashion as part of the identity and actions of that substance; the inseparable integration and action of all features of a substance; unified interplay of component parts.

Sama-Veda: One of the four primary *Vedas* consisting of 1,549 songs or verses that accompanied the preparation and offering of ritual sacrifices.

Samhanana: Bodily conformation and structural integrity.

Samhita: A unified collection; usually a collection of sacred, philosophical, or medical teachings.

Samidhanya: Legumes, beans, and lentils.

Samkalpa: Conception, will, motivation, intention, synthesis.

Samma sati: Buddhist term denoting right or balanced mindfulness.

Sammurchanna: The pathological amalgamation of *Ama* and *dushya* (vitiated tissues, organs, and channels).

Samprajnata-samadhi: In Classical Yoga, it is the form of meditation wherein the subject continues to experience an object; see *Nirvikalpa-samadhi*.

Samprapti: Pathogenesis; the stages of the disease process.

Samsara: Cycles of repetition; pulsed cyclic rebirth; the impermanent, and dynamic phenomenal world.

Samsarga: A disease state characterized by the involvement of two vitiated *doshas*.

Samshaya: Doubt.

Samskara: Conditioning: the impressions, changes, and layers of modification and habit produced by thoughts and actions; conditioning reflects material and psychological impermanence.

samsarjana krama: A specific, graduated dietary intake used after formal *Panchakarma* is completed.

Samvarana: Gross or dense covering.

Samvritti-satya: Conventional and relative truth ascertained by ordinary, discursive but nonreflective mentation; "partial mind."

Samya: Equilibrium.

Samyak smriti: Sanskrit term denoting right or balanced mindfulness.

Samyama: Self-discipline through rigorous physical and mental constraint.

Samyoga: Combination; also *sama yoga.*

Sanatana Dharma: Hinduism characterized as imperishable and eternal, and revealed (*sruti*) to the sages (*rishis*).

Sanchaya: Accumulation or buildup of *doshas* in the initial stages of the disease process.

Sanchoc: Constriction, spasm.

Sandhis: Bony joints.

Sandra: Dense; congealing.

Sanga: Obstruction, stagnation, blockage; may also denote socializing in groups.

Sankhya: One of the six major orthodox systems (*darshanas*) of Hindu philosophy that enumerates details of the process of cosmic evolution; also spelled *Samkhya.*

Sannikrustha: Agents that cause the instantaneous manifestation of a disease.

Sannipatta: A disease state characterized by involvement of three vitiated *doshas.*

Sara: Optimal quality; mobile, steady flow.

Sarangadhara Samhita: Fourteenth century text presenting the Ayurvedic technique of pulse diagnosis.

Sarasvati: The companion of *Brahma;* the deity associated with the development of speech, learning, scholarship, music, and the arts; associated with the *Muladhara Chakra.*

Sarga: Creation.

Sarpagati: Snakelike pulse movements characteristic of *Vata.*

Sarva arthata: Ordinary, conventional consciousness.

Sat: Absolute, eternal, and unchanging Being.

Sati: Meditative awareness.

Satipatthana: Sitting meditation; a Pali Buddhist term.

Satkaryavada: The doctrine that states that all effects already reside within that which causes them.

Satmya: Wholesome; see *Kushala.*

Satsanga: Associating with those who are wholesome.

Sattva: One of the three *Maha gunas;* the highly rarefied principle of consciousness, intelligence, harmony, equilibrium, optimal balance, clarity, purity, luminosity, and lightness.

Sattvic: Having the quality of *Sattva.*

Satya: Truth.

Satya Buddhi: The ascertainment of truth; the state of *samadhi.*

Satyam: Truth.

Saumya: The cool, cold, and wet seasons; in the United States, usually fall and winter; also *Visarga*.

Savikalpa-samadhi: In *Vedanta,* it is the meditative form of witnessing wherein subject and object dualisms continue to exist; see *Samprajnata-samadhi*.

Sesame: Nutritive and medicinal oil (*Sesamum indicum*).

Shabda: Sound; a *Tanmatra*.

Shakha: The limbs or extremities; the peripheral compact tissues.

Shakha Marga: The bodily pathway within which disease travels to reach the compact tissues, especially those of the four limbs.

Shakti: Power, force, energy; the companion (*Devi*) of Shiva.

Shalakyatantra: Otolaryngology and Ophthalmology as branches of Ayurveda.

Shalyatantra: Surgery, one of the eight branches of Ayurveda.

Shamana: Therapeutic techniques that reduce toxic *Ama* and excess vitiated *doshas*.

Shankara: Esteemed Hindu teacher (A.D. 788–822) born in Kerala, South India, and advocate of *Advaita-Vedanta*.

Sharira: Physical body that experiences wear and tear.

Shastra: Treatise or textbook consisting of ideas, beliefs, theories, rituals, or scientific formulations.

Shatavari: Herb (*Asparagus racemosus*).

Shila: Buddhist equivalent of Yogic *Yama,* ethical, interpersonal guidelines of conduct; mental disposition.

Shirobasti: Therapeutic oil retention on the top of the head.

Shirodhara: Therapeutic oil drip to the forehead.

Shishya: pupil; disciple.

Shita: Cool.

Shiva: One of the triune deities in Hinduism; the deity of dissolution and transformation; for example, from impurity into purity, and from ignorance into understanding.

Shlakshna: Smooth.

Shlathana: Softening and loosening.

Shleshaka: Kapha.

Shleshaka Kapha: The subdosha of *Kapha* composed of joint and synovial fluids.

Shlesma: Ancient name for *Kapha*.

Shlesmadhara kala: The special membrane associated with the plasma; also spelled *sleshakadhara kala*.

Shodhana: Radical Ayurvedic purification therapy.

Shoshana: Absorption.

Shraddha: Faith; faithfulness.

Shramana: The aspirant or striver on the path to expanded consciousness, self-realization, and salvation who uses means alternate to the primary use of Vedic rituals; Buddhism and Jainism are primary *shramanas.*

Shravana: The first stage of study and observation, especially listening, in the process of attaining right knowledge according to *Vedanta.*

Shrotra: Ears.

Shuddha: Purity, unadulterated; a principal feature of *Sattva;* also spelled *shuddhi, suddhi.*

Shuddhi Kriya: The purification techniques unique to Yoga practice.

Shudra: One of the Vedic social classes composed of skilled and unskilled laborers.

Shukra: Reproductive fluids; semen.

Shukra Beej: Paternal seed or genetic material.

Shukradhara kala: The special membrane of the reproductive system.

Shukravaha Srotas: The male reproductive system.

Shunyata: Emptiness and Void as the ultimate nature of being; the central proposition within Buddhism, especially Mahayana Buddhism.

Siddhi: Success; exceptional abilities or powers that may appear as by-products of spiritual practices.

Sira: Blood vessels; veins.

Sira Granthi: Dilation, swelling.

Siravyadha: Therapeutic blood letting using sterile syringes.

Skandhas: A Sanskrit term used in Buddhism and Zen to denote an individual in the sense of an embodied person or personality whose being is ephemeral and merely an impermanent aggregation of five ever-changing and mutually dependent components (*skandhas*). These are (1) the physical body (*rupa*); (2) emotional reactions (*vedana*) to the five sensory experiences and to *Manas;* (3) the mind's capacity for perception and concept formation; developing the seeds for pleasurable attractions and painful repulsions (*samja*); (4) consolidated habits, memories, conditioned thinking and behavior, and passive responsivity (*samskaras*); and (5) individualized consciousness and knowing (*vijnana*) whose default state of cognition pivots on the duality of subject versus object thought processing. The *skandhas* are the matrix for an individual's proclivity toward attachment and clinging (*upadana*).

Sleshakadhara kala: The membrane of the plasma (*rasa*) tissue; also spelled *sleshakadhara kala.*

Smartas: Around the fourth century A.D., those Brahmins who followed the secondary (*smriti*) revelation literature (especially *Puranas*), which placed personal deities and combinations of them such as Vishnu, Shiva, and Devi as central to worship; this contrasted with the *srautas* who continued to hold the *Vedas,* primary revelation (*sruti*), as central.

Smriti: Memory or recollection associated with knowledge derived from tradition; the bulk of commentaries on the primary *Vedas;* insights achieved through contemplation and meditation; also spelled *smruti.*

Snayus: Ligaments.

Snehana: Therapeutic procedures using oils and fats as in massage or therapeutic ingestion.

Snigdha: Oily.

Soma: In the *Rig-Veda,* a sacred plant and its juice used by the Brahmins for ritual purposes; the exact nature of *Soma,* in current times, is ambiguous.

Spandana Sankhya: Pulse rate.

Sparsha: Touch; a *Tanmatra.*

Sparshana: Contact by touch; examination by palpation.

Srotas: The channels of circulation through which the seven bodily tissue elements (*dhatus*) dynamically move and perfuse the bodily tissues.

Srotorhodha: Obstruction of the channels of circulation.

Sruti: Revelation; the revealed sacred Vedic scriptures originally "heard" by the *rishis;* the orthodox *Vedas;* also spelled *shruti.*

Stambhana: Astringent reductions; constriction.

Stanyavaha Srotas: The channels of circulation of the female lactation system.

Sthana-Samshraya: The pathological deposition of *Ama* into vitiated tissue.

Sthanya: Breast milk.

Sthayi: Stable, mature, fully processed; similar to *poshada, posada,* and *poshaka.*

Sthira: Stable.

Sthula: Gross; coarse; physical; and material.

Sthula sharira: The physical body.

Sukadhanya: Cereals and grains.

Sukha: Happiness.

Sukha Sadhya: Disease that has a favorable prognosis.

Sukshma: Subtle; energetic.

Surya Namaskara: The "sun salutation" yogic exercise; also *suryasana.*

Sushruta: Ancient Ayurvedic surgeon (c. seventh century B.C.) who composed the standard Ayurvedic text, *Sushruta Samhita.*

Sushruta Samhita: The classic Ayurvedic textbook written by *Sushruta* that highlights the significance of the blood and the importance of surgical in additional to other medical techniques.

Sushumna: The primary and central energy channel running along the spine and brain that contains the *Kundalini* and along which the seven *chakras* are located.

Sushupti: The state of deep sleep.

Susukshma: Having the highest degree of immateriality or subtlety within created nature.

Sutra: A terse aphorism that summarizes sacred knowledge.

Svadhisthana Chakra: The energy node at the root of the genital region.

Svadhyaya: The study of sacred scripture.

Svapna: Sleep in general; the state of dreaming in particular; also *taijasa*.

Svarga: Heaven.

Sveda (Sweda): Sweat.

Svedavaha Srotas: Channels of circulation that carry sweat.

Swami: Reverend; an appellation of respect toward a religious or spiritual figure; also spelled *svamin*.

Swastha: Health and well-being.

Swasthavritta: Ayurvedic lifestyle regimens for promoting optimal health.

Swedhana: Ayurvedic procedure to promote therapeutic sweating; also referred to as sudation therapy; also spelled *svedhana* or *svedana*.

Syadvada: The expression in language of the infinite attributes or partial facets of the whole of reality, though not perceived at the moment of knowing; the fact of the relativity feature within human cognition.

Taijasa: The state of dream sleep.

Tail: Medicated oil.

Tamas: One of the three *Maha gunas;* the highly rarefied principle that engenders inertia, density, and dulling.

Tamasic: Having the quality of *Tamas.*

Tanmatra: One of the five subtle or energetic (*sukshma*) states that act as precursor to the formation of the Five Great Gross Elements, especially as they contribute to the formation of the five senses. They are called the five *Vishishtha gunas.* There are five *Tanmatras: Sparsha* (touch), *Shabda* (sound), *Rupa* (vision), *Rasa* (taste), and *Gandha* (smell).

Tantra: Technique, method, mechanism; a development in Hinduism specifically concerned with the transformative power of *Kundalini* energy to unite all opposites; the dialogues between Shiva and his companion, Shakti or Devi; Charaka uses this term in describing the structure of Ayurveda as compiled in his classic treatise, *Charaka Samhita.*

Tao: In Chinese Taoism, founded by Lao Zi (c. sixth century B.C.), *Tao* has several meanings. First, it is *Wu* or the Void; second, it is *Tai Yi* or the Supreme Ultimate out of which the *Yin* and the *Yang* and *Qi* arise. *Wu* is closest in meaning to *Avyakta* and the Buddhist concept of *Shunyata; Tai Yi* is closest in meaning to *Prakriti.*

Tapas: Rigorous spiritual cultivation that involves an amalgam of fierce efforts aimed toward self-discipline, austerity, mortification, and internally heat-generating impulses; inner fire driving self-development.

Tarka: Inquiry; examination.

Tarpaka Kapha: The subdosha of *Kapha* located in the cerebrospinal fluids and white matter of the nervous system.

Tarpana: Observances and exercise that address recognition of one's ancestral heritage in an attempt to disengage from bondage to a predetermined legacy.

Tat: A cryptic reference to the Absolute.

Tathagatagarbha: The Buddha-nature, Buddha-Self, Buddha-dhatu; *Atman.*

Tattva: A fundamental principle, category, or truth within a *darshana* or worldview.

Te: The Chinese Taoist term connoting the energy of Tao that gives birth to *wan wu,* the "ten thousand things" that comprise the created universe. *Te* is akin to *Prakriti.*

Tejas: Brilliance; the subtle energetic form of *Pitta;* the Fire Element. *Tejas* works through *Sadhaka Pitta* and is the intelligence pervading cellular, tissue, *srota,* organ, and Mind, especially *Buddhi.*

Theravada Buddhism: The branch of Buddhism, arising between the sixth and first centuries B.C., that emphasizes individual self-development through ascetic renunciation as a means to liberation (*Moksha*) from desire and the transitory attachments of the material world.

Tikshna: Penetrating; sharp.

Tikshna Agni: The pathologically high state of the digestive fire or *Agni.*

Tikta: The Bitter taste.

Tonification: Term denoting increasing the nourishment of the body and *dhatus* (tissues), especially by using enriching foods and strengthening herbs; increasing the Earth and Water Elements in the body.

Tridosha: The three *doshas: Vata, Pitta,* and *Kapha* (VPK).

Triguna: The three *Maha gunas: Sattva, Rajas,* and *Tamas.*

Triphala: Famous Ayurvedic triple herbal combination: *Haritaki, Amalaki,* and *Bibhitaki.*

Tripti: Contentment, satiation.

Trishna: Desire, craving, and excessive thirst; this encompasses desire for sense objects, for existence, and even for nonexistence.

Trit: Fluid restriction.

Tulsi: Indian holy basil (*Ocimum sanctum*).

Turiya: The fourth and most refined state of consciousness described in the Manduka/Mandukya *Upanishad,* part of the *Atharva-Veda,* as the true experience of the *atman-Brahman* unity.

Turmeric: Spice (*Curcuma longa*).

Tvak: Skin.

Tzu jan: In Chinese Taoism, it is the ontological nature of the Tao, the spontaneous activation that is motivated by its own internal disposition. It is akin to the concept of *Prakriti.*

Udaka: Water.

Udakavaha Srotas: The channels of circulation that carry water.

Udana Vata: The subdosha of *Vata* associated with upward movement and expiration.

Udgitha: Primal chant; AUM or OM.

Umada: Mental disorders.

Upadana: Attachment, desire, and the formation of bonds to material and worldly experience; the five *skandhas* that compose the personality are the source of this clinging.

Upadhatu: The secondary or accessory tissue elements that result from the formation of the seven primary bodily tissues (*dhatus*).

Upadrava: Complications of a disease.

Upamana: Analogy.

Upanishads: Ancient Hindu scriptures that are termed *Vedanta* or the later parts of the *Vedas* written roughly between the ninth and fourth centuries B.C.

Upashaya (Upasaya): Relief of symptoms after a suitably appropriate treatment intervention.

Upastha: Genitalia.

Upaveda: One of the subsidiary, subsequent, or secondary *Vedas,* i.e., Ayurveda, an accessory to the *Atharva-Veda.*

Upayoga samstha: Dietary and nutritional guidelines.

Upchaya: Physical build; suitability.

Upeksha: Mental equanimity.

Up-pa-sad: Sanskrit term describing the seating of a pupil across from a teacher when engaged in the study of ancient scripture.

Ushna: Hot.

Utkleshana: Liquefied vitiated *doshas* that are ready to be eliminated via *Panchakarma.*

Utpadaka: Vitiation, impairment, and disturbance, especially of a *dosha.* See *Prakopa.*

Utsaha: Endurance, vitality.

Uttarakarma: Procedures used after formal *Panchakarma* is completed.

Uttara-Mimamsa: *Vedanta.*

Vac: Speech; see *Vak.*

Vagbhata: Ayurvedic physician who wrote major medical text *Asthanga Hridaya* (c. A.D. 700–500).

Vahni: Fire.

Vaidya: Physician.

Vaigunya: Defective.

Vairagya: Dispassion; nonattachment.

Vaisamya: Disequilibrium.

Vaisheshika: One of the oldest of the six major orthodox Hindu worldviews (*darshanas*) that attempts to delineate a scientific categorization of nature.

Vaishvanara: The state of awake or wakeful consciousness; also *jagrat.*

Vaishya: The Vedic social class of merchants and agriculturists that provided materials and goods within that society.

Vajikarana: Reproductive and aphrodisiac medicine, one of the eight branches of Ayurveda; also an aphrodisiac substance or substance that contributes to enhancing one's capacity to produce progeny.

Vajra: Thunderbolt; diamond; connotes phallic power.

Vajrayana: A form of *Mahayana* Buddhism, especially common in Tibet. It encompasses deeply psychological practices, Tantric rituals, and yoga. The *Vajra* connotes the indestructible emptiness (*shunyata*) that is unborn and uncreated; it cannot be understood in a cognitive sense, but only experienced in states of enlightenment (*Turiya*).

Vak: Mouth, speech, voice, language; goddess of words in the *Vedas;* also spelled *vac, vach.*

Valli: Specifically refers to the leaning like creeping plants of the *Upanishads* against the *Vedas.*

Vamana: One of the five *Panchakarma* purification treatments that involve therapeutic emesis.

Varna: Color with symbolic meaning; complexion.

Vasa: Muscle fat.

Vata: The bioenergetic *dosha* of Air; one of the body's three fundamental regulatory principles whose main function is that of propulsion and movement.

Vataja: That which is caused by vitiated *Vata.*

Vatshamak: That which controls and regulates aggravated *Vata.*

Vaya: Age.

Vayas: Lifespan.

Vayayama Shakti: Energy level.

Vayu: In the *Vedas,* the deity of air; the Air Element; synonymous with *Vata dosha.*

Vedana: Emotional reactions such as those that are pleasant, unpleasant, or neutral.

Vedanga: Limbs of the *Vedas;* supplementary texts to the ancient *Vedas.*

Vedanta: The end of the *Vedas;* found in texts such as the *Upanishads.*

Vedas: The knowledge, wisdom, and sacred teachings revealed to the ancient seers. The primary *Vedas* comprise the four main Vedic texts: *Rig-Veda, Sama-Veda, Yajur-Veda,* and *Atharva-Veda.*

Vega-dharana: Natural, physiological urges.

Vibhuti: The broad range of empowerments arising from the modulation of desire and the refinement of consciousness: magnanimity, compassionate charisma, and spiritual radiance.

Vidahi: Overly stimulating.

Vihara: Lifestyle practices; a set of lifestyle choices deliberately chosen.

Vijnana: Intelligence; consciousness of reality in everyday living; individualized knowing as a function both of *Manas* and of *Chitta;* the default dualistic state of cognition that pivots on subject versus object thought processing.

Vijnanomaya Kosha: The intelligence-wisdom sheath; the fourth of five layers or sheaths that compose the individual human being.

Vikalpa: Unruly; disordered; false imagination; the attributes of a *dosha* that are abnormally increased in disease; may also connote imagination and fantasy.

Vikara: Diversification; the differing manifestations that develop as a disease progresses.

Vikruti: The current, imbalanced state of one's *prakruti* or constitution that results from doshic imbalances and the accumulation of toxicity in the body.

Vikruti Pariksha: The examination of the imbalanced constitution.

Vikshepa: False covering, a scattering of or distraction away from correct understanding.

Vilepi: Thick rice soup.

Vilodana: Liquefying and dissolving.

Vimarga gamana: The pathological flow of bodily substances outside of their proper channels of circulation.

Vimukti: Buddhist term virtually synonymous with Hindu term *Moksha*.

Vipaka: Ripening; the postdigestive effect of an ingested substance; cellular and tissue assimilation after primary digestion in the gastrointestinal tract.

Viparita-Bhavana: The ordinary and erroneous belief that the visible world of appearances constitutes the whole of reality; a function of *Manas*.

Vipassana: Meditative insight; Buddhist concept, Pali dialect; also spelled *vipashyana*.

Viprakrushta: Agents that produce disease after a long incubation period.

Viraga: Nonattachment.

Virechana: Ayurvedic purgation therapy as one aspect of *Panchakarma* purification.

Virya: The energetic power of a substance characterized on a spectrum ranging from hot to cold; *virya* is rooted in the *Jatharagni*.

Visada: Clear.

Visarga: Releasing.

Visarga Kala: The wet seasons; generally fall and winter in the United States; also *saumya*.

Vishama Agni: The pathologically variable, inconsistent, or irregular state of the digestive fire or *Agni;* also spelled *vishrama Agni*.

Vishaya: Object of experience through the senses.

Vishaya-Shakti: The intrinsic power of *Manas* that impels ordinary attention toward an alluring attraction to the world of sensory objects; the hypnotic pull and glamour of the material world.

Vishaya Gunas: The *Tanmatras*. *Vishaya* (or *vishistha*) denotes the force of the world of the senses.

Vishesha: Opposites balance each other; one of the two fundamental principles of Ayurvedic treatment. *Vishesha* means distinction, differentiation, differences, particulars, and specifically different attributes. It is the fifth of the six *padarthas* (categories) of *Vaisheshika,* the oldest of the six *ashtika darshanas* of orthodox Hindu philosophy.

Vishishtha gunas: The five *Tanmatras.*

Vishnu: Deity mentioned in the *Rig-Veda;* later, viewed as the second of the three major Hindu deities (Brahma, Vishnu, and Shiva) and considered the sustainer of the universe.

Vishrama: Displacement, especially of *Ojas;* inconsistent and irregular state of the digestive fire, *Agni;* connotes any erratic fluctuations that are usually precipitated by unstable *Vata;* sometimes spelled as *visama* or *visrama.*

Vishuddha Chakra: The energy node located in the region of the throat.

Vishva: The waking state of an individual; connotes the cosmos in its entirety.

Vitiation: Impairment, disturbance, spoiling, marring, impairing, aggravation, excitation, or imbalance of a *dosha* that may act as a factor leading to the development of disease. See *Prakopa, Dosha Dushti.*

Vivarana: Rapid pervasive and dispersive action.

Viveka: The capacity to properly discriminate, separate out, or split out that which is real and enduring from the illusory, superficial, and transient phenomena of experience; distinction.

Vriddha: Older age.

Vritti: The unstable and irregular oscillations and fluctuations of thoughts within mental processes; a negative connotation describing the untamed mind.

Vruddhi: Quantitative increase.

Vrukkau: Kidney.

Vyabhichari: Very mild stimuli that may cause disease.

Vyadhi: Disorder; sickness.

Vyadhikshamatva: Immunity.

Vyakta: Manifest reality; the level of phenomena; appearance.

Vyakti: The stage of manifestation of a disease.

Vyana Vata: The subdosha of *Vata* that propels bodily materials in an outward direction; the subdosha that energizes circulation and outward movements.

Vyapat: Impairment, vitiation; see *Dushti.*

Vyapi: Distributed throughout the body as, for example, *apara ojas.*

Vyavaharika: The ordinary default state of mind; the assumption that an individual is only his/her material organism, and that the entire whole can correctly be perceived and known in a simple and direct manner; conventional, relative reality.

Vyayama: Physical exercise.

Wan wu: The Taoist phrase: "the ten thousand things," which connotes the infinite multiplicity emerging out of *Prakriti* that comprises the created universe.

Wu: The Chinese Taoist term connoting the immense Void or nothingness aspect of the Tao that contains all potentialities.

Wu hsing: Chinese designation for the five elemental movers in nature, the Five Great Gross Elements; also spelled *wu xing.*

Wu nien: Chinese and Zen Buddhist concept of empty or clear mind; also called *mushin.*

Wu wei: A concept believed to have been formalized in the fourth century B.C. by the Chinese Taoist, Chuan Tzu. It connotes the attitude of "being in the world, but not of the world"; an attitude marked by the *bodhichitta* orientation that quietly strives toward enlightenment by a social engagement devoid of harm and the imposition of unnecessary karma to self and to others; it is moving within the world in an unmolesting and unmolested fashion, allowing natural events to happen, witnessing them in their flow, and riding the wave of *Prakriti.*

Yajamana: The one who offers a ritual sacrifice.

Yajna: Sacrificial offering.

Yajur-Veda: One of the four primary *Vedas* (c. 1000 B.C.) that contains sacrificial formulas to be chanted during the performance of sacred rituals.

Yajus: Ritual prayers and formulas, especially those derived from the *Rig-Veda.*

Yakrut: Liver.

Yama: Self-control and self-restraint virtues; the self-discipline, especially in regard to others, achieved through the practice of the five *behavioral guidelines* in the form of abstentions enumerated in the first level of Yoga practice known by the same name.

Yang: A fundamental concept in Chinese medicine connoting the principles of outward movement, solidity, heat, and masculine qualities.

Yappa: Diseases that are chronic but manageable over time.

Yatna: Effort.

Yin: A fundamental concept in Chinese medicine connoting the principles of inward movement, fluidity, coolness, and female qualities.

Yoga: In Sanskrit means yoke or union; one of the six major, orthodox Hindu *darshanas;* a system of practice in which an individual strives, through strict self-discipline, to achieve ever greater degrees of connectedness or harnessing to God; a major system of Hindu self-development formulated in the *Yoga Sutras* of Patanjali.

Yoga Sutras: The collection of *sutras* (c. second century B.C. to fourth century A.D.) associated with the name of Patanjali that delineate the Classical Yoga system.

Yogatattva: Famous Yoga *Upanishad* (c. 100 B.C.–A.D. 300) that describes the earliest known forms of varied, preclassical Yoga practices.

Yu: The Chinese Taoist term connoting the Being or everythingness aspect of the Tao.

Yuan chi: The power of Prakriti to drive creation.

Yukti: The creation of a substance, process, or effect resulting from the confluence of a wide variety of etiological factors; for example, the conjunction of materials, place, and timing that results in a finished product.

Zazen: Sitting meditation; a Japanese Buddhist term.

Zen: Japanese Buddhism.

Zephirum: Emptiness, the Void, *shunyata, wu, Avyakta.*

REFERENCES

Acharya, N.R., & Pandurang, S. (Eds.). (1945). *Sushruta Samhita*. Bombay: Nirnaya Sagar Press.

Allchin, B., & Allchin, R. (1982). *The rise of civilization in India and Pakistan*. Cambridge: Cambridge University Press.

Anandamurti, S.S. (1993). *Discourses on Tantra* (Vol. 1). Bombay: Ananda Marga Publications.

———. (1994). *Discourses on Tantra* (Vol. 2). Bombay: Ananda Marga Publications.

Apte, V.S. (1993). *The student's Sanskrit-English dictionary*. Delhi: Motilal Banarsidass. (Original work published 1970)

Aurobindo, S. (1976). *The synthesis of Yoga*. Pondicherry, India: Sri Aurobindo Ashram.

Bedekar, V.M., & Palsule, G.B. (Eds.). (1995). *Sixty Upanishads of the Veda*. Delhi: Motilal Banarsidass.

Bender, E. (1967). *Hindi grammar and reader*. Philadelphia: University of Pennsylvania Press.

Bhishagratna, K.L. (Trans.). (1968). *Sushruta Samhita*. Varanasi, India: Chowkhamba Sanskrit Series.

Biardeau, M. (Ed.). (1989). *Hinduism, the anthropology of a civilization*. New Delhi: Oxford University Press.

Bion, W.R. (1959). Attacks on linking. *International Journal of Psycho-Analysis,* Vol. 40, Parts 5–6.

Block N., Flanagan O., & Guzeldere, G. (1997). *The nature of consciousness*. Boston: MIT Press.

Bloomfield, M. (1967). *Hymns of the Athara Veda,* SBE 42. Delhi: MLBD. (Original work published 1897)

Bryant, E. (2001). *The quest for the origins of Vedic culture*. New York: Oxford University Press.

Bryant, E., & Patton, L.L. (2005). *Indo-Aryan controversy: Evidence and inference in Indian history*. London: Routledge.

Buitenen, J.A.B. (Trans.). (1973–1978). *The Mahabharata* (Vols. 1–3). Chicago and London: University of Chicago Press.

————. (1981). *The Bhagavadgita in the Mahabharata.* Chicago and London: University of Chicago Press.

Cairns-Smith, A.G.G. (1996). *Evolving the mind: On the nature of matter and the origin of consciousness.* Cambridge: Cambridge University Press.

Chen, K. (1984). *Buddhism in China.* Princeton, NJ: Princeton University Press.

Clifford, T. (1984). *Tibetan Buddhist medicine and psychiatry.* York Beach, ME: Samuel Weiser.

Condron, D.R. (1991). *Dreams of the soul: The Yogi Sutras of Patanjali.* Windyville: MI: SOM Publishing.

Corcos, A.F. (1984). Reproduction and heredity beliefs of the Hindus based on their sacred books. *Journal of Heredity, 75* (2), 152–154.

Coward, H.G., & Raja, K.K. (1990). *The philosophy of the grammarians, Encyclopedia of Indian philosophies* (Vol. 5). Princeton, NJ: Princeton University Press.

Dales, G., & Kenoyer, J.M. (1993). *Excavations at Mohenjo Daro, Pakistan.* Philadelphia: University of Pennsylvania Museum Monograph.

Das, S. (1984). Shusruta of India: Pioneer in vesicolithotomy. *Urology, 23* (3), 317–319.

Dasgupta, S. (1975). *A history of Indian philosophy* (Vols. 1–5). Delhi: Motilal Banarsidass.

————. (1989). *A study of Patanjali.* Delhi: Motilal Banarsidass.

Douillard, J. (2000). *The 3-season diet: Solving the mysteries of food cravings, weight loss, and exercise.* New York: Random House.

Dube, K.C. (1979). Nosology and therapy of mental illness in Ayurveda. *Comparative Medicine East West, 6* (3), 208–209.

Dumont, L. (1980). *Homo Hierarchicus: The caste system and its implications.* Chicago and London: University of Chicago Press.

Dwight, W. (1984). *Athara Veda Samhita.* Delhi: Motilal Banarsidass.

Edney, M.H. (1997). *Mapping an empire: The geographical construction of British India, 1765–1843.* Chicago & London: University of Chicago Press.

Eliade, M. (1973). *Yoga: Immortality and freedom.* Princeton, NJ: Princeton University Press.

————. (1978). *History of religious ideas: Vol. 1. From the Stone Age to the Eleusinian Mysteries.* Chicago & London: University of Chicago Press.

————. (1982). *History of religious ideas: Vol. 2. From Gautauma Buddha to the triumph of Christianity.* Chicago & London: University of Chicago Press.

Fairservis, W.A. (1975). *The roots of ancient India.* Chicago & London: University of Chicago Press.

Fallon, S. (1999). *Nourishing traditions.* Washington, DC: New Trends.

Feuerstein, G. (1989). *The Yoga-Sutra of Patanjali: A new translation and commentary.* Rochester, VT: Inner Traditions International.

————. (1998). *The Yoga tradition: Its history, literature, philosophy, and practice.* Prescott, AR: Hohm Press.

————. (1990). *Encyclopedic dictionary of Yoga.* New York: Paragon House.

Fischer-Schreiber, I., Ehrhard, F.K., & Friedrichs, K. (1994). *The encyclopedia of Eastern philosophy and religion.* Boston: Shambhala.

Forte, A.O. (1990). *The self and its states: A state of consciousness doctrine in Advaita Vedanta.* Delhi: Motilal Banarsidass.

Frawley, D., & Lad, V. (1986). *The Yoga of herbs.* Twin Lakes, WI: Lotus Press.

Freud, S. (1938a). Splitting of the Ego in the process of defense. *Standard edition of the complete psychological works of Sigmund Freud* (Vol. XXIII). London: Hogarth Press, 1964.

———. (1938b). An outline of psychoanalysis. *Standard edition of the complete psychological works of Sigmund Freud* (Vol. XXIII). London: Hogarth Press, 1964.

Fuller, C. J. (2004). *The camphor flame*. Princeton, NJ: Princeton University Press.

Ganapati, S. V. (1992). *Samaveda*. Delhi: Motilal Banarsidass. (Original work published 1982)

Gardner, A., & Boles, R. G. (2005). Is a "mitochondrial psychiatry" in the future? A review. *Current Psychiatry Review*. 1:257–272.

Garfield, J. (1995). *The fundamental wisdom of the middle way: Nagarjuna's Mulamadhyamakakarika*. New York & Oxford: Oxford University Press.

Griffith, R. T. H. (1973). *The Rig-Veda*. Delhi: Motilal Banarsidass. (Original work published 1896)

Grossman, J. (1994). The evolution of inhaler technology. *Journal of Asthma, 31* (1), 55–64.

Gurdjieff, G. I. (1963). *Meetings with remarkable men*. London: Routledge & Kegan Paul.

Hajicek-Dobberstein, S. (1995). Soma siddhas and alchemical enlightment: psychedelic mushrooms in Buddhist tradition. *Journal of Ethnopharmacology, 48* (2), 99–118.

Haldipur, C. V. (1984). Madness in ancient India: Concept of insanity in Charaka Samhita (1st century A.D.). *Comprehensive Psychiatry, 25* (3), 335–344.

———. (1989). Psychiatric nosology and taxonomy in ancient India. *Acta Psychiatrica Scandinavia, 80* (2), 148–150.

Hameroff, S. R., Kaszniak, A. W., & Scott, A. C. (Eds.). (1996). *Toward a science of consciousness*. Boston: MIT Press.

Hardman, J. G., & Limbird, L. E. (Eds.). (2001). *Goodman's & Gillman's: The pharmacological basis of therapeutics*. New York: McGraw-Hill.

Harishastri, B. (Ed.). (1939). *Vagbhata-Ashtanga Hridaya*. Bombay: Nirnaya Sagar Press.

Harris, D. S., Wolkowitz, O. M., & Reus, V. I. (2005). Psychoneuroendocrinology. In B. J. Sadock and V. A. Sadock (Eds.). *Kaplan & Sadock's Comprehensive Textbook of Psychiatry. 8th ed.* Vol. II. Baltimore: Lippincott Williams and Wilkins, 126–137.

Hauben, D. J., Baruchin, A., & Mahler, A. (1982). On the history of the free skin graft. *Annals of Plastic Surgery, 9* (3), 242–245.

Heesterman, J. C. (1993). *The broken world of sacrifice: Essays in ancient Indian ritual*. Chicago & London: University of Chicago Press.

Hiltebeitel, A. (1999). *Rethinking India's oral and classical epics*. Chicago & London: University of Chicago Press.

Jamison, S. W. (1991). *Ravenous hyenas and the wounded sun: Myth and ritual in ancient India*. Ithaca, NY: Cornell University Press.

Jee, H. H. Bhagvat Sinh (1993). *Aryan medical science*. New Delhi: D. K. Publishers. (Original work published 1895)

Jha, G. (Trans.). (1984). *The Nyaya-Sutras of Gautama*. Delhi: Motilal Banarsidass.

Johnson, W. (1994). *The Bhagavadgita*. Oxford: Oxford University Press.

Joshi, S. V. (1996). *Ayurveda and Panchakarma*. Twin Lakes, WI: Lotus Press.

Kadar, S. (1996). *The colors of violence: Cultural identities, religion, and conflict.* Chicago & London: University of Chicago Press.

Kaelber, W.O. (1989). *Tapta Marga: Asceticism and initiation in Vedic India.* Albany: State University of New York Press.

Kak, S. (1987). On the chronology of ancient India. *Indian Journal of the History of Science, 22* (3), 51–62.

Kalupahana, D.J. (1986). *Nagarjuna: The philosophy of the middle way.* Albany: State University of New York Press.

Kane, P.V. (1930–1962). History of *Dharmasastra*, 5 vols. (7 parts). Poona: Bhandarkar Oriental Research Institute.

Kansupada, K.B., & Sassani, J.W. (1997). Sushruta: The father of Indian surgery and ophthalmology. *Doctoral Ophthalmology, 93* (1–2), 159–167.

Kaviratna, A.C. (1902–1925). *Charaka Samhita* (Vols. 1–4). Calcutta: Girish Chandra Chakravarti Deva Press.

Klein, M. (1946). Notes on some schizoid mechanisms. *International Journal of Psycho-Analysis*, Vol. 27 [III].

Klostermaier, K.K. (1994). *A survey of Hinduism.* Albany: State University of New York Press.

Kripal, J. (1998). *Kali's child: The mystical and the erotic in the life and teachings of Ramakrishna.* Chicago & London: University of Chicago Press.

Lad, V. (1984). *Ayurveda: The science of self-healing.* Twin Lakes, WI: Lotus Press.
———. (1996). *Secrets of the pulse: The ancient art of Ayurvedic pulse diagnosis.* Albuquerque, NM: Ayurvedic Press.
———. (2002). *Textbook of Ayurveda.* Albuquerque, NM: Ayurvedic Press.

Lamm, N. (1986). *Faith and doubt: Studies in traditional Jewish thought.* New York: Ktav Publishing House.

Larsen, G.J. (1969). *Classical Sankhya.* Delhi: Motilal Banarsidass.

Lele, A., Ranade, S., & Qutab, A. (1997). *Pancha-Karma and Ayurvedic massage.* Pune, India: International Academy of Ayurveda.

Lele, R.D. (1986). *Ayurveda and modern medicine.* Bombay: Bharratiya Vidya Bhavan.

Lindtner, C. (1997). *Master of wisdom: Writings of the Buddhist Master Nagarjuna.* Berkeley, CA: Dharma Publishing.

Lipner, J. (1994). *Hindus: Their religious beliefs and practices.* London: Routledge.

Mahdihassan, S. (1981). The tradition of alchemy in India. *American Journal of Chinese Medicine, 9* (1), 23–33.
———. (1985a). Cinnabar-gold as the best alchemical drug of longevity, called Makaradhwaja in India. *American Journal of Chinese Medicine, 13* (1–4). 93–108.
———. (1985b). Indian and Chinese cosmologies reconsidered. *American Journal of Chinese Medicine, 13* (1–4), 5–12.
———. (1989). The five cosmic elements as depicted in Indian and Chinese cosmologies. *American Journal of Chinese Medicine, 17* (3–4), 245–252.

Manyam, B.V. (1990). Paralysis agitans and levodopa in "Ayurveda": Ancient Indian medical treatise. *Movement Disorders, 5* (1), 47–48.

Mead, G.R.S. (1895). *Selected works of Plotinus.* London: G. Bell & Sons.
———. (1913). *Quests old and new.* London: G. Bell & Sons.

Mehta, P.M. (Ed.). (1949). *Charaka Samhita.* Jamnagar, Gujarat: Gulab Kunverba Society.

Miller, L., & Miller, B. (1995). *Ayurveda and aromatherapy*. Twin Lakes, WI: Lotus Press.

Mishra, Lakshmi Chandra (Ed.). (2004). *Scientific basis for Ayurvedic therapies*. Boca Raton, FL: CRC Press.

Mishra, R.S. (1959). *Fundamentals of Yoga*. New York: Julian Press.

———. (1963). *The textbook of Yoga psychology*. New York: Julian Press.

Moos, Vayaskara N.S. (Ed. & Trans.). (1984). *Vagbhata's Ashtanga Hridaya Samhita*. Kerala: Vaidyasarathy Press.

Morningstar, A., & Desai, U. (1990). *The Ayurvedic cookbook*. Twin Lakes, WI: Lotus Press.

Mukerjee, A.B. (1974). The concept of nutrition—Ancient and modern. *Journal of Indian Medical Association*, 62 (7), 250–251.

Muller, M. (1899). *The six systems of Indian philosophy*. London: Longmans, Green.

Murkherjee, P.K. (2001). Evaluation of Indian traditional medicine. *Drug Information Journal*, 35, 631–640.

Murthy, K.R. Srikanta (Trans.). (1987). *Madhava Nidanam*. Varanasi, India: Chaukhambha Orientalia.

——— (Trans.). (2004). *Vagbhata's Astanga Hridayam*. Varanasi, India: Chaukhambha Orientalia.

——— (Trans.). (2005). *Astanga Samgraha of Vagbhata*. Varanasi, India: Chaukhambha Orientalia.

Narang, S. (1984). *The Vaisnava philosophy*. Delhi: Nag Publishers.

Narasimhan, C.V. (Ed.). (1997). *The Mahabharata*. New York: Columbia University Press.

Neumann, E. (1954). *The origins and history of consciousness*. Princeton, NJ: Princeton University Press.

Nichter, L.S., Morgan, R.F., & Nichter, M.A. (1983). The impact of Indian methods for total nasal reconstruction. *Clinical Plastic Surgery, 10* (4), 635–647.

Ninivaggi, F.J. (1999). Attention/Deficit-Hyperactivity Disorder in children and adolescents: Rethinking diagnosis and treatment implications for complicated cases. *Connecticut Medicine, 63* (9), 515–521.

———. (2001). *An elementary textbook of Ayurveda: Medicine with a six thousand year old tradition*. Madison, CT: International Universities/Psychosocial Press.

———. (2005a). BioPsychoSpiritual Psychiatry. *Vision, 15* (2), 8–9.

———. (2005b). The BioPsychoSpiritual perspective in contemporary clinical Psychiatry. *Elements, 3* (1), 6–8.

———. (2005c). Borderline intellectual functioning and academic problem. In B.J. Sadock and V.A. Sadock (Eds.). *Kaplan & Sadock's Comprehensive Textbook of Psychiatry. 8th ed*. Vol. II. Baltimore: Lippincott Williams and Wilkins; 2272–2276.

———. (2007). Diagnostic manual-intellectual disabilities: A textbook of diagnosis of mental disorders in persons with intellectual disabilities. Book review. *Journal of Autism and Developmental Disorders, 37* (11), 2223–2229.

Oberoi, H. (1995). *The construction of religious boundaries*. Chicago & London: University of Chicago Press.

O'Flaherty, W.D. (1981). *The Rig Veda: An anthology*. London: Penguin Books.

Olivelle, P. (1992). *The Samnyasa Upanishads, Hindu scriptures on asceticism and renunciation*. New York & Oxford: Oxford University Press.

Osho, R. (1994). *Heartbeat of the absolute: Discourses on the Ishavasya Upanishad.* Boston: Element.

———. (1995). *Returning to the source: Talks on Zen.* Boston: Element.

———. (1996). *Meditation: The first and last freedom: A practical guide to meditation.* New York: St. Martins Press.

Parpola, A. (1994). *Deciphering the Indus script.* Cambridge: Cambridge University Press.

Pillai, N.K. (1998). *History of Siddha medicine.* Chennai, India: Department of Indian Medicine and Homeopathy.

Porter, R. (1997). *The greatest benefit to mankind: The history of medicine.* New York: W.W. Norton.

Potter, K.H. (Ed.). (1994). *Indian philosophical analysis: Nyaya-Vaisesika from Gangesa to Raghunatha Siromani: Vol. 6. Encyclopedia of Indian philosophies.* Princeton, NJ: Princeton University Press.

Prabhupada, Swami (A.C. Bhaktivedanta). (1997). *Bhagavad-Gita as it is.* New York & Los Angeles: Baktivedanta Book Trust.

Prakash, U.B. (1978). Sushruta of ancient India. *Surgical Gynecology & Obstetrics, 146* (2), 263–272.

Radhakrishnan, S. (Trans.) (1953). *The principal Upanishads.* London: Unwin Hyman.

Ranade, S. (1993). *Natural healing through Ayurveda.* Salt Lake City, UT: Passage Press.

———. (2003). *Ayurvedic Panchakarma.* Delhi: Chaukhamba Ayurvijan.

Ranade, S., Ranade, S., Qutab, A., & Deshpande, R. (1997). *Health and disease in Ayurveda and Yoga.* Pune, India: Anmol Prakashan.

Ray, P., & Gupta, H.N. (1965). *Charaka Samhita: A scientific synopsis.* New Delhi: National Institute of Sciences of India.

Russo-Neustadt, A. (2003). Brain-derived neurotrophic factor, behavior, and new directions for the treatment of mental disorders. *Seminars Clinical Neuropsychiatry, 8* (2), 109–118.

Sankalia, H.D. (1962). *Indian archaeology today.* New York: Asia Publishing House.

———. (1972). *The prehistory and protohistory of India and Pakistan.* Pune, India: Deccan College Postgraduate and Research Institute.

Sarkar, S.P.R. (1993). *Yogic treatments and natural remedies.* Calcutta: Ananda Marga Publications.

Savithri, S.R. (1987). Speech pathology in ancient India: A review of Sanskrit literature. *Journal of Communication Disorders, 20* (6), 437–445.

Shaffer, J. (1984). The Indo-Aryan invasions: Cultural myth and archaeological reality. In J.R. Lukacs (Ed.). *The people of South Asia: The biological anthropology of India, Pakistan and Nepal.* New York: Plenum Press, pp. 77–88.

Shahar, M. (2001). Ming-Period evidence of Shaolin martial practice. *Harvard Journal of Asiatic Practice, 61* (2): 359–413.

Sharma, P.V. (1976). *Introduction to Dravyaguna.* Varanasi, India: Chaukhambha Orientalia.

———. (1977). *Yogaratnamala of Nagarjuna.* Varanasi, India: Chaukhambha Orientalia.

———. (1995). *Caraka-Samhita* (Vols. 1–4). Varanasi, India: Chaukhambha Orientalia.

Siegel, G.J., Albers, R.W., Brady, S.T., and Price, D.L. (Eds.) (2006). *Basic Neurochemistry: Molecular, Cellular and Medical Aspects.* 7th ed. Boston: Elsevier Academic Press.

Sigerist, H.E. (1951). *A history of medicine: Vol. 1. Primitive and archaic medicine.* New York: Oxford University Press.

———. (1961). *A history of medicine: Vol. 2. Early Greek, Hindu, and Persian medicine.* New York: Oxford University Press.

Singer, C., & Underwood, E.A. (1962). *A short history of medicine* (2nd ed.). New York: Oxford University Press.

Sivaraman, K. (1973). *Saivism in philosophical perspective: A study of the formative concepts, problems and methods of Saiva Siddhanta.* Delhi: Motilal Banarsidass.

Solso, R.L. (1999). *Mind and brain sciences in the 21st century.* Boston: MIT Press.

Somvanshi, R. (2006). Veterinary medicine and animal keeping in ancient India. *Asian Agri-History, 10* (2), 133–146.

Staal, F. (1963). Sanskrit and Sanskritization. *Journal of Asian Studies, 23* (3), 261–275.

———. (1983). *Agni. The Vedic Ritual of the Fire Altar (Vols. 1–2).* Berkeley: University of California Press.

———. (1989). *Rules without meaning, ritual, mantras and the human sciences.* NewYork: Peter Lang.

Steiner, R. (1964). *The philosophy of freedom.* New York: Anthroposophic Press. (Original work published 1884)

———. (1968). *A theory of knowledge.* New York: Anthroposophic Press. (Original work published 1886)

Stoll, A. (2002). An Elementary Textbook of Ayurveda: Medicine with a Six Thousand Year Old Tradition, Book Review; *Psychosomatics* 43: 345–346.

Svoboda, R.E. (1989). *Prakruti: Your Ayurvedic constitution.* Albuquerque, NM: Geocom.

———. (1992). *Ayurveda: Life, health and longevity.* London: Arkana Penguin-Books.

Trikamji, J., & Ram, N. (1980). *Sushruta Samhita of Sushruta.* Varanasi, India: Chaukhambha Orientalia.

Unschuld, P.U. (1979). The Chinese reception of Indian medicine in the first millennium A.D. *Bulletin of the History of Medicine, 53* (3), 329–345.

———. (1985). *Medicine in China.* Berkeley: University of California Press.

Urbach, E.E. (1979). *The sages: Their concepts and beliefs.* Cambridge, MA: Harvard University Press.

Varma, V.P. (1968). *Modern Indian political thought.* Agra: Laksnmi Narain Agrawala.

Vesci, U. (1992). *Heat and sacrifice in the Vedas.* Delhi: Motilal Banarsidass.

Vishnudevananda, S. (1960). *The complete illustrated book of Yoga.* New York: Julian Press.

White, D.G. (1996). *The alchemical body: Siddha traditions in medieval India.* Chicago & London: University of Chicago Press.

Whitney, W.D., & Lanman, C.R. (1996). *Athara Veda Samhita: Translation with critical and exegetical commentary.* Delhi: Motilal Banarsidass. (Original work published 1905).

Williams, P. (1989). *Mahayana Buddhism: The doctrinal foundations*. London & New York: Routledge.

Wiseman, N., & Ellis, A. (1985). *Fundamentals of Chinese medicine*. Brookline, MA: Paradigm Publications.

Wohlberg, J. (1990). Haoma-Soma in the world of ancient Greece. *Journal of Psychoactive Drugs, 22* (3), 333–342.

Wolkowitz, O.M., & Rothschild, A.J. (2003). *Psychoneuroendocrinology*. Washington, DC: American Psychiatric Publishing.

Yarema, T., Rhoda, D., & Brannigan, J. (2006). Eat-Taste-Heal: An Ayurvedic Cookbook for Modern Living. Kapaa, HI: Five Elements Press.

Yogananda, P. (1946). *Autobiography of a Yogi*. Los Angeles: Self Realization Fellowship.

Yukteswar, S. (1990). *The holy science*. Los Angeles: Self-Realization Fellowship. (Original work published 1894)

Zaehner, R.C. (1961). *Mysticism sacred and profane*. New York: Oxford University Press.

———. (1966). *Hinduism*. New York: Oxford University Press.

Zimmer, H. (1951). *Philosophies of India*. Princeton, NJ: Princeton University Press.

INDEX

secondary digestion (*dhatuagni*), 96–
97, 100–101, 288
secondary tissues (*upadhatus*), 59, 75–
76, 309
second nature, 107
self, 48–49, 106, 245–49
self-development: and Ayurveda, xviii,
14, 17, 56; *BioPsychoSpiritual* perspective on, 245, 253; and meditation, 238–40, 257; and *Moksha*, 82,
226; and psychotherapy, 253; and
suffering, 222; and will to change,
229–31; and Yoga, 93, 196–97
self-discipline (*Samyama*), 194, 196–
97, 303
self-examination (*aham tarka*), 233–
34, 238, 280
self-integration, 80, 243, 248, 250–52
semen, 305
semen (*retas*), 301. *See also*
reproductive fluids
sense organs (*jnanendriyas*), 14, 47–
48, 124–27, 148, 291
sensory perception (*pratyaksha*), 36–
37, 41–42
sesame, 304. *See also* herbs and spices;
oils and fats
seven bodily tissues (*sapta dhatusi*),
71–74
sexual activity, 189–92, 293
Shabda, 33, 52, 125–26, 301, 304
Shad Darshanas, 32
Shad Upakramas, 206
shakha, 77, 207, 304
shakha marga, 304
Shakti (Devi), 16, 304
shalakyatantra, xxii, 304
shalyatantra, xxii, 19, 304
shamana, 42, 203–5, 207, 304
shamshaya, 228
Shankara, 15, 35, 304
Shao-lin Monastery, 18
sharira, 59–65, 77, 80–81, 107, 121,
304
sharira karana, 80–81
sharira krija, 87
sharira malas, 75–76
sharira rachana, 59–65
sharira sthula, 59, 80–81, 107, 121

sharira sukshma, 81
sharp (*tikshna*), 40, 42, 308
shastra, 154, 304
shatavari, 304. *See also* herbs and
spices
shavasana, 199. *See also* Yoga
sheaths (*koshas*): definition of, 59, 72,
287, 292; bliss sheath, 81, 96, 281;
breath sheath, 81, 96, 299; food
sheath, 81, 96, 281; intelligence-
wisdom sheath, 81, 96, 311; mental
and emotional sheath, 81, 96, 294;
muscle sheath, 73, 294; omentum
sheaths, 76
Shen Nong's Materia Medica, 21
shila, 196, 304
shira, 77
Shira Marma, 78
shirobasti, 210, 304
shirodhara, 210, 304
shishya, 304. *See also chela*
shita, 40–41, 304
shitali kumbhaka, 199
Shiva, 8, 16, 83–84, 304
shlakshna, 40, 42, 304
shlathana, 42, 304
Shleshaka, 304
Shleshaka Kapha, 66–67, 304, 305
Shlesma, 304. *See also* Kapha
shlesmadhara kala, 304. *See also rasa*
(plasma)
shodhana, 42, 203, 205, 235–36, 304.
See also Panchakarma
shonitam. *See* blood
shoshana, 41, 304
shraddha, 304
Shramana schools, 31
Shramanas, 35, 305
shravana, 231–32, 305
shrotra, 54, 125–26, 305
shuddha, 46, 57, 184, 197, 305
shuddhi kriya, 198, 305. *See also*
purification; Yoga
shudra, 10, 305
shukra, 74, 76, 305
shukra beej, 106, 305
shukradhara kala, 74, 305
Shukravaha Srotas, 88, 90–91, 146,
305

Shunyata, 241, 305
Siddha system, 26
Siddhartha Gautama. *See* the Buddha
siddhasana, 296
siddhi, 305
sight (*Rupa*), 52, 69, 126, 137, 139,
    147, 301
silence, 190, 196, 233, 237–38, 252
Silk Road, 22
sira, 76, 88, 305. *See also* blood
sira granthi, 88, 305
siravyadha, 219, 305. *See also* blood
sishada (or *visada*), 40, 42, 311
skandhas, 48, 305
skeletal system (*asthi dhatu*), 74
skin (*tvacha* or *tvak*), 54, 76, 308. *See
    also Bhrajaka Pitta*
slakshna, 40
sleep, 153, 186, 189–92. *See also
    doshas; sushupti; svapna; taijasa*
sleshakadhara kala, 72–73, 305. *See
    also rasa* (plasma)
slimy (*slakshna*), 40, 42, 304
small intestine (*grahani*), 78, 96, 183,
    289
Smartas, 16, 305
smell (*Gandha*), 52, 69, 127, 158–59,
    289
smooth (*slakshna*), 40, 42, 304
smriti (or *smruti*), 13, 15, 32, 122, 238,
    305
snayus, 76, 306
snehana, 73, 202–3, 209–11, 296,
    306
Snehana Kapha, 66–67
snigdha, 40–41, 306
soft (*mridu*), 40, 42
solidifying (*prasadana*), 42, 299
soma, 12–13, 44, 306. *See also* ritual
    and sacrifice
soteriology, 224–26
soul (*atman*), 33. *See also Purana*
sound (*Sabda* or *Shabda*), 33, 52, 125–
    26, 301, 304
Sour taste (*amla*), 100, 134; definition
    of, 281; overview of, 165–66; and
    diet and nutrition, 129, 159, 161–65;
    and *doshas,* 181–83
spandana sankhya, 150, 306

Sparsha, 52, 150, 306
sparshana, 306
sparsha pariksha, 150
spices. *See* herbs and spices
spicy taste. *See* Pungent taste
spirit. *See Purana*
spirituality, man's need for, 224
spiritualized state. *See karana*
spleen, 78–79, 183
spreading (*prasara*), 135, 299
spring and diet and nutrition, 180
Sri Aurobindo, 197
srotas, 59; definition of, 306; overview
    of, 87–91; and diet and nutrition,
    89–90; and diseases, 144–47; and
    Panchakarma, 211; vitiation of,
    130, 144–47. *See also specific srotas
    by name*
sroto dushti, 88
srotorhodha, 88, 136, 306
sruti, 10, 14, 32, 306
stabilization (*dharana*), 42, 196, 287
stable (*sthira*), 40, 42, 306
stable tissue (*sthayi dhatus*), 75
stambhana, 202–3, 306
Stanyavaha srotas, 88, 146–47, 306
static (*sthira*), 40, 42, 306
sthana-samshraya, 134, 135–37, 306.
    See also Ama
sthanya, 306
sthayi, 155, 306
sthayi dhatu, 75, 97, 155
sthira, 40, 42, 306
sthula, 40, 42, 306
sthula mala, 75, 77
sthula sharira, 59–65, 77, 80–81, 107,
    121, 306
sticky (*picchila*), 40, 42, 297
stimulating (*prerana*), 42, 299
Stoll, Andrew, 261
stomach (*amashaya*), 78, 96, 183,
    198–99, 280, 288
stress, 95, 131, 227
subatomic particles (*paramanu*), 45,
    297
subtle (*sukshma*), 40, 48, 60, 69, 94,
    306
subtle waste products (*kleda*), 75, 76,
    292. *See also malas*

About the Author

FRANK JOHN NINIVAGGI, M.D., is an Associate Attending Physician at Yale-New Haven Hospital, an Assistant Clinical Professor of Child Psychiatry at Yale University School of Medicine, Yale Child Study Center, and a member of the Yale-New Haven Community Medical Group. He is the Medical Director for the Devereux Glenholme School in Washington, Connecticut. He is Board Certified in Psychiatry and Neurology, and in 2004 was certified as a Fellow of the American Psychiatric Association. He received his training at Johns Hopkins School of Medicine. He currently holds university and hospital appointments at the Yale Child Study Center, where he earlier received Fellowship specialty training in child and adolescent psychiatry. He received training at the New England Institute for Ayurveda in Boston and, in 1999, was credentialed with a formal Diploma of Ayurveda (D. Ay.) authorized by the Open International University whose center is in Colombo, Sri Lanka.